T0195453

Creasy and Resnik's
STUDY GUIDE FOR
MATERNAL-FETAL MEDICINE

Creasy and Resnik's
STUDY GUIDE FOR
MATERNAL-FETAL
MEDICINE

A Companion to the 9th Edition

EDITORS

Charles J. Lockwood, MD, MHCM
Dean
Morsani College of Medicine;
Executive Vice President
USF Health;
Professor of Obstetrics and Gynecology and Public Health
University of South Florida;
Executive Vice President
Tampa General Hospital
Tampa, Florida

Joshua A. Copel, MD
Professor and Vice Chair, Clinical Operations
Department of Obstetrics, Gynecology
   and Reproductive Sciences,
Professor
Department of Pediatrics,
Assistant Dean for Clinical Affairs
Yale School of Medicine
New Haven, Connecticut

Lorraine Dugoff, MD
Professor,
Director, Reproductive Genetics
Department of Obstetrics and Gynecology
University of Pennsylvania Perelman School of Medicine
Philadelphia, Pennsylvania

Judette Louis, MD, MPH
Professor and Chair
Department of Obstetrics and Gynecology
Morsani College of Medicine
University of South Florida
Tampa, Florida

Thomas R. Moore, MD
Professor and Chair Emeritus
Department of Obstetrics, Gynecology and Reproductive
   Sciences
UC San Diego School of Medicine
La Jolla, California

Robert M. Silver, MD
Professor and Chair
Department of Obstetrics and Gynecology
University of Utah Health
Spencer Fox Eccles School of Medicine
Salt Lake City, Utah

Robert Resnik, BA, MD
Professor and Chair Emeritus
Department of Obstetrics and Gynecology and Reproductive
   Sciences
UC San Diego School of Medicine
La Jolla, California

ELSEVIER

Elsevier
1600 John F. Kennedy Blvd.
Ste 1800
Philadelphia, PA 19103-2899

CREASY AND RESNIK'S STUDY GUIDE FOR MATERNAL-FETAL MEDICINE   ISBN: 978-0-323-83497-1
Copyright © 2024 by Elsevier Inc. All rights reserved.

No part of this publication may be reproduced or transmitted in any form or by any means, electronic or mechanical, including photocopying, recording, or any information storage and retrieval system, without permission in writing from the publisher. Details on how to seek permission, further information about the Publisher's permissions policies, and our arrangements with organizations such as the Copyright Clearance Center and the Copyright Licensing Agency can be found at our website: www.elsevier.com/permissions.

This book and the individual contributions contained in it are protected under copyright by the Publisher (other than as may be noted herein).

Notice

Practitioners and researchers must always rely on their own experience and knowledge in evaluating and using any information, methods, compounds, or experiments described herein. Because of rapid advances in the medical sciences, in particular, independent verification of diagnoses and drug dosages should be made. To the fullest extent of the law, no responsibility is assumed by Elsevier, authors, editors, or contributors for any injury and/or damage to persons or property as a matter of product liability, negligence or otherwise, or from any use or operation of any methods, products, instructions, or ideas contained in the material herein.

Content Strategist: Nancy Duffy
Content Development Specialist: Mary O'Brien
Publishing Services Manager: Shereen Jameel
Project Manager: Beula Christopher
Design Direction: Margaret M. Reid

Printed in India

Last digit is the print number: 9 8 7 6 5 4 3 2 1

Working together
to grow libraries in
developing countries

www.elsevier.com • www.bookaid.org

Sonya S. Abdel-Razeq, MD
Associate Professor
Department of Obstetrics, Gynecology, and Reproductive
    Sciences
Yale School of Medicine
New Haven, Connecticut

Vikki M. Abrahams, PhD
Professor
Department of Obstetrics, Gynecology and Reproductive
    Sciences
Yale School of Medicine
New Haven, Connecticut

Reem S. Abu-Rustum, MD
Associate Professor,
Director of Ultrasound Education and Research
Division of Maternal Fetal Medicine
Department of Obstetrics and Gynecology
University of Florida
Gainesville, Florida

Dalal S. Ali, MD, FRCPI
Clinical Fellow
Division of Endocrinology and Metabolism
McMaster University
Hamilton, Ontario, Canada

Laith Alshawabkeh, MD, MSc
Associate Professor of Medicine
Division of Cardiovascular Medicine
University of California, San Diego, School of Medicine;
Director
University of California, San Diego
Adult Congenital Heart Program
La Jolla, California

Michael J. Aminoff, MD, DSc
Distinguished Professor of Neurology
Department of Neurology
School of Medicine
University of California San Francisco School of Medicine
San Francisco, California

Tooba Anwer, MD
Clinical Fellow
Brigham and Women's Hospital
Boston, Massachusettes

Mert Ozan Bahtiyar, MD
Professor
Department of Obstetrics, Gynecology and Reproductive
    Sciences,
Director
Yale Fetal Care Center
Yale University School of Medicine
New Haven, Connecticut

Caitlin Baptiste, MD
Assistant Professor
Maternal Fetal Medicine-Genetics
Columbia University Irving Medical Center
New York, New York

Linda Anne Barbour, MD, MSPH
Professor of Medicine and Obstetrics and Gynecology
Department of Medicine and Obstetrics and Gynecology
University of Colorado Anschutz Medical Campus School of
    Medicine
University of Colorado School of Medicine
Aurora, Colorado

Marie Beall, MD
Practicing Physician
Los Angeles Perinatal Associates
Los Angeles, California

Richard Beigi, MD, MSc
Professor of Reproductive Sciences
Department of Obstetrics, Gynecology and Reproductive
    Sciences
University of Pittsburgh School of Medicine
Pittsburgh, Pennsylvania

Vincenzo Berghella, MD
Director
Division of Maternal-Fetal Medicine,
Professor
Department of Obstetrics and Gynecology
Sidney Kimmel Medical College, Thomas Jefferson University
Philadelphia, Pennsylvania

Kristin Bixel, MD
Assistant Professor
Division of Gynecologic Oncology
Department of Obstetrics and Gynecology
The Ohio State University
Columbus, Ohio

Daniel G. Blanchard, MD
Professor of Medicine
Division of Cardiovascular Medicine
University of California, San Diego, School of Medicine;
Director
University of California San Diego
Fellowship Program
La Jolla, California

Lisa M. Bodnar, PhD, MPH, RD
Professor of Epidemiology
University of Pittsburgh School of Public Health
Pittsburgh, Pennsylvania

Rupsa C. Boelig, MD
Assistant Professor
Department of Obstetrics and Gynecology
Division of Maternal Fetal Medicine
Sidney Kimmel Medical College, Thomas Jefferson University
Philadelphia, Pennsylvania

D. Ware Branch, MD
James R. and Jo Scott Research Chair and Professor
    of Obstetrics and Gynecology
University of Utah School of Medicine and
    University of Utah Health
Salt Lake City, Utah

Bryann Bromley, MD
Professor, Part-Time
Department of Obstetrics and Gynecology and Reproductive
    Biology
Massachusetts General Hospital, Harvard Medical School
Boston, Massachusetts

Catalin S. Buhimschi, MD, MBA
Department Head
University of Illinois at Chicago,
Department of Obstetrics and Gynecology
College of Medicine
Chicago, Illinois

Mary Catherine Cambou, MD
Department of Medicine
University of California, Los Angeles
Los Angeles, California

Katherine H. Campbell, MD, MPH
Associate Professor
Department of Obstetrics, Gynecology, and Reproductive
    Sciences
Yale School of Medicine
New Haven, Connecticut

Patrick Catalano, MD
Professor
Mother Infant Research Institute
Tufts Medical Center
Boston, Massachusetts

Janet Catov, PhD, MS
Associate Professor
Departments of Obstetrics, Gynecology and Reproductive
    Sciences and Epidemiology
University of Pittsburgh School of Medicine
Pittsburgh, Pennsylvania

Christina Chambers, PhD, MPH
Professor,
Co-Director
Center for Better Beginnings
Division of Environmental Science and Health
Department of Pediatrics
University of California, San Diego
La Jolla, California

Beth Christian, MD
Professor of Clinical Internal Medicine
Division of Hematology
The Ohio State University
Columbus, Ohio

Rebecca K. Chung, MD
Fellow Physician
Department of Reproductive Endocrinology and Infertility
University Hospitals, Cleveland
Cleveland, Ohio

David E. Cohn, MD, MBA
Professor
Division of Gynecologic Oncology
Department of Obstetrics and Gynecology
Ohio State University College of Medicine;
Chief Medical Officer
Arthur G. James Cancer Hospital and Solove Research
    Institute
Columbus, Ohio

Joshua A. Copel, MD
Professor and Vice Chair, Clinical Operations
Department of Obstetrics, Gynecology and Reproductive
    Sciences,
Professor
Department of Pediatrics,
Assistant Dean for Clinical Affairs
Yale School of Medicine
New Haven, Connecticut

David Crosby, MD, MBA
Consultant Obstetrician and Gynaecologist
Subspecialist in Reproductive Medicine, Surgery and Genetics,
Head
Department of Reproductive Medicine
National Maternity Hospital;
Clinical Director
Merrion Fertility Clinic;
Assistant Clinical Professor
University College Dublin
Dublin, Ireland

Mary E. D'Alton, MB, BCh, BAO
Willard C. Rappleye Professor, Chair
Department of Obstetrics and Gynecology
Columbia University, College of Physicians and Surgeons;
Director
Obstetrics and Gynecology Services
Columbia University Irving Medical Center
New York, New York

Karel Dandurand, MD, FRCPC
Clinical Fellow
Division of Endocrinology and Metabolism
McMaster University
Hamilton, Ontario, Canada

Lori B. Daniels, MD, MAS
Professor of Medicine
Division of Cardiovascular Medicine
University of California, San Diego, School of Medicine;
Director
Cardiac Care Unit
University of California, San Diego
Sulpizio Cardiovascular Center
La Jolla, California

Viviana De Assis, DO
Fellow
Division of Maternal Fetal Medicine
Department of Obstetrics and Gynecology
Morsani College of Medicine
University of South Florida
Tampa, Florida

Vanja C. Douglas, MD
Sara and Evan Williams Foundation Endowed
  Neurohospitalist Chair and Professor of Neurology
Department of Neurology
University of California, San Francisco School of Medicine
San Francisco, California

Lorraine Dugoff, MD
Professor
Director, Reproductive Genetics
Department of Obstetrics and Gynecology
University of Pennsylvania Perelman School of Medicine
Philadelphia, Pennsylvania

Jose R. Duncan, MD
Assistant Professor
Division of Maternal Fetal Medicine
Department of Obstetrics and Gynecology
Morsani College of Medicine
University of South Florida
Tampa, Florida

Jeffrey R. Fineman, MD
Professor
Department of Pediatrics
University of California, San Francisco
San Francisco, California

Ariadna Forray, MD
Associate Professor
Department of Psychiatry
Yale School of Medicine;
Section Chief
Department of Psychological Medicine
Yale New Haven Hospital
New Haven, Connecticut

Jan M. Friedman, MD, PhD, FAAP, FABMG, FCCMG, FRCPC
Professor
Department of Medical Genetics
University of British Columbia;
Senior Clinician Scientist
BC Children's Hospital Research Institute
Vancouver, British Columbia, Canada

Rosemary J. Froehlich, MD
Assistant Professor
Division of Maternal Fetal Medicine
Department of Obstetrics and Gynecology
University of Pittsburgh Medical Center
Pittsburgh, Pennsylvania

Lauryn C. Gabby, MD
Fellow
Division of Maternal-Fetal Medicine
Department of Obstetrics, Gynecology, and Reproductive
  Sciences
University of California, San Diego
La Jolla, California

Alessandro Ghidini, MD
Director
Antenatal Testing Center
Inova Alexandria Hospital
Alexandria, Virginia;
Professor
Department of Obstetrics and Gynecology
Georgetown University Medical Center
Washington, District of Columbia

Kelly S. Gibson, MD, FACOG
Division of Maternal-Fetal Medicine
Department of Obstetrics and Gynecology
The MetroHealth System;
Associate Professor
Department of Reproductive Biology
Case Western Reserve University
Cleveland, Ohio

Jennifer Gilner, MD, PhD
Assistant Professor
Department of Obstetrics and Gynecology
Duke University
Durham, North Carolina

James M. Greenberg, MD
Professor of Pediatrics
Division of Neonatology
University of Cincinnati College of Medicine;
Co-Director
Perinatal Institute
Cincinnati Children's Hospital Medical Center
Cincinnati, Ohio

Anthony R. Gregg, MD, MBA
Maternal Fetal Medicine and Clinical Genetics
Department of Obstetrics and Gynecology
Prisma Health
Columbia, South Carolina

William Grobman, MD, MBA
Professor
Department of Obstetrics and Gynecology
The Ohio State University
Columbus, Ohio

Christina S. Han, MD
Division Director
Associate Clinical Professor
Department of Maternal-Fetal Medicine, Obstetrics and
    Gynecology
David Geffen School of Medicine at UCLA
Los Angeles, California

Spencer Hansen, MD
Psychiatrist
Department of Psychiatry
University of Utah
Salt Lake City, Utah

Lorie M. Harper, MD, MSCI
Associate Professor,
Chief
Division of Maternal Fetal Medicine
Department of Obstetrics and Gynecology
University of Texas at Austin, Dell Medical School
Austin, Texas

Joy L. Hawkins, MD
Professor
Department of Anesthesiology
University of Colorado School of Medicine;
Director of Obstetric Anesthesia
Department of Anesthesiology
University of Colorado Hospital
Aurora, Colorado

Robert Phillips Heine, MD
Professor and Frank R. Lock Chair
Department of Obstetrics and Gynecology
Wake Forest University
Winston Salem, North Carolina

Katherine P. Himes, MD, MS
Associate Professor
Department of Obstetrics, Gynecology, and Reproductive
    Sciences
University of Pittsburgh School of Medicine
Pittsburgh, Pennsylvania

**Andrew D. Hull, BMedSci, BM BS, FRCOG,
FACOG**
Professor
Department of Obstetrics, Gynecology and Reproductive Sciences
University of California, San Diego
La Jolla, California

Meredith Humphreys, MD
Fellow
Department of Obstetrics and Gynecology
University of Utah
Salt Lake City, Utah

Claire E. Jensen, MD, MSCR
Assistant Professor
Division of General Obstetrics and Gynecology
Department of Obstetrics and Gynecology
University of North Carolina at Chapel Hill School of
    Medicine
Chapel Hill, North Carolina

Gregory Jones, MD
Family Medicine
Upper Great Lakes Family Health Center
Marquette, Michigan

Anjali Kaimal, MD, MAS
Professor and Vice Chair, Clinical Operations
Departments of Obstetrics and Gynecology
Morsani College of Medicine and College of Public Health
University of South Florida
Tampa, Florida

S. Ananth Karumanchi, MD
Professor of Medicine
Department of Medicine
Harvard Medical School
Boston, Massachusetts;
Staff Physician
Department of Medicine and Biomedical Sciences
Cedars-Sinai Medical Center
Los Angeles, California

Thomas F. Kelly, MD
Clinical Professor and Chief
Division of Maternal Fetal Medicine
Department of Obstetrics, Gynecology and Reproductive
    Sciences
University of California, San Diego
La Jolla, California

Anne Kennedy, MB, BCh
Chief of Ultrasound
Department of Radiology and Imaging Sciences
University of Utah
Salt Lake City, Utah

Aliya A. Khan, MD, FRCPC, FACP, FACE, FASBMR
Clinical Professor of Medicine
Divisions of Endocrinology and Metabolism
McMaster University
Hamilton, Ontario, Canada

Sarah J. Kilpatrick, MD, PhD
Chair
Department of Obstetrics and Gynecology
**Helping Hand of Los Angeles Endowed Chair,
Associate Dean for Faculty Development and Diversity**
Cedars-Sinai Medical Center
Santa Monica, California

Sumire Kitahara, MD
Associate Professor of Pathology,
Associate Director, Hematopathology Fellowship Program
Department of Pathology and Laboratory Medicine
Cedars-Sinai Medical Center
Los Angeles, California

Michelle A. Kominiarek, MD, MS
Associate Professor
Department of Obstetrics and Gynecology
Northwestern University Feinberg School of Medicine
Chicago, Illinois

Jeffrey A. Kuller, MD
Professor of Obstetrics and Gynecology
Division of Maternal-Fetal Medicine
Duke University School of Medicine
Durham, North Carolina

Stephen Lapinsky, MB BCh, MSc, FRCPC
Professor of Medicine
Department of Medicine
University of Toronto
Toronto, Ontario, Canada

Robert M. Lawrence, MD
Adjunct Clinical Professor of Pediatrics
Department of Pediatrics
University of Florida
San Diego, California

Ruth A. Lawrence, MD
Distinguished Alumna Professor Emeritus of Pediatrics and
    Obstetrics and Gynecology
Division of Neonatology
Department of Pediatrics
Founding Director
Breastfeeding and Human Lactation Study Center,
Director (Emeritus)
Finger Lakes Children's Environmental Health Center
University of Rochester
Rochester, New York

James H. Liu, MD
Arthur H. Bill Professor and Chair
Department of Reproductive Biology and Obstetrics and
    Gynecology
UH Case Medical Center
Cleveland, Ohio

Ming Y. Lim, MBBChir, MSCR
Associate Professor
Division of Hematology and Hematologic Malignancies
Department of Internal Medicine
University of Utah
Salt Lake City, Utah

Adetola Louis-Jacques, MD
Assistant Professor of Obstetrics and Gynecology and
    Maternal-Fetal Medicine
Department of Obstetrics and Gynecology
University of Florida
Gainesville, Florida

Stephen J. Lye, PhD
Senior Investigator
Lunenfeld-Tanenbaum Research Institute
Sinai Health System;
Professor
Department of Obstetrics and Gynecology,
Department of Physiology
University of Toronto
Toronto, Ontario, Canada

George Macones
Professor and Chair
Department of Women's Health
Dell Medical School-UT Austin
Austin, Texas

Mala S. Mahendroo, PhD
Professor
Department of Obstetrics and Gynecology
Green Center for Reproductive Biology Sciences
University of Texas Southwestern Medical Center
Dallas, Texas

Fergal D. Malone, MD
Professor and Chairman
Department of Obstetrics and Gynecology
Royal College of Surgeons in Ireland;
Chief Executive Officer/Master
Rotunda Hospital, Parnell Square
Dublin, Ireland

Emin Maltepe, MD, PhD
Professor
Departments of Pediatrics, Biomedical Sciences,
    Developmental and Stem Cell Biology
University of California, San Francisco
San Francisco, California

Giancarlo Mari, MD, MBA
The Ruhlman Family Chair in Maternal Fetal Medicine
Department of Obstetrics and Gynecology
The University Hospitals
Cleveland, Ohio

Joan M. Mastrobattista, MD
Professor of Obstetrics and Gynecology, Ultrasound Clinic
    Chief
Department of Obstetrics and Gynecology
Baylor College of Medicine
Houston, Texas

Ann McHugh, MB BCh, BAO, MA, PhD
Consultant Obstetrician and Gynaecologist
Department of Obstetrics and Gynaecology
Rotunda Hospital
Dublin, Ireland

Christina J. Megli, MD, PhD
Assistant Professor
Department of Obstetrics, Gynecology and Reproductive
    Sciences
University of Pittsburgh School of Medicine
Pittsburgh, Pennsylvania

Dora J. Melber, MD
Fellow
Division of Maternal-Fetal Medicine
Department of Obstetrics, Gynecology, and Reproductive
 Sciences
University of California, San Diego
La Jolla, California

Brian M. Mercer, MD, FACOG, FRCSC
Division of Maternal-Fetal Medicine
Department of Obstetrics and Gynecology
The MetroHealth System;
Professor
Department of Reproductive Biology
Case Western Reserve University
Cleveland, Ohio

C. Noel Bairey Merz, MD, FACC, FAHA, FESC
Director
Barbra Streisand Women's Heart Center;
Professor of Medicine
Smidt Heart Institute, Cedars-Sinai Medical Center
Los Angeles, California

Giacomo Meschia, MD
Emeritus Professor
Department of Pediatrics
University of Colorado
Aurora, Colorado

Sam Mesiano, PhD
William H. Weir, MD Professor
Department of Reproductive Biology
Case Western Reserve University;
Vice Chair for Research
Department of Obstetrics and Gynecology
University Hospitals of Cleveland
Cleveland, Ohio

Torri D. Metz, MD, MS
Associate Professor
Department of Obstetrics and Gynecology
University of Utah Health
Salt Lake City, Utah

Erin E. Moise, PA-C
Health Professional Specialist
Department of Women's Health
Dell Medical School - UT Austin,
Comprehensive Fetal Care Center
Dell Children's Medical Center
Austin, Texas

Manju Monga, MD
Professor and Vice Chair (Clinical Affairs)
Department of Obstetrics and Gynecology
Baylor College of Medicine
Houston, Texas

Laura A. Montaney, RDMS, RDCS, BA
Sonographer
Department of Maternal Fetal Care and Genetics
University of California San Diego Health
San Diego, California

Ana Monteagudo, MD
Carnegie Imaging for Women,
Clinical Professor
Department of Obstetrics, Gynecology and Reproductive
 Science
Icahn School of Medicine at Mount Sinai
New York, New York

Thomas R. Moore, MD
Professor and Chair Emeritus
Department of Obstetrics, Gynecology and Reproductive
 Sciences
UC San Diego School of Medicine
La Jolla, California

Gil Mor, MD, PhD
Professor and Director
C.S. Mott Center for Human Development
Wayne State University
Detroit, Michigan

Louis J. Muglia, MD, PhD
President and CEO
Office of the President
Burroughs Wellcome Fund
Research Triangle Park, North Dakota;
Adjunct Professor
Department of Pediatrics
University of Cincinnati and Cincinnati Children's Hospital
Cincinnati, Ohio

Karin Nielsen-Saines, MD, MPH
Professor of Pediatrics
David Geffen UCLA School of Medicine
Los Angeles, California

Joshua F. Nitsche, MD, PhD
Associate Professor
Division of Maternal-Fetal Medicine
Department of Obstetrics and Gynecology
Wake Forest School of Medicine
Winston Salem, North Carolina

Sarah Obican, MD
Associate Professor, Division Director
Division of Maternal Fetal Medicine
Department of Obstetrics and Gynecology
Morsani College of Medicine
University of South Florida
Tampa, Florida

Anthony Odibo, MD
Virginia S. Lang Professor of Obstetrics and Gynecology
Department of Obstetrics and Gynecology
Washington University in St. Louis
St. Louis, Missouri

Koyelle Papneja, MD, FRCPC, FAAP, FACC
Assistant Clinical Professor
Division of Pediatric Cardiology
David Geffen School of Medicine at UCLA
Los Angeles, California

Mana Parast, MD, PhD
Professor
Department of Pathology
University of California San Diego
La Jolla, California

Christian Pettker, MD
Professor
Department of Obstetrics, Gynecology, and Reproductive
    Sciences
Yale School of Medicine
New Haven, Connecticut

Jessica L. Pippen, MD
Division of Maternal Fetal Medicine
Department of Obstetrics and Gynecology
The MetroHealth System;
Assistant Professor
Department of Reproductive Biology
Case Western Reserve University
Cleveland, Ohio

Lauren A. Plante, MD, MPH
Professor
Departments of Obstetrics and Gynecology and Public Health
    Sciences
Penn State College of Medicine
Penn State Milton S. Hershey Medical Center
Hershey, Pennsylvania

Camille Elise Powe, MD
Co-Director, Diabetes in Pregnancy Program
Diabetes Unit, Endocrine Division, Department of Medicine
Massachusetts General Hospital;
Assistant Professor
Department of Medicine,
Assistant Professor
Department of Obstetrics, Gynecology and Reproductive
    Biology
Harvard Medical School
Boston, Massachusetts

Dolores H. Pretorius, MD
Professor Emeritus of Radiology
UCSD Center for Maternal Fetal Care and Genetics
Univeristy of California, San Diego
San Diego, California

Aleksandar Rajkovic, MD, PhD
Professor
Department of Pathology, Obstetrics, Gynecology and
    Reproductive Sciences
University of California, San Francisco
San Francisco, California

Bhuvaneswari Ramaswamy, MD, MRCP
Professor
Internal Medicine
The Ohio State University
Columbus, Ohio

Uma M. Reddy, MD, MPH
Professor of Obstetrics and Gynecology
Columbia University Irving Medical Center
New York, New York

Robert Resnik, BA, MD
Professor and Chair Emeritus
Department of Obstetrics and Gynecology and Reproductive
    Sciences
UC San Diego School of Medicine
La Jolla, California

Drucilla Jane Roberts, MD, MS
Professor of Pathology
Department of Pathology
Harvard Medical School;
Pathologist
Department of Pathology
Massachusetts General Hospital
Boston, Massachusetts

Stephanie T. Ros, MD, MSCI
Associate Professor of Maternal Fetal Medicine
Department of Obstetrics and Gynecology
University of South Florida
Tampa, Florida

Michael G. Ross, MD, MPH
Distinguished Professor
Department of Obstetrics and Gynecology
Geffen School of Medicine at UCLA;
Distinguished Professor
Community Health Sciences
Fielding School of Public Health at UCLA
Los Angeles, California

Jane E. Salmon, MD
Collette Kean Research Chair and Professor of Medicine
Hospital for Special Surgery - Weill Cornell Medicine
New York, New York

Lisa R. Sammaritano, MD
Professor of Clinical Medicine
Hospital for Special Surgery—Weill Cornell Medicine
New York, New York

Thomas Savides, MD
Distinguished Professor of Clinical Medicine
Division of Gastroenterology
Department of Medicine
University of California, San Diego School of Medicine
La Jolla, California

Claudio Schenone, MD
Fellow Physician
Division of Maternal Fetal Medicine
Department of Obstetrics and Gynecology
Morsani College of Medicine
University of South Florida
Tampa, Florida

Anna Katerina Sfakianaki, MD, MPH
Associate Professor
Department of Obstetrics, Gynecology and Reproductive
    Sciences
University of Miami Miller School of Medicine
Miami, Florida

Matthew A. Shear, MD
Clinical Fellow
Department of Obstetrics, Gynecology and Reproductive
    Sciences
University of California, San Francisco
San Francisco, California

Thomas D. Shipp, MD
Associate Professor of Obstetrics, Gynecology and
    Reproductive Biology
Harvard Medical School;
Department of Obstetrics and Gynecology
Brigham and Women's Hospital
Boston, Massachusetts

Robert M. Silver, MD
Professor and Chair
Department of Obstetrics and Gynecology
University of Utah Health
Spencer Fox Eccles School of Medicine
Salt Lake City, Utah

Hyagriv N. Simhan, MD, MS
Professor
Department of Obstetrics, Gynecology, and Reproductive
    Sciences
University of Pittsburgh School of Medicine;
Executive Vice Chair for Obstetrics
Department of Obstetrics, Gynecology and Reproductive
    Sciences
UPMC
Pittsburgh, Pennsylvania

Mark Steven Sklansky, MD
Professor and Chief
Division of Pediatric Cardiology
David Geffen School of Medicine at UCLA
Los Angeles, California

Jordan Stone, MD
Resident
Department of Obstetrics and Gynecology
Northwestern University Feinberg School of Medicine
Chicago, Illinois

Lena C. Sweeney, MD
Fellow, Maternal Fetal Medicine
Department of Obstetrics, Gynecology, and Reproductive
    Sciences
Yale School of Medicine
New Haven, Connecticut

Ravi I. Thadhani, MD, MPH
Chief of Nephrology
Department of Medicine
Massachusetts General Hospital
Boston, Massachusetts

Ilan E. Timor-Tritsch, MD
Professor
Department of Obstetrics and Gynecology
NYU Grossman School of Medicine
New York, New York

Alan T. N. Tita, MD, PhD
Professor
Department of Obstetrics and Gynecology
University of Alabama at Birmingham
Birmingham, Alabama

Methodius Tuuli, MD, MPH, MBA
Chace-Joukowsky Professor and Chair
Department of Obstetrics and Gynecology
Warren Alpert School of Medicine at Brown University;
Chief of Obstetrics and Gynecology
Women and Infants Hospital of Rhode Island
Providence, Rhode Island

Amy Miyoshi Valent, DO
Associate Professor
Department of Obstetrics and Gynecology
Oregon Health and Science University
Porland, Oregon

Ronald J. Wapner, MD
Professor
Department of Obstetrics and Gynecology
Columbia University Medical Center
New York, New York

Randall Wilkening, MD
Professor
Department of Pediatrics
University of Colorado School of Medicine
Aurora, Colorado

Isabelle Wilkins, MD
Professor and Vice Chair
Department of Obstetrics and Gynecology
University of Pittsburgh
Pittsburgh, Pennsylvania

Richard B. Wolf, DO, MPH
Clinical Professor
Department of Obstetrics, Gynecology, and Reproductive
  Sciences
Division of Maternal-Fetal Medicine
University of California San Diego
La Jolla, California

Paula Woodward, MD
Vice Chair for Education,
Professor of Radiology and Imaging Sciences
University of Utah
Salt Lake City, Utah

Blair Johnson Wylie, MD, MPH
Virgil G. Damon Professor of Obstetrics and Gynecology
Division of Maternal-Fetal Medicine
Department of Obstetrics and Gynecology
Columbia University Vagelos College of Physicians and
  Surgeons
New York, New York

Kimberly A. Yonkers, MD
Professor
Department of Psychiatry, Obstetrics and Gynecology
UMass Chan School of Medicine
Worceter, Massachusetts

Brett C. Young, MD
Assistant Professor
Department of Maternal Fetal Medicine, Obstetrics and
  Gynecology
Beth Israel Deaconess Medical Center
Boston, Massachusetts

We live in an age of astonishing progress in medical knowledge. Thus, continued mastery of the discipline of maternal-fetal medicine requires a commitment to lifelong learning. And while a physician's approach to disease prevention, diagnosis, and treatment must be fluid, changing as new evidence is accumulated, it must also rest on a solid foundation of basic biological principles, validated clinical paradigms, and explicit knowledge needed to build and maintain clinical mastery. Constructing that framework for lifelong learning in perinatology is the focus of the 9th edition of *Creasy & Resnik's Maternal-Fetal Medicine: Principles and Practice*. However, since modern pedagogical theory holds that assessment is a cornerstone of learning, to complement this renowned textbook we are excited to introduce the *Creasy and Resnik's Study Guide for Maternal-Fetal Medicine*.

This new study guide covers all 6 parts and 73 chapters of the textbook. The former include the scientific basis of perinatal biology; principles and practice of obstetrical imaging; diagnosis and treatment of fetal disorders, as well as those at the maternal-fetal interface (e.g., preterm delivery, preeclampsia); and the etiology, pathogenesis, and management of maternal and neonatal complications. Each study guide chapter includes a summary of the corresponding textbook chapter with key highlights followed by a comprehensive set of multiple-choice questions to allow you to confirm your mastery of a topic or indicate areas that may need a bit more consideration.

We believe that the *Creasy and Resnik's Study Guide for Maternal-Fetal Medicine* will be of great use for trainees but equally valuable to established MFM practitioners who want to refresh and reinforce their foundation in the principles and practice of perinatology to ensure that lifelong learning efforts rest on sound biological and clinical bases. We are very grateful to the authors of both the parent textbook and new study guide for their outstanding contributions and exhaustive efforts to ensure the accuracy, relevance, and completeness of each chapter. Taken together, these chapters span the breadth and depth of the discipline, and their mastery will help ensure the best possible outcome for mothers and babies.

CONTENTS

Scientific Basis of Perinatal Biology

1

Human Basic Genetics and Patterns of Inheritance

ANTHONY R. GREGG | JEFFREY A. KULLER

(see *Creasy and Resnik's Maternal-Fetal Medicine, 9e: Ch 1*)

Summary

The practicing maternal-fetal medicine physician must acquire an understanding of the human genome. Doing so facilitates necessary interactions with patients, genetic counselors, and colleagues who may have foundational knowledge of human genetics. It is no longer sufficient to be facile with a superficial distinction between meiosis and mitosis, the number of chromosomes in a euploid cell, and basic principles of Mendelian inheritance. The 21st-century maternal-fetal medicine physician must understand the human genome at a higher resolution while applying newer technologies to achieve earlier diagnoses that can positively impact patient care.

DNA STRUCTURE

DNA sequences are prone to change. Sequence variation typically occurs during gamete development and after conception within somatic cells. A rubric for classifying sequence variation within genes has been established according to its impact on human development. Five possibilities exist: Pathogenic (P), Likely Pathogenic (LP), Benign (B), Likely Benign (LB), and Variant of Uncertain Significance (VUS). This nomenclature permeates the laboratory reports from molecular genetics laboratories. Recombination occurs when portions of the maternal and paternal homologue of a chromosome exchange material. This creates some of the diversity seen within families; however, when perturbed, this can result in pathologic conditions identified at the time of fetal ultrasound or across the lifespan. Unequal crossing over, or a failure of equal sharing, can result in microdeletions or microduplications, also called copy number variations (CNVs). A rubric has been used to classify this type of variation and the nomenclature used is identical.

CELL DIVISION

Normal fertilization takes place when a single sperm permeates the zona pellucida of the oocyte. Meiosis is a cell division mechanism wherein the chromosome number within the primordial germ cells is reduced from 46 to 23. In females, meiosis begins during fetal development, pauses during meiosis I, and is completed monthly after menarche. The pause from fetal life to menarche in females takes place during prophase of meiosis I. In males, meiosis starts with puberty and can continue across the lifespan. Aneuploidy results most commonly from either of two processes: anaphase lag or nondisjunction during meiosis I after puberty in females. The 45X and trisomy 21 karyotypes derive from these mechanisms, respectively. When somatic cells divide, the chromosome number (46) is intended to be conserved. However, mitotic abnormalities can lead to tissues whose cells are of different genetic makeups (mosaicism). Rapidly dividing somatic tissues (e.g., cancers, placenta) are prone to mosaicism.

IMPRINTING

Imprinting refers to gene expression that depends on parental origin. Most genes are expressed from the maternal and paternal chromosome in roughly equal amounts (biparental expression). However, genes within identified regions are subject to imprinting. Imprinted regions are specific for either maternal or paternal expression but not both. Imprinted genes are turned off by methylation of the promoter regions' CpG islands. Imprinted regions are reset (demethylated) during gametogenesis and reestablished at the earliest stages of embryonic development. When an allele from one parent is deleted, there can be only uniparental gene expression. If that remaining gene is imprinted, there can be an abnormal phenotype because there is no expression of the remaining gene from the other parent. Prader-Willi and Angelman syndrome are examples of imprinting disorders. They can occur as a result of having both members of the chromosome 15 pair derived from one parent, a condition known as uniparental disomy.

TRISOMIC RESCUE

Trisomic rescue is a mechanism that serves to "rescue" the early embryo from trisomies that result from abnormal meiosis or mitosis. During cell division within the early embryo, the extra chromosome is extruded, resulting in preferential survival of euploid cells, which then expand normally. Trisomic rescue may be incomplete, resulting in mosaicism. When the rescue process results in a euploid cell line with both chromosomes derived from a single parent (isodicentric), there is a risk of abnormal imprinting if the chromosome is one that is associated with imprinting (e.g., chromosome 11 and 15). Heterodisomy (chromosomes from both parents) after trisomy rescue is not predicted to result in conditions associated with abnormal imprinting.

STRUCTURAL VARIATION

Structural variation is a nonspecific term that refers to large and small changes within the genome. Translocation marker chromosomes and CNVs are examples. Robertsonian translocations occur between acrocentric chromosomes as a result of joining at the centromere. Collected data allow one to predict the outcomes of pregnancies where one parent is a carrier of a Robertsonian translocation. The gametes that result from insertional translocations and inversions can also be predicted. Predicting the phenotype when a marker chromosome (piece of stray DNA) is identified can be difficult but possible when the genomic material that makes up the marker can be identified. CNVs are common in the general population (1%–2%), and when de novo, they appear to arise during meiosis II of sperm development. DiGeorge syndrome results from one of the most common pathogenic CNVs in nature (22q11.2 del). This autosomal dominant condition is usually de novo but can be inherited from a parent. The phenotype varies depending on the specific genes deleted.

GERMLINE MOSAICISM

Mosaicism refers to the presence of cells within a tissue or organism that are not identical with respect to their genetic makeup. When a dominant condition recurs within a nuclear family and neither parent expresses the condition, one explanation is the possibility of germline mosaicism. Some portion of primordial germ cells acquired a genetic change before giving rise to affected gametes that participated in fertilization.

CONFINED PLACENTAL MOSAICISM

Mosaicism is identified in 1%–2% of chorionic villus sampling (CVS) specimens. Placental mosaicism arises from mitotic nondisjunction. To confirm the diagnosis of confirmed placental mosaicism (CPM), the abnormal cell line must not be seen in the embryo, fetus, or neonate. Fetal sampling (amniocentesis or fetal blood sampling) or sampling of the neonate (buccal smear or blood) can facilitate this diagnosis. CPM has been associated with impaired placental function and in some cases may be associated with fetal growth restriction.

MENDELIAN INHERITANCE

Mendelian inheritance provides the probability of a phenotype associated with dominant, recessive, or X-linked conditions. CNVs within families typically transmit in a Mendelian fashion. Dominant conditions are passed to 50% of the offspring. Recessive conditions are passed to 25% of offspring, and 50% become carriers like the parents. One-fourth of offspring from a recessive mating are neither a carrier nor affected. Semidominant inheritance is associated with phenotypes that are more severe when homozygous compared with heterozygous. Achondroplasia is an example. The homozygous conception is lethal. Factor V Leiden is another example, since homozygous individuals tend to be much more severely impacted.

Penetrance refers to the proportion of people with a genomic change that exhibit signs or symptoms of the genetic condition. When inheriting an abnormal allele does not always result in an abnormal phenotype, there is incomplete penetrance.

Age-related penetrance is seen in autosomal dominant polycystic kidney disease. Variable expressivity refers to the range of signs or symptoms that can occur in different people with the same genetic condition (e.g., neurofibromatosis). Variable expressivity is seen in common aneuploidies such as Down syndrome and Turner syndrome.

X-LINKED INHERITANCE

In females with two or more X chromosomes, there is a potential for an excess of gene expression when compared with males with one X chromosome. X inactivation, also called Lyonization, is nature's response to this imbalance. In females, one X chromosome within cells is randomly inactivated. The distal end of each sex chromosome harbors genes that are expressed as would be in autosomes (non–sex chromosomes). These follow Mendelian inheritance for recessive and dominant genes and escape X-inactivation. This region of the X and Y chromosome is called the pseudoautosomal region. Like the autosomes, these regions are subject to recombination (thus copy number variation) and translocation.

MITOCHONDRIAL INHERITANCE

The mitochondrial genome is distinct from the nuclear genome. The mitochondrial genome encodes mostly transfer RNAs. Although some proteins required for energy production are encoded in the mitochondria, these organelles also require nuclear gene-derived proteins for proper function. The organelles are found exclusively in the oocyte at fertilization and are thus maternally derived. Usually, mitochondrial DNA is identical (homoplasmy), although changes in DNA sequence can occur, resulting in cells, organs, or the entire fetus carrying varied percentages of normal and abnormal mitochondrial genome (heteroplasmy). Heteroplasmy of 60%–90% is thought necessary for a mitochondrial disorder to result in a phenotype.

TRINUCLEOTIDE REPEATS

Trinucleotide repeats are repetitive sequences of the same three nucleotides. The nucleotides that make up the repeat and the number of times the sequence is repeated are condition specific. Anticipation is the phenomenon where a trinucleotide tract expands during gametogenesis, leading to successively earlier ages of onset, more severe symptoms, or both across generations. Predisposition for expansion is sex specific for many trinucleotide repeat disorders. Fragile X syndrome is the most common trinucleotide repeat disorder. It is an X-linked condition associated with severe developmental delay. Expansion of premutation alleles occurs during oogenesis.

QUESTIONS

1. Which of the following describes primary DNA structure?
   a. Base pairing; A to T and G to C
   b. The double helix
   c. DNA sequence
   d. Histone modification

2. Which is true about primordial germ cells?
   a. When not dividing, have 2N (23) chromosomes
   b. When not dividing, have 2N (46) chromosomes
   c. When not dividing, have N (23) chromosomes
   d. When not dividing, have 4N (92) chromosomes

3. Which is true about the conclusion of normal meiosis I?
   a. DNA is 4N
   b. DNA is 3N
   c. DNA is 2N
   d. DNA is 1N

4. Which is true about the conclusion of normal meiosis II?
   a. DNA is 4n
   b. DNA is 3N
   c. DNA is 2N
   d. DNA is 1N

5. Which is true about homologous recombination within germ cells?
   a. It occurs during metaphase of meiosis II
   b. It occurs during prophase–pachytene of meiosis I
   c. It occurs during prophase–leptotene of meiosis I
   d. It occurs during prophase–leptotene of meiosis II

6. When comparing meiosis in males and females, which of the following is true?
   a. Completion occurs over years in both.
   b. It is completed over years in males and is arrested in utero in females.
   c. It is short in males and arrested during meiosis I in females.
   d. It is short in males and arrested during meiosis II in females.

7. When alleles of the same gene segregate into separate gametes, this is
   a. Mendel's law of segregation
   b. Mendel's law of dominance
   c. Mendel's law of random assortment
   d. Starling's law of segregation

8. Triploidy results from
   a. An error in homologous recombination
   b. Nondisjunction of a chromosome
   c. Dispermy
   d. Early extrusion of the polar body

9. Nondisjunction
   a. Derives from an abnormality in metaphase
   b. In meiosis I results in heterodisomy
   c. Derives from an abnormality in telophase
   d. In meiosis I results in isodisomy

10. All of the following are true about CNVs except
    a. Clinically relevant CNVs occur in 1%–2% of healthy people.
    b. Pathogenic CNVs are visible on conventional karyotype.
    c. A CNV can be pathogenic when only a regulatory subunit is affected.
    d. A CNV can be pathogenic when a gene product is lost or gained.

11. All are true about Robertsonian translocations except
    a. Are a type of structural variation
    b. Occur only with acrocentric chromosomes
    c. Involve autosomes and the X chromosome
    d. 13:14 is the most common

12. All the following represent structural variations in the genome except
    a. Microdeletion/microduplication
    b. Robertsonian translocation
    c. Pericentric inversion
    d. Transition/transversion

13. All the following are true about imprinted genes except
    a. Results in unequal expression of parental genes
    b. Methylation is a mechanism
    c. Sequence variation is a mechanism
    d. Takes place during gametogenesis

14. All the following are true about trisomic rescue except
    a. Cannot result in uniparental disomy
    b. Follows nondisjunction in meiosis
    c. Follows nondisjunction in mitosis
    d. Results in euploid cells

15. All of the following are true about germ line mosaicism except
    a. Arises from somatic cell nondisjunction.
    b. Describes a population of gametes with more than one genetic constitution.
    c. Risk to offspring is independent of when in embryogenesis the mosaicism occurs.
    d. Risk to offspring is highest when the mosaicism occurs in oocytes.

16. All of the following are true about confined placental mosaicism except
    a. Arises from somatic cell nondisjunction.
    b. It will not be identified with chromosome microarray.
    c. It occurs in 1%–2% of chorionic villous samples.
    d. When suspected, amniocentesis should be offered.

17. All of the following are true about Mendelian inheritance except:
    a. Describes that for an affected offspring; one parent must be a carrier to result in a phenotype
    b. Allows one to predict the genotype phenotype outcomes
    c. Describes how when one parent carries a pathogenic dominant gene, 50% of offspring are predicted to have the associated phenotype
    d. CNVs within a family follow the rules of Mendelian inheritance

18. All of the following are true about X inactivation except
    a. Serves to compensate for an imbalance in the number of genes located on the X chromosome in males and females
    b. Is permanent (once inactive, a chromosome stays inactive)
    c. Is a function of the gene *XIST*
    d. Is random

19. All of the following are true about mitochondrial inheritance except
    a. It is maternal, since the oocyte contains mitochondria and sperm do not.
    b. Homoplasmy refers to mitochondria within an organ that are of the same genetic constitution.
    c. Heteroplasmy occurs when sperm are abnormal and also make contributions to the mitochondrial pool within an organ.
    d. Three-parent in vitro fertilization allows families to reduce the risk of having a child with a mitochondrial disorder.

20. All of the following are true about trinucleotide repeat disorders except
    a. The number of repeats that cause disease is unique to each condition.
    b. Anticipation is the phenomenon of expansion from one generation to the next.
    c. Anticipation occurs during gametogenesis.
    d. Anticipation occurs equally during spermatogenesis and oogenesis for all disorders.

Molecular Genetic Technology

JENNIFER GILNER | ALEKSANDAR RAJKOVIC | JEFFREY A. KULLER

(see Creasy and Resnik's Maternal-Fetal Medicine, 9e: Ch 2)

Summary

Each human being's complete genetic sequence reveals a significant amount of genetic variation. Naturally occurring differences in the DNA sequence are called single nucleotide polymorphisms (SNPs). To be classified as a SNP, two or more versions of the nucleotide sequence must be present in at least 1% of the general population. In addition to individual sequence variation through SNPs, comparative genome studies between individual sequences have revealed a far more pervasive form of genetic variation termed *copy number variants* (CNVs). A CNV can be benign (no known effect on the phenotype) or pathogenic (well-documented effect on the phenotype), and a significant proportion of identified CNVs have as yet unknown significance.

Genetic risk assessment begins with evaluation of the biologic parents. Family history and prior obstetric history may reveal indications for targeted testing, such as assessment for single-gene disorders such as cystic fibrosis or parental karyotyping in the setting of recurrent pregnancy loss. Certain populations have an increased risk of specific, identifiable genetic diseases. The goal of carrier screening is to provide individuals with information that will allow them to make informed reproductive decisions. Screening for spinal muscular atrophy (SMA) and cystic fibrosis status and for hematologic diseases such as the thalassemias is recommended for all patients. Additional screening may be tailored to family history and ethnicity. Ethnic and panethnic carrier screening have limitations. With the development of SNP-based and sequencing technologies, expanded carrier screening can now detect at least 200 conditions. As with all screening tests, expanded carrier screening is risk reducing rather than risk eliminating because not all variants for any disorder can be identified.

The American College of Obstetricians and Gynecologists (ACOG) and the Society for Maternal-Fetal Medicine (SMFM) recommend that all pregnant patients be counseled about the opportunities for prenatal genetic assessment consisting of aneuploidy screening and testing. This recommendation is not dependent on maternal age or other risk factors. Furthermore, prenatal ultrasound is recommended for accurate determination of gestational age, fetal number, placental location, and diagnosis of fetal anomalies. The most commonly used forms of genetic testing are chorionic villus sampling (CVS) and amniocentesis to obtain cellular samples from the placenta and fetus, respectively, for cytogenetic analysis and molecular genetic testing where appropriate. Procedure-related risk of miscarriage is low; for amniocentesis it is 0.1% and for CVS, 0.2%. The cells in the amniotic fluid derive from extraembryonic ectoderm and include cells from the fetal skin, respiratory tract, gastrointestinal tract, and amnion. Amniotic fluid after 15−16 weeks may be analyzed directly by extraction of DNA from the amniocytes for hybridization-based DNA analysis using microarray or polymerase chain reaction (PCR). Alternatively, or in parallel, the amniocytes may be cultured for cytology-based methods of chromosomal analysis such as traditional karyotyping. As with amniocyte culture, DNA may be extracted from cultured cytotrophoblasts or villus mesenchymal cells from CVS, allowing for application of DNA analysis. Most biochemical diagnoses that can be made from amniotic fluid can be made from chorionic villi as well. Mosaicism occurs in approximately 1% of CVS samples and may require follow-up testing by amniocentesis.

The predominant use for fetal cells obtained by amniocentesis or CVS has traditionally been cytogenetic analysis. Chromosomal microarray analysis (CMA) is a powerful technology with the ability to survey the entire genome and identify not only chromosomal abnormalities detected by conventional cytogenetic techniques but also submicroscopic deletions and duplications (CNVs). The resolution of CMA is on the order of 10 to 400 kb or more than 100-fold greater resolution than traditional G-banding karyotyping. Even in the absence of an identified anomaly on fetal ultrasound, CMA should be offered for any patient undergoing invasive sampling because CMA has been demonstrated to detect a pathogenic or likely pathogenic CNV in approximately 1% of patients with a normal fetal ultrasound and a normal karyotype. The rate of a pathogenic CNV in a fetus with a structural abnormality and normal karyotype is higher at approximately 6%. All providers offering prenatal CMA should be aware of the reporting criteria of the laboratory; CNVs are assigned to one of four main categories: normal, benign, pathogenic, and variant of uncertain clinical significance (VUS). Although CMA is designed to access genetic imbalance, it does not reach the resolution of smaller deletions and therefore single-gene disorders such as cystic fibrosis or most skeletal dysplasias will not be detected by CMA. Moreover, balanced rearrangements, such as inversions or translocations, are not detected by CMA. Commonly identified "pitfalls" of CMA include VUS, identification of adult-onset disease or parental presymptomatic disorders, revelation of nonpaternity, unsuspected consanguinity, findings linked to diseases with variable expressivity and penetrance, and microdeletions involved with a predilection for cancer development.

Next-generation sequencing has revolutionized genetic sequencing capabilities. Next-generation sequencing involves preparation of a full DNA "library" by amplifying and fragmenting the DNA source of interest. Clinical sequencing including exome sequencing, which includes only the protein-coding region of DNA, and genome sequencing have well-established efficacy as diagnostic techniques in the pediatric setting and represent the next frontier in prenatal genetic diagnostic techniques for appropriately selected clinical presentations. Data generated from sequencing methods are vast; widespread use of prenatal sequencing technology currently remains limited by long turnaround times, prohibitive cost, and the high rate of VUS. In addition, prenatal genotyping remains challenging to interpret in the setting of limited phenotyping offered by prenatal ultrasound. Current consensus guidelines from the International Society of Prenatal Diagnosis and SMFM support pursuit of exome sequencing in selected cases of fetuses with patterns of anomalies suggestive of a single-gene disorder or nondiagnostic standard genetic testing or in cases of recurrent fetal anomalies or stillbirth for which standard testing has been nondiagnostic.

Noninvasive prenatal screening refers to a class of genetic tests designed to detect fetal aneuploidy by quantitation of small fragments of cell-free DNA (cfDNA) circulating in the maternal plasma. The cfDNA performance statistics for detection of the common aneuploidies (trisomies 21, 18, and 13) are far better than any other standard screening method. It is important to note that the aneuploidy rate is increased in cfDNA samples with an inadequate fetal fraction. The recommendation is to follow up no-call cfDNA results with counseling regarding the increased aneuploidy risk and discussion about detailed fetal ultrasound and diagnostic testing options. The current SMFM recommendation is that screening for microdeletions or single-gene disorders by cfDNA is not indicated at this time because clinical validation is lacking and the positive and negative predictive values of these rare microdeletion syndromes are unknown. In recent years, there has been more widespread utilization of embryo testing during IVF. Preimplantation genetic testing (PGT) is now divided into two general categories: high-risk PGT, also known as *preimplantation genetic diagnosis*, and low-risk PGT-A (for aneuploidy). Low-risk PGT-A is generally reserved for infertility patients undergoing in vitro fertilization (IVF) with the theoretical goal of increasing take-home pregnancy rates by screening for aneuploidy. However, its efficacy remains controversial but its use has become common in the United States. PGT-M is a term used to describe genetic testing for Mendelian disorders performed before an embryo is implanted in the uterus. In order for PGT-M to be performed, carrier status of the parents and identifiable pathogenic variants are required for testing. The most common monogenetic disorders evaluated by PGT-M are autosomal recessive diseases including cystic fibrosis, B-thalassemia, and SMA; autosomal dominant conditions such as myotonic dystrophy and Huntington disease; and X-linked conditions such as fragile X syndrome, Duchenne and Becker muscular dystrophy, and hemophilia. A parent who is a carrier of a balanced chromosomal rearrangement has a higher risk of producing unbalanced embryos, leading to recurrent miscarriage or a fetus with an unbalanced rearrangement. PGT-SR permits the transfer of only embryos with a normal or balanced chromosomal complement and has been demonstrated to significantly improve outcomes.

Finally, much controversy has been generated surrounding the use of newly available genome editing technologies such as clustered regularly interspaced short palindromic repeats (CRISPR) to edit embryo genomes. Because of this, routine application of genome editing in humans is unlikely to occur clinically in the near future.

QUESTIONS

1. Naturally occurring differences in the genetic code that are not typically associated with disease are best termed:
   a. CNVs
   b. SNPs
   c. Duplications
   d. Inversions

2. CNVs are best described as:
   a. Always pathogenic
   b. Always benign
   c. May have an as yet unknown significance
   d. Smaller than SNPs

3. Which genetic carrier screening modality is recommended by the ACOG?
   a. Ethnicity based
   b. Panethnic
   c. Expanded
   d. All of the above

4. In which of the following genetic diseases is carrier screening of all populations recommended?
   a. Fragile X syndrome
   b. Cystic fibrosis
   c. Hemophilia
   d. Achondroplasia

5. Which of the following criteria best applies to expanded carrier screening panels?
   a. The carrier frequency should be 1 in 200 or greater.
   b. The disease should have a well-defined phenotype.
   c. The disease should be amenable to prenatal treatment.
   d. The disease should be lethal in the pediatric period.

6. According to the ACOG, which best describes which patients should be offered aneuploidy screening and testing?
   a. Patients older than or equal to 35 years of age
   b. Patients with previous pregnancies complicated by aneuploidy
   c. All patients
   d. Patients with abnormal cell-free DNA screening results

7. A 35-year-old G2P1 at 16 weeks' gestation wants to pursue diagnostic amniocentesis for aneuploidy. Which figure best describes the modern-day procedure-related loss rate?
   a. 1/100
   b. 1/200
   c. 1/500
   d. 1/1000

8. A 37-year-old G3P2 at 12 weeks' gestation undergoes CVS testing for aneuploidy. The risk of a mosaic result is best described as:
   a. 0.1%
   b. 0.5%
   c. 1%
   d. 2%

9. Which patients undergoing diagnostic amniocentesis should be offered chromosomal microarray analysis (CMA)?
   a. Those 35 years and older
   b. Those with a fetal anomaly on fetal ultrasound examination
   c. Any patient undergoing diagnostic testing
   d. None; it is not indicated by current guidelines

10. A 35-year-old G3 P2 has a normal 18-week detailed fetal ultrasound examination and undergoes amniocentesis. The karyotype returns as normal. What is the likelihood of a pathogenic CNV on chromosomal microarray (CMA)?
    a. 0.1%
    b. 1%
    c. 5%
    d. 10%

11. What are known limitations of CMA for prenatal diagnosis?
    a. It cannot detect single-gene disorders.
    b. It cannot detect balanced chromosomal rearrangements.
    c. It may detect a VUS.
    d. All of the above.

12. What are known limitations of exome sequencing for prenatal diagnosis?
    a. Long turnaround times
    b. Prohibitive costs
    c. Generation of high numbers of VUSs
    d. All of the above

13. A 36-year-old G2 P1 had a previous pregnancy complicated by multiple fetal structural abnormalities and growth restriction. Karyotype and CMA were normal. She presents at 18 weeks' gestation, and fetal ultrasound detects a constellation of abnormalities similar to her last pregnancy. Which prenatal test is most appropriate?
    a. Karyotype
    b. CMA
    c. Exome sequencing
    d. Skeletal dysplasia gene panel

14. A 40-year-old G1 patient at 12 weeks' gestation declines invasive testing for aneuploidy but wants to pursue noninvasive aneuploidy screening. Which screening test is most appropriate?
    a. Cell-free DNA screening
    b. Quad screen
    c. First-trimester nuchal screening with serum analytes
    d. Assessment of the fetal nasal bone

15. A 37-year-old G2P1 at 12 weeks' gestation undergoes cfDNA screening and the fetal fraction is reported as low. What is the best next step?
    a. Counseling regarding the increased aneuploidy risk with discussion of detailed ultrasound and diagnostic testing
    b. Assessment of body fat composition
    c. CMA
    d. First-trimester screening with nuchal translucency and serum analytes

16. Microdeletion screening during cfDNA screening is indicated for which of the following indications?
    a. Fetal heart defects
    b. All patients
    c. Not currently recommended
    d. If a constellation of fetal abnormalities is noted suggestive of a syndromic diagnosis

17. A 35-year-old G2P1 undergoes IVF and wishes to have preimplantation genetic testing. Which PGT (preimplantation genetic testing) modality is most appropriate?
    a. PGT-A (aneuploidy)
    b. PGT-M (Mendelian)
    c. PGT-SR (structural chromosomal rearrangement)
    d. PGT-P (polygenic risk)

18. A 28-year-old G2 P1 patient had a previous pregnancy complicated by cystic fibrosis with two identifiable parental mutations. Which PGT modality is most appropriate?
    a. PGT-A
    b. PGT-M
    c. PGT-SR
    d. PGT-P

19. A 34-year-old G3P2 carries a known 14;21 balanced chromosomal rearrangement discovered with delivery of a trisomy 21 child. Which PGT modality is most appropriate?
    a. PGT-A
    b. PGT-M
    c. PGT-SR
    d. PGT-P

20. Genomic editing such as CRISPR is currently indicated for:
    a. Patients with a structural fetal abnormality
    b. Patients with a metabolic fetal defect
    c. A patient wanting to decrease the change of their child developing an infectious disease such as HIV
    d. Not currently clinically indicated

3

Normal Early Development

DRUCILLA JANE ROBERTS | MANA PARAST

(see Creasy and Resnik's Maternal-Fetal Medicine, 9e: Ch 3)

Summary

This chapter explores human placentation and embryogenesis from fertilization through development of the body plan and early organogenesis from a molecular developmental perspective.

The placental epithelium develops from trophectoderm, the earliest specified tissue type in the embryo. During the transition from morula to blastocyst, the outermost cells of the compact morula differentiate into specialized extraembryonic cells termed *trophectoderm*, which subsequently gives rise to the three trophoblast lineages: cytotrophoblast (CTB), syncytiotrophoblast (STB), and extravillous trophoblast (EVT). These epithelial cells have distinct properties necessary for survival of the embryo and placental development/function.

The CTB is the stem cell of the trophoblast lineage and can differentiate into either STB or EVT. CTBs are mononuclear proliferative cells and relatively hormonally inert. The STB is a true syncytium formed by differentiation and fusion of CTB cells in floating villi. The STB is a terminally differentiated cell, which lines the placenta like a glove and performs many of the unique functions of the placenta, including hormone production and transportation of factors between the mother and the fetus. EVTs arise from CTB in anchoring villi and have two subtypes. The interstitial EVT anchors the placenta to the decidualized endometrium by invading the decidua and the inner third of the myometrium. Endovascular EVTs invade the spiral arterioles and help transform them into low-resistance, high-capacitance vessels. EVTs also transiently occlude the lumen of spiral arterioles, preventing maternal perfusion of the early developing placenta until around the end of the first trimester, when they detach and allow maternal blood flow. The early developing embryo and placenta are nourished by histotrophic secretions from the endometrial glands until then.

EVTs are intimately associated with maternal tissues, including the endomyometrium and decidual immune cells with which they coordinate via cell surface receptors and secreted factors, allowing a semiallogeneic embryo to implant in the uterus. To survive within the maternal environment, all trophoblasts lack classical human leukocyte antigen (HLA) molecules, with EVT expressing only nonclassical HLA molecules, allowing crosstalk with maternal immune cells.

In addition to trophoblast, the placenta is also composed of extraembryonic mesoderm and resident macrophages, termed *Hofbauer cells,* arranged in villous structures formed by branching morphogenesis. Vascularization of the villi occurs by both vasculogenesis and angiogenesis, each regulated by changes in oxygen tension. Villous morphology adapts throughout gestation, from early chorionic villi composed of loose stroma and two layers of trophoblast (inner CTB and outer STB) with centrally placed vasculature, to late-gestation predominance of small "terminal" villi with a discontinuous CTB layer and a thin STB layer with syncytiotrophoblastic knots. Terminal villi have characteristic peripheral capillaries with close adherence of fetal endothelium to the STB layer, forming the vasculosyncytial membranes, which facilitate gas exchange and minimize diffusion distances.

Implantation is a process by which the blastocyst burrows into the decidua (specialized endometrial stroma altered in phenotype by progesterone, among other factors). Implantation occurs in a window from 6–10 days post fertilization and requires trophoblast, maternal immune cells, and a receptive uterus. Receptivity is a poorly understood phenomenon but is a function of estrogen- and progesterone-responsive factors among others. Key factors include leukemia inhibitory factor (a secreted cytokine), IHH (a morphogen), and HOXA10 and HOXA11 (transcription factors). Nonreceptive endometrium is an important cause of implantation failure (early pregnancy loss).

Following implantation, the trophoblast differentiates first to primitive syncytium and then to the three sublineages described earlier. During this time the blastocyst's inner cell mass (the primitive embryo) begins to undergo gastrulation, giving rise to three tissue types: endoderm, mesoderm, and ectoderm. During this process the embryo is patterned such that there is ventral (endoderm side) and dorsal (ectoderm side) polarity. The primitive streak from which the endoderm and mesoderm are formed also sets up the anterior-posterior (AP) axis. The right-left axis is formed by factors at the primitive node. Early events after gastrulation involve increased patterning along these three axes.

Early neurulation involves formation of a dually open-ended tube. Specialized cells undergo epithelial-to-mesenchymal transition and delaminate from the folds to form neural crest cells, important in cranial, cardiac, and intestinal development. The tube then undergoes a series of subdivisions to form the regions of central nervous system. Neurulation is patterned along the AP axis by the *HOX* genes giving positional identity to the different regions of the central nervous system. The *HOX* code is also important in AP patterning of the vertebrae, gut, and limb. Neurulation results in folding and turning of the embryo.

Cardiac formation starts in two inverted horseshoe-shaped zones anterior to the node: the primary and secondary heart fields. The heart is formed by mesoderm and neural crest cells. Ventricular myocardium is primarily derived from primary heart field, and outflow tract is formed from the secondary heart field with neural crest cell contribution. As the embryo lengthens and folds during neurulation, the heart is brought posteroventrally to its position in the thoracic cavity. The primitive heart starts to function at about 4 weeks' developmental age, long before maternal perfusion of the placenta.

Mesodermal patterning regions include paraxial, lateral plate, and intermediate mesoderm. Paraxial mesoderm is adjacent to the notochord and will form the vertebra and ribs, extracranial skeletal muscles, and dermis. Lateral plate mesoderm has a splanchnic layer and a somatic layer. The splanchnic lateral plate mesoderm forms the pleura and heart fields, as well as the smooth muscle of the gut. The somatic layer forms the sternum and skeleton of the limbs, as well as all the connective tissue of the lateral and ventral body wall. The intermediate mesoderm forms the genitourinary system. Paraxial mesoderm forms somites—balls of cells developing in an anterior-to-posterior sequence using oscillating gene expression described as a "clock-and-wavefront model." An oscillatory clock results in segmentation by wavefronts of critical secreted factors and morphogens. After somitogenesis, the cell populations of each somite are regionalized into a medial sclerotome, giving rise to the skeletogenic cells of the vertebrae and ribs and a dermomyotome that produces the dorsal dermis and all postcranial striated muscles. Signals controlling this process come from the notochord, dorsal neural tube, and surface ectoderm.

Limb development has been well described and is produced by the somatic lateral plate and migrating somitic myoblasts. Limb position is directed by mesodermal expression of specific transcription factors. The limb bud has specialized signaling regions that control pattern in the AP, dorsal (ectoderm side) polarity, and outgrowth using growth factors and morphogens. Individual digits are formed by apoptosis of cells the interdigital regions coordinated by secreted factors—BMPs. The ZPA (zone of proliferating activity) and its morphogen SHH coordinate AP pattern by inducing nested *HOX* gene expression for digit specification. The AER (apical ectodermal ridge) and its secreted factors are critical in limb outgrowth.

Organogenesis begins after gastrulation and neurulation, occurring rapidly such that development of all organs and tissues is well under way by the end of the first trimester, when maternal perfusion of the placenta begins.

QUESTIONS

1. Which is the first cell type to differentiate in the zygote?
   a. Extraembryonic mesoderm
   b. Neural epithelium
   c. Endoderm
   d. Trophectoderm
   e. Cardiac mesoderm

2. During what time window (day post fertilization [dpf]) does the blastocyst implant in the uterus?
   a. 3-5 dpf
   b. 4-6 dpf
   c. 6-10 dpf
   d. 8-12 dpf
   e. 12-15 dpf

3. What are the three main sublineages that arise from trophectoderm?
   a. Primitive syncytium, extravillous trophoblast, syncytiotrophoblast
   b. Cytotrophoblast, syncytiotrophoblast, extravillous trophoblast
   c. Interstitial trophoblast, endovascular trophoblast, cytotrophoblast

4. What is considered the stem cell of the trophoblast lineage?
   a. Syncytiotrophoblast
   b. Interstitial extravillous trophoblast
   c. Primitive syncytium
   d. Endovascular extravillous trophoblast
   e. Cytotrophoblast

5. Which trophoblast lines the villi and "faces" the maternal blood in the maternal lakes?
   a. Syncytiotrophoblast
   b. Interstitial extravillous trophoblast
   c. Primitive syncytium
   d. Endovascular extravillous trophoblast
   e. Cytotrophoblast

6. What is the function of the extravillous trophoblast?
   a. Secrete hormones to maintain the pregnancy
   b. Anchor the placenta to the uterus
   c. Transform the spiral arterioles to high-capacitance, low-resistance vessels
   d. All of the above
   e. b and c

7. What features are important for development of a receptive uterus for successful implantation?
   a. Estrogen and progesterone responsive factors (e.g., IHH, HAND2, LIF)
   b. Nonhormone responsive factors (e.g., MSX2, BMP2, and HOXA10)
   c. bHCG
   d. a and b
   e. All of the above

8. Successful implantation involves all of the below except
   a. Optimally a fundal location
   b. Remodeling the spiral arterioles
   c. A receptive uterus
   d. Interplay between extravillous trophoblast and specialized immune cells in the decidua
   e. The presence of an embryo

9. Maternal perfusion of the placenta starts
   a. At the end of the first trimester
   b. At implantation
   c. At gastrulation
   d. When the fetal heart functions
   e. When the placenta has formed a disk

10. Molecules that control embryonic development include
    a. Morphogens
    b. Signaling molecules
    c. Transcription factors
    d. All of the above
    e. None of the above

11. Which is not true about chorionic villous development?
    a. Uses branching morphogenesis
    b. Continues through the second trimester
    c. Adapts to hypoxic signals
    d. Occurs over the entire blastocyst in the early gestation but then degenerates over the chorion laeve
    e. Forms vasculosyncytial membranes in the first trimester

12. Errors in implantation can result in all the following except:
    a. Spontaneous abortion
    b. Development of preeclampsia
    c. Abnormal placentation as in circumvallation
    d. Delayed villous maturation
    e. Placenta membranacea

13. Gastrulation
    a. Results in formation of these three axes: anterior/posterior, dorsal/ventral, and left/right
    b. Occurs before implantation
    c. Is controlled by maternal effect genes
    d. Forms the placental disk
    e. Controls position of the umbilicus

14. Which is not true about limb development?
    a. Interdigital apoptosis, coordinated by BMPs, results in individual digits
    b. Nested *HOX* gene expression induced by SHH controls anterior/posterior pattern
    c. Secreted factors from the AER control limb outgrowth
    d. The ZPA expresses SHH
    e. Axial positions are determined by secreted morphogens from the notochord

15. Which is an example of a transcription factor?
    a. BMP2
    b. HOXA11
    c. FGF4
    d. WNT3
    e. Retinoic acid

16. The process of neurulation involves
    a. Folding the ectoderm into a spherical shape
    b. Signals from the mesoderm
    c. Regionally restricted expression of *HOX* genes
    d. Formation of a closed end tube
    e. Migration of the neural crest cells into the neural folds

17. Somitogenesis is controlled in part by
    a. Clocklike action/ periodic expression of factors in the presomitic/paraxial mesoderm
    b. The *HOX* code
    c. Endodermal signals to the mesoderm
    d. Ectodermal signals to the mesoderm
    e. Morphogens

18. Heart formation occurs from specialized mesodermal tissue in two "fields": primary and secondary. The primary heart field
    a. Is also known as the cardiac crescent and is an inverted U-shaped field anterior to the primitive node
    b. Is formed in part from pharyngeal mesoderm
    c. Forms the atria and outflow tracts
    d. Forms part of the heart tube, which functions at around 10 weeks' gestational age
    e. Includes neural crest tissue

19. The urogenital system is formed from
    a. Lateral plate mesoderm
    b. Somites
    c. Intermediate mesoderm
    d. Endoderm
    e. Notochord

20. Extravillous trophoblast must evade maternal immunologic rejection, as they are semiallogeneic. They achieve immune privilege by using all these techniques except:
    a. Lack of expression of the classical HLA-A and HLA-B proteins
    b. Expression of nonclassical HLA proteins including HLA-G, HLA-C, and HLA-E
    c. Increasing the Treg pool in the maternal decidua
    d. Facilitating cross-talk with maternal natural killer cells and macrophages
    e. Avoiding maternal immune cells by secreting inhibitory factors

4

Amniotic Fluid Dynamics

MICHAEL G. ROSS | MARIE BEALL

(see Creasy and Resnik's Maternal-Fetal Medicine, 9e: Ch 4)

Summary

Amniotic fluid (AF) is necessary for normal human fetal growth and development. The fluid volume cushions the fetus, protecting it from mechanical trauma, and its bacteriostatic properties may help maintain a sterile intrauterine environment. The space created by the AF allows fetal movement and aids in the normal development of both the lungs and limbs. AF volume increases progressively between 10 and 30 weeks' gestation. After 30 weeks the increase slows, and AF volume may remain unchanged until 36 to 38 weeks' gestation, when it tends to decrease, resulting in an increased incidence of oligohydramnios in postterm gestations.

In the first trimester of pregnancy, AF is isotonic with maternal or fetal plasma likely arising from a transudate of plasma from either the fetus or mother. Beginning near the end of the first trimester, the major contributors to AF volume are fetal urine and fluid lung liquid with AF resorption via fetal swallowing and intramembranous flow. Evidence suggests that the entire volume of AF turns over daily, making this a highly dynamic system.

Fetal urine is the major contributor to AF volume, with the amount of urine produced increasing progressively with advancing gestation. Near term the fetus may produce nearly 1000 mL per day. Reduction or absence of fetal urine flow is commonly associated with oligohydramnios. Fetal urine production may decrease in response to maternal and fetal dehydration, fetal renal or bladder anomalies, or potentially fetal hypoxemia.

The fetal lung is a secondary source of AF, as evidenced by the finding of pulmonary phospholipids (lecithin, sphingomyelin, and phosphatidylglycerol) in the AF. Approximately half of the fluid exiting the lungs enters the AF, and half is swallowed, resulting in a net AF contribution only about one-sixth that of urine. Almost all fetal stimuli (hypoxia, hormones) have been demonstrated to reduce production of fetal lung liquid, indicating that lung liquid production functions at maximal capacity. Rather than regulating AF volume, fetal lung fluid secretion is likely most important in providing for pulmonary expansion, which promotes airway and alveolar development.

The major route of AF resorption is fetal swallowing, accounting for up to 760 mL/day near term. Swallowing may increase near term, contributing to a reduction in AF volume. Fetal swallowing may increase in response to dehydration and decreases with hypotension or hypoxia. In addition to fetal swallowing, AF is resorbed across the intramembranous (IM) pathway: the route of absorption from the amniotic cavity directly across the amnion into the fetal vessels. Although IM flow has never been directly detected in humans, indirect evidence supports its presence. In nonhuman primates, IM flow would explain the absorption of AF technetium and vasopressin in fetuses after esophageal ligation. Thus water and compounds can cross directly from the AF to the fetal circulation with water crossing via cellular aquaporin channels. The combination of fetal swallowing and IM flow balances fetal urine and lung liquid production under homeostatic conditions.

Although most of the major sources of AF inflow and outflow can be influenced by the fetus, only IM flow can be shown to undergo modulation in response to primary changes in AF volume, suggesting IM flow as the candidate mechanism for AF volume homeostasis. Whereas polyhydramnios and oligohydramnios often can be explained by fetal anatomic or functional anomalies, it is likely that idiopathic amniotic fluid volume abnormalities are due to alterations in IM flow, perhaps a result of differences in aquaporin water channels.

QUESTIONS

1. A 36-year-old woman, G4 P2 at 32 weeks' gestation, arrives in Labor and Delivery complaining of dizziness, headache, and uterine contractions for the past 48 hours. Outdoor temperatures have been up to 40°C, and she complains that the air conditioning is "out" in her building. Fetal heart rate is 160 bpm, with variability. Accelerations and decelerations are absent. An ultrasound reveals a normally grown fetus in a breech presentation with a deepest amniotic fluid pocket of 1.8 cm. What is the best next step in management?
   a. Antenatal corticosteroids and delivery in 48 hours
   b. Deliver immediately without waiting for steroids
   c. 1 L of oral hydration with water
   d. Intravenous hydration with a 500 mL bolus of D5LR

2. What do you think is the mechanism of the reduced amniotic fluid?
   a. This amount of fluid is normal for some fetuses.
   b. The fetus is likely hypoxic, and the low fluid is a consequence of this, with fetal blood flow being diverted away from the fetal kidneys.
   c. The mother is ill, and her blood flow has been redistributed. The fetus is not getting sufficient blood flow or oxygen and is redistributing blood flow away from the kidneys.
   d. The mother is dehydrated, and water is not flowing to the fetus across the placenta, as the normal osmotic gradient is not present. Subsequently the fetus reduces urine flow, the effect of which is to preserve fetal blood volume.

3. A 27-year-old woman G2P0 at 33 weeks' gestation with a known anencephalic fetus presents with known polyhydramnios. She is symptomatic, and on ultrasound her deepest pocket of fluid is 18 cm, indicating severe polyhydramnios. When counseling her about an amnioreduction, which of the following most accurately describes the expected time for reaccumulation?
   a. One day. The fetus, on average, replaces the fluid every 24 hours.
   b. Four days. The fetus, on average, generates 1000 mL fluid daily.
   c. The fluid will not reaccumulate.
   d. Not predictable. The release of the intrauterine pressure will have an unpredictable effect on fetal urine output.

4. A 17-year-old G3P0 with no prenatal care presents to Labor and Delivery for uterine contractions. A limited bedside ultrasound reveals a single fetus at 36 weeks' gestation in a vertex presentation with an estimated fetal weight of 2800 g. The amniotic fluid index is 25 cm with a single deepest pocket of 8.5 cm.
   What is the most likely etiology of polyhydramnios in this pregnancy?
   a. Duodenal atresia
   b. Gestational diabetes
   c. Maternal malnutrition
   d. Tracheal-esophageal fistula

5. A 32-year-old G3P2 at 27w 4d presents to Labor and Delivery due to decreased fetal movement. She had prenatal care elsewhere and is here on a visit; records are not immediately available. She states that her fetus had a severe diaphragmatic hernia and has had a tracheal balloon placed.
   How will the tracheal balloon affect the amniotic fluid volume?
   a. The amniotic fluid will be decreased, as lung fluid is not reaching the amniotic cavity, and this should be considered in interpreting the ultrasound results.
   b. The amniotic fluid will be increased due to pressure of the balloon on the esophagus, but this effect is minor and does not change the interpretation of the ultrasound results.
   c. The amniotic fluid will be decreased, but this effect is minor and does not change the interpretation of the ultrasound results.
   d. The amniotic fluid will be increased due to pressure of the balloon on the esophagus, and this should be considered in interpreting the ultrasound results.

6. Intramembranous flow is thought to make up about what proportion of amniotic fluid resorption in normal fetal sheep?
   a. 10%
   b. 33%
   c. 66%
   d. 90%

7. Water crosses biologic membranes via:
   a. Simple diffusion
   b. Through membrane channels
   c. By facilitated diffusion
   d. By active transport

8. To calculate diffusion across the maternal/placental interface, a number of factors are needed. Which of these may be difficult to obtain and often results in a calculation of filtration coefficient rather than the volume water flow?
   a. Reflection coefficient
   b. Osmotic pressure on the fetal side of the membrane
   c. Hydraulic conductance
   d. Membrane surface area

5

Multiple Gestation: The Biology of Twinning

CLAUDIO SCHENONE | SARAH OBICAN

(see *Creasy and Resnik's Maternal-Fetal Medicine*, 9e: Ch 5)

Summary

Twin birth rates doubled between 1971 and 2014 largely due to older maternal age distribution and expanded use of assisted reproductive technology, accounting for 3% of all births.

Twin pregnancies are categorized on the basis of their zygosity or chorionicity. Zygosity is determined based on the type of conception. Dizygotic twins (70% of cases) are the result of multiple ovulations with fertilization of two separate ova by two separate sperm cells. These babies have the same genetic relationship as non-twin siblings sharing approximately 50% of their genes. Monozygotic twins are thought to occur following the division of a zygote that originated from the fertilization of one ovum by a single sperm cell. While the prevalence of dizygotic twinning has geographical variations, monozygotic twinning occurs at a constant rate. Rates are also influenced by maternal age, body mass index, height, parity, tobacco use, levels of circulating follicle-stimulating hormone, the use of assisted reproductive technology, and other factors.

Chorionicity refers to the type of placentation. While dizygotic pregnancies almost always have dichorionic placentas (separate fetoplacental circulations for each twin), the type of placentation in monozygotic twins depends primarily on the timing at which the zygote splits. In short, early division leads to two separate placentas while those that divide later are more likely to have a shared fetoplacental circulation (monochorionic). In dichorionic placentas, the intertwin membrane comprises two amnion layers separated by a fused layer of two chorions with separate chorionic vascular beds. In contrast, monochorionic placentas have a thin, semitranslucent, two-layered intertwin membrane that lacks interposed chorion and is loosely attached to the chorionic plate. This type of placenta usually exhibits intertwin vascular connections crossing the intertwin membrane, including artery-to-artery (AA), vein-to-vein, and artery-to-vein (AV) anastomoses. AV anastomoses are obligatorily unidirectional, while the blood flow direction within AA and vein-to-vein anastomoses depends on pressure gradients between the twins and has a compensatory role for flow imbalances generated by AV anastomoses.

Twin pregnancies are susceptible to complications that may or may not be related to their twin status, and the death of one twin may affect the outcome of the other. Fetal growth discordance can affect both dichorionic and monochorionic pregnancies and is defined as more than 20–25% discrepancy between estimated fetal weights, including severe intrauterine growth restriction of one twin. Potential contributors to this complication include differing genetic growth potential, structural or chromosomal fetal anomalies, congenital infection, uneven placental sharing, and discordant cord insertion types.

Monochorionic pregnancies have a higher incidence of preterm birth, low birth weight, and prolonged stay in the neonatal intensive care unit. Furthermore, perinatal mortality rates are significantly higher in this cohort when compared with dichorionic pregnancies. This is explained at least partly due to complications that are more frequently seen in this population, such as twin-twin transfusion syndrome, twin anemia-polycythemia syndrome (TAPS), and twin reversed arterial perfusion (TRAP) sequence.

Twin-twin transfusion syndrome entails chronic fetofetal blood transfusion from one twin (donor) to the other (recipient) through placental vascular communications across unbalanced unidirectional AV anastomoses that induce dysregulation of a variety of hormonal and biochemical regulators, leading to an exaggerated hemodynamic response to fluid shifts in both twins. The frequency of uneven placental sharing and marginal or velamentous cord insertion of at least one twin is significantly higher in this population, likely contributing to its pathophysiology.

TAPS occurs when a few small anastomoses allow chronic transfusion of blood at a slower rate from donor to recipient twin, leading to a large intertwin difference in hemoglobin and reticulocyte levels. TAPS donors tend to have a larger placental share, even though that twin is usually smaller than the recipient twin. These observations suggest that fetal growth in TAPS may be primarily driven by intertwin blood transfusion rather than placental share, and there is no consensus regarding marginal cord insertion as a potential contributor to this condition.

Twin reversed arterial perfusion sequence relates to the presence of an acardiac twin with circulatory failure that is entirely dependent on the healthy co-twin (donor or pump twin) to provide blood supply through retrograde flow into its umbilical arteries via intertwin AA anastomoses shunting partially deoxygenated blood preferentially to the lower half of the acardiac twin, resulting in predominant lower body growth with concurrent anomalies in other parts.

Monoamniotic twinning pertains to monochorionic pregnancies with fetuses sharing a single amniotic sac. In these cases, the umbilical cords are typically inserted close to each other on the chorionic plate and connected by large-caliber superficial vascular anastomoses. In the case of conjoined twins, placentas may have a single umbilical fused cord with a variable number of vessels that may range from three to eight.

Complete hydatidiform moles may coexist with a healthy "co-twin." Placental pathology in these cases reveals a sharp contrast between grapelike clusters of cysts in the molar component and the age-appropriate normal-appearing placenta of the normal pregnancy.

Finally, spontaneous loss of an embryo or fetus during the first trimester of a twin pregnancy is known as vanishing twin syndrome. This is also termed *fetus papyraceus* when the same phenomenon occurs during the early second trimester (12–20 weeks).

In summary, multiple gestations involve an array of complex biological interactions. As a clinical entity, the incidence of twin pregnancies has risen over the past four decades, and they portray a significantly higher risk of perinatal morbidity and mortality, especially in monochorionic pregnancies because of a set of complications that are specific to this type of placentation.

QUESTIONS

1. A 30-year-old woman, gravida 2, para 1, comes for her first prenatal visit at 18 weeks' gestation. Ultrasonography reveals two separate fetuses in two separate sacs divided by a triangular projection extending up to the base of the dividing membrane. Assuming this is a monozygotic twin pregnancy, the number of days at which the split most likely occurred following fertilization is:
   a. 0–3 days
   b. 4–8 days
   c. 9–12 days
   d. >12 days

2. When compared with singleton pregnancies, the likelihood of congenital anomalies in twins is:
   a. Higher
   b. Lower
   c. Equivalent
   d. Difficult to estimate

3. A 26-year-old woman, gravida 3, para 2, comes for a detailed anatomy scan at 22 weeks due to suspicion of twin-twin transfusion syndrome (TTTS) on an earlier ultrasound by the referring physician. As you discuss the implications of this condition, you explain to the patient that TTTS traditionally refers to:
   a. Exsanguination from the surviving twin into the circulation of the dead or dying co-twin
   b. Chronic fetofetal blood transfusion from one twin to the other through placental vascular communications
   c. Postpartum placentofetal blood transfusion to the remaining twin through vascular anastomoses
   d. The phenomenon of bidirectional flow across AA anastomoses

4. A 28-year-old woman, gravida 2, para 1 with monochorionic diamniotic twin pregnancy complicated by TAPS comes for a follow-up ultrasonographic evaluation. Fetal biometry of both twins revealed fetal growth discordance of 26% and newly diagnosed selective fetal growth restriction of Twin B (third percentile). As you counsel the patient and family members, you explain that the highest contributor to growth discordance in monochorionic pregnancies complicated by TAPS is likely:
   a. Unequal placental sharing
   b. Cord insertion differences
   c. Intertwin blood transfusion
   d. Postzygotic genetic changes

5. A 22-year-old woman, gravida 1, para 0 with a monochorionic diamniotic twin intrauterine pregnancy is diagnosed with twin reverse arterial perfusion (TRAP) sequence. As part of your counseling, you disclose the presence of several congenital anomalies in the acardiac twin and the rationale behind this phenomenon. Given the pathogenesis and angioarchitecture of pregnancies complicated by TRAP, the body part of the acardiac twin most likely to grow is:
   a. Head
   b. Thorax and upper extremities
   c. Abdomen
   d. Pelvis and lower extremities

6. A 21-year-old woman, gravida 1, para 0 comes for her first prenatal visit at 18 weeks' gestation. During an ultrasonographic survey, you notice two separate fetuses. A triangular projection extending up to the base of the dividing membrane is seen. Estimated fetal weight using Hadlock's formula is obtained for both twins. Regarding multiple gestations, which of the following is the correct definition of severe fetal growth discordance?
   a. >20–25% discordance between estimated fetal weights (EFW)
   b. EFW <10th percentile in both twins
   c. EFW <10th percentile in one or both twins
   d. >20–25% discordance between estimated fetal weights (EFW), with one twin measuring <10th percentile based on EFW

7. A 34-year-old woman, gravida 7, para 4 with dichorionic diamniotic twin intrauterine pregnancy presents for a follow-up ultrasonographic evaluation. The estimated fetal weight of Twin A is 920 g (39th percentile), and Twin B 728g (3rd percentile) using Hadlock's formula. Which of the following is the correct percentage of fetal weight discordance based on the above estimated fetal weights?
   a. 21%
   b. 26%
   c. 36%
   d. 42%

8. A 26-year-old woman, gravida 3, para 2, comes for a detailed anatomy scan at 25 weeks' gestation due to suspicion of twin-twin transfusion syndrome on an earlier scan by the referring provider. As you discuss the implications of this condition, you explain to the patient that the blood flow imbalance causing the findings on ultrasound is mainly caused by the following type of vascular anastomosis:
   a. Artery-artery
   b. Vein-vein
   c. Artery-vein
   d. All of the above

9. A 32-year-old woman, gravida 3, para 2, comes for a detailed anatomy scan at 18 weeks' gestation. You notice the presence of two separate fetuses and two separate amniotic sacs. Which of the following is an ultrasonographic sign suggestive of a monochorionic pregnancy?
   a. Triangular projection extending up to the base of the dividing membrane
   b. The presence of two distinct placental masses
   c. A thin dividing membrane that approximates the placenta at a 90-degree angle
   d. Discordant sex

10. A 32-year-old woman, gravida 3, para 2, is diagnosed with a monochorionic monoamniotic twin intrauterine pregnancy. The patient asks about potential complications pertaining to this type of pregnancy. Which of the following complications is specific to monoamniotic pregnancies?
   a. Severe fetal growth discordance
   b. Fetus papyraceous
   c. Coexistent complete hydatidiform mole
   d. Cord entanglement

6

Biology of Parturition

MALA S. MAHENDROO | STEPHEN J. LYE

(see Creasy and Resnik's Maternal-Fetal Medicine, 9e: Ch 6)

Summary

- The timing of birth is a critical determinant of perinatal outcome. The fetoplacental unit is in control of the timing of labor in humans, and maternal factors are also involved.
- It is likely that a parturition cascade is responsible at term for the removal of mechanisms maintaining uterine quiescence and for the recruitment of factors acting to promote uterine activity.
- Inflammatory signals and an influx of maternal immune cells into uterine tissues play a key role in the process of parturition.
- Contractile activity of the myometrium is mediated by depolarization of the myocyte cell membrane. This depolarization induces an influx of calcium into the myocytes and the activation of the contractile protein machinery leading to an energy-dependent interaction of myosin and actin molecules and shortening of the cell.
- Stimulatory hormones, such as prostaglandins and oxytocin, act in part to promote myocyte membrane depolarization and calcium influx, whereas myometrial relaxants inhibit these processes and the signals that lead to actin-myosin interaction. These pathways are targeted by clinical therapeutics aimed at induction or inhibition of labor.
- The myometrium exhibits a program of differentiation during pregnancy including an initial phase of myocyte proliferation (mediated by estrogen and androgen) followed by a phase of cellular hypertrophy (mediated by myometrial tension in the presence of progesterone). A final differentiation induced by progesterone receptor withdrawal, posttranslational modification, or isoform switching leads to a contractile phenotype in which the myometrium becomes activated (as a result of increased *CAP* gene expression), endogenous stimulants drive contractions, and the myocytes anchor to the underlying matrix proteins so that cellular shortening translates into uterine contraction.
- Local metabolism of progesterone and dominance of progesterone receptor A over progesterone receptor B isoforms represent mechanisms by which a functional progesterone may occur in human pregnancy even in the presence of elevated peripheral progesterone levels at term.
- Cervical remodeling in preparation for parturition begins early in pregnancy and culminates with loss of mechanical integrity at term.
- Timely completion of cervical remodeling requires sustaining both immunologic and barrier protection by the epithelia and structural reorganization of collagen in the stroma.
- Hormone-regulated biochemical changes alter the structure and mechanical strength of the cervical extracellular matrix from early pregnancy to parturition.

QUESTIONS

1. As pregnancy progresses, there is a redistribution of blood flow within the uterus with 80%—90% of the flow going to the:
   a. cervix
   b. myometrium
   c. placenta
   d. endometrium

2. Genetic defects in genes encoding which type of component are associated with cervical insufficiency?
   a. Steroid hormone synthesis
   b. Extracellular matrix components
   c. Prostaglandin synthesis
   d. Proinflammatory cytokines

3. In the human, functional withdrawal of progesterone action is not achieved by which of the following?
   a. A decline in progesterone synthesis
   b. Increased progesterone metabolism
   c. Decreased expression of progesterone receptor (PR) coactivators
   d. A change in the ratio of the PR nuclear receptors, PR-A and PR-B

4. Which of the following molecules does not enhance uterine contractility?
   a. Prostaglandins
   b. Oxytocin
   c. Connexin 43
   d. Relaxin

5. A key mediator of cervical softening during pregnancy is:
   a. a decline in collagen crosslinks
   b. collagen degradation
   c. increased synthesis of hyaluronan
   d. decline in the peptide hormone relaxin

6. Which phase of cervical remodeling is a slow progesterone dominant phase?
   a. Postpartum repair
   b. Ripening
   c. Softening
   d. Dilation

7. Current research supports all but one of the following as a contributor to the timing of labor.
   a. Social determinants of health
   b. Functional estrogen withdrawal
   c. Functional progesterone withdrawal
   d. Cervical insufficiency

8. The human placenta is an incomplete steroidogenic organ. What fetal tissue and steroid serve as a substrate for estrogen biosynthesis?
   a. Lung, estriol
   b. Adrenal, dehydroepiandrosterone sulfate (DHEAS)
   c. Liver, DHEAS
   d. Adrenal, cortisol

9. Prostaglandins have numerous proposed roles in the process of labor, and their levels in fetal membranes and the reproductive tract are regulated by a balance between synthesis and catabolism. What enzyme is a key regulator of catabolism?
   a. PGHS1
   b. PGHS2
   c. PGDH
   d. PLA2

10. Cellular stress can trigger both fetal membrane weakening and labor onset in term and preterm birth through activation of danger-associated molecular patterns (DAMPs). Which of the following is NOT a DAMP molecule?
    a. Matrix metalloproteases
    b. Heat shock proteins
    c. Cell-free DNA
    d. HMGB1

7

Pathogenesis of Spontaneous Preterm Birth

CATALIN S. BUHIMSCHI | SAM MESIANO | LOUIS J. MUGLIA

(see Creasy and Resnik's Maternal-Fetal Medicine, 9e: Ch 7)

Summary

Preterm birth (PTB) is defined as birth between 20 0/7 weeks' gestation and 36 6/7 weeks' gestation. This syndrome is caused by various pathologic processes leading to decidual activation, increased myometrial contractility, cervical remodeling, and membrane rupture.

Recent advancements in technology demonstrate transition of the myometrium from quiescence to contractile status involves tightly controlled transcriptional events as shown by variation in the expression of specific genes whose products increase contractibility and excitability. Transcriptomics shows that the more significantly expressed genes induced by the primary mediator of inflammation, interleukin-1β, were coding sequences for chemokines, cytokines, prostaglandin-synthesizing enzymes, microsomal prostaglandin E synthase, transcriptional regulators, and MMP-1. The process of parturition is blocked by progesterone, at least in part by repressing responsiveness to proinflammatory and prolabor stimuli, and functional progesterone withdrawal may play a role in PTB. Changes in the net transcriptional activity of the progesterone receptor isoforms, PR-A and PR-B, are a phenomenon leading to excess unliganded PR-A promoting expression of genes encoding contraction-associated proteins.

Prostaglandins are viewed as crucial mediators for the onset of labor because they can induce myometrial contractility and promote proteolysis of cervical and fetal membrane extracellular matrices to cause cervical ripening and fetal membrane rupture. An increase in the expression of prostaglandin endoperoxide synthase 2 (PTGS-2) activity induced by inflammation-induced NF-κB activity in the myometrium and fetal membrane may play a central role. Although relatively distinct from other causes of prematurity, placental abruption can trigger molecular events responsible for decidual activation that are inflammatory in their nature.

Because amniotic fluid is normally sterile and most pathologic intraamniotic bacteria are genital tract microorganisms, the current paradigm of intrauterine infection posits that bacteria originate from the lower genital tract and invade the pregnant uterus via an ascending route. The past decade has been characterized by forceful debate whether or not the gestational sac and placenta are sterile reproductive compartments. Most evidence points toward very low bacterial levels harbored by the placenta and favors the premise that a naturally harbored microbiome carries a minimal role in triggering inflammation and preterm parturition. In contrast, cytokines and various proinflammatory and antiinflammatory factors, including complement and lipoxin, respectively, can activate the myometrial contractility, leading to early birth.

Stress has been proposed as an important risk factor for PTB. This is a complex etiologic factor to analyze because it involves complex biochemical and neurohormonal interactions among maternal, fetal, and placental compartments. A series of physiologic adaptive responses can be triggered by stress subsequent to malnutrition, infection, ischemia, vascular damage, and psychosocial factors, and women who are stressed but unable to mount an adequate stress response could be at particular risk for PTB. The exponential rise in maternal plasma corticotropin-releasing hormone (CRH) concentrations is associated with a concomitant fall in levels of CRH-binding protein, leading to a rapid increase in bioavailable CRH. High circulating levels of CRH early in pregnancy are predictive of PTB. Recently, it was demonstrated that increased decidual cell expression of the transcription factor FK506-binding protein 51 (FKBP51), which is induced by glucocorticoids and impedes both glucocorticoid and progesterone receptor transcriptional activity, was present in women with idiopathic PTB. This may help explain the link between maternal or fetal stress and normal fetal HPA maturation and both term labor and stress-induced PTB, respectively.

Several lines of evidence suggest that genetic factors contribute to the risk of PTB, particularly through variants in the maternal genome. Discovery of specific genetic variants that lead to PTB has proven to be challenging, likely due to the heterogeneous phenotype of PTB, its environmental contributors, evolutionary pressure against such mutations, and contributions from both maternal and fetal genomes.

While the traditional classification systems categorize prematurity as either spontaneous or provider initiated, most recently PTB was largely categorized on the basis of clinical phenotype. In this chapter we review the most common pathways leading to PTB, specifically premature activation of the maternal or fetal hypothalamic-pituitary-adrenal axis, exaggerated inflammatory response/infection and/or an altered genital tract microbiome, abruption (decidual hemorrhage), excessive uterine distention, genetic factors, and cervical insufficiency. The debate about which (if any) of these events is the master regulator controlling the timing of preterm parturition and which is the main factor without which parturition cannot occur continues. Regardless, all these processes converge into a common pathway of parturition, which includes anatomic, biochemical, immunologic, endocrinologic, and inflammatory changes. It is largely expected that molecular phenotyping of parturition syndrome will represent the next significant step necessary to complement clinical medicine toward a better understanding of PTB's pathophysiology and designing targeted therapies to prevent prematurity.

QUESTIONS

1. Evidence of a role for prostaglandins in the initiation of human parturition includes all of the following except:
   a. Administration of prostaglandins induces termination of pregnancy.
   b. Concentrations of prostaglandins in plasma and amniotic fluid increase during labor.
   c. Expression of myometrial prostaglandin receptors increases in labor.
   d. Prostaglandins induce the fetal hypothalamus to release corticotropin-releasing hormone (CRH), which increases myometrial contractility.

2. What enzyme is considered a rate-limiting step in the production of prostaglandins in the fetal amnion?
   a. Cyclooxygenase-2 (COX-2)
   b. Cyclooxygenase-1 (COX-1)
   c. Thromboxane synthase
   d. 11ß-hydroxysteroid dehydrogenase

3. Metagenomic studies of amniotic fluid show that:
   a. Bacterial diversity of the amniotic fluid microbiome is rich.
   b. Uncultivable bacteria are present in the amniotic fluid.
   c. Most frequent amniotic fluid infections are multibacterial.
   d. All of the above.

4. What enzyme does the human placenta lack?
   a. 3β-hydroxysteroid dehydrogenase (3β-HSD)
   b. P450c17 enzyme
   c. Alkaline phosphatase
   d. Catalase

5. Which of the following statements is correct?
   a. Congenital heart defects are not associated with spontaneous preterm birth.
   b. Right ventricular outflow tract obstructions are associated with an increased risk of spontaneous PTB.
   c. Anomalies of the cardiac system are not the most common nonchromosomal anomalies.
   d. There are no in-utero interventions available to treat congenital heart defects.

6. Characterization of the cortisol effect on placental CRH and preterm parturition includes:
   a. Cortisol stimulates CRH synthesis, which is responsible for increased prostaglandin production in the fetal membranes that can access the adjacent decidua and myometrium.
   b. Cortisol inhibits CRH synthesis, which is responsible for estrogen synthesis via increased maternal adrenal DHEA.
   c. CRH and its receptor, CRH-R1, are decreased in the placentas of pregnancies complicated by pPROM and chorioamnionitis.
   d. Cortisol does not interact with placental CRH, which was never identified in the human placenta.

7. Cervical collagen:
   a. is substituted entirely by myometrial cells toward the end of gestation.
   b. is actively synthesized during pregnancy and remodeled by the interplay of neutrophils, fibroblasts, and various enzymatic pathways.
   c. is responsible for inhibition of trophoblast penetration in placenta previa.
   d. does not interact with decorin during the process of collagen reorganization and cross-linking.

8. During pregnancy the process of cervical ripening involves all of the following except:
   a. decline in the collagen type I mRNA.
   b. gradual decrease in cervical collagen fluorescence with advancing gestation.
   c. reliance on negatively charged glycosaminoglycans and levels of VEGF.
   d. relaxin decreases collagenase activity and decreases glycosaminoglycan synthesis.

9. The process of decidual activation and bleeding involved molecular mechanisms that involve the following factors except:
   a. thrombin
   b. tissue factor
   c. progesterone
   d. thyroid-stimulating releasing factor

10. All of the following are mechanisms of preterm birth except:
    a. premature activation of the maternal or fetal hypothalamic-pituitary-adrenal axis
    b. exaggerated inflammatory response/infection and/or an altered genital tract microbiome
    c. abruption (decidual hemorrhage)
    d. overinnervation of the myometrium

11. Observations that suggest a genetic component to preterm birth risk include:
    a. Sisters of women having had a preterm infant are at increased risk for preterm birth.
    b. Mothers born preterm are at increased risk for having an infant born preterm.
    c. There is an increased risk of preterm birth to a mother with a prior preterm birth.
    d. All of the above

12. Family-based, twin, and epidemiologic studies demonstrate that genetic factors contributing to birth timing are:
    a. limited to the fetal genome
    b. limited to the maternal genome
    c. from both the maternal and fetal genomes, with a larger contribution from the maternal genome
    d. from both the maternal and fetal genomes, with a larger contribution from the fetal genome

13. A pathway (s) recently implicated in control of birth timing in genome-wide association studies in the maternal genome is:
    a. WNT4
    b. interleukin-1
    c. both WNT4 and interleukin-1
    d. neither WNT4 nor interleukin-1

14. Rare variants increasing the risk for preterm birth have been identified in:
    a. androgen receptor
    b. IGF1 receptor
    c. HSPA1L
    d. all of the above

15. Gene–environment interactions likely contribute to preterm birth risk as demonstrated for:
    a. the association of polymorphisms in COL24A1 interacting with maternal prepregnancy overweight/obesity
    b. the association of polymorphisms in PTPRD interacting with maternal prepregnancy overweight/obesity
    c. the association of polymorphisms in PTPRD interacting with maternal lifetime stress
    d. both a and c

16. The human placenta synthesizes progesterone:
    a. from pregnenolone supplied by the maternal corpus luteum
    b. de novo from maternal cholesterol beginning at around the end of the first trimester
    c. from pregnenolone supplied by the fetal adrenals
    d. from cholesterol derived from amniotic fluid

17. The human placenta synthesizes estrogens:
    a. de novo from maternal cholesterol
    b. by the aromatization of androgens supplied by the fetal gonads
    c. by the aromatization of androgens supplied by the fetal adrenals
    d. in response to chorionic gonadotropin

18. Human parturition is triggered by:
    a. a systemic decrease in maternal circulating total progesterone levels
    b. increased production of oxytocin by the fetal pituitary
    c. cortisol produced by the fetal adrenal glands
    d. none of the above

19. Estriol levels in human pregnancy:
    a. directly reflect activity of the fetal hypothalamic-pituitary-adrenal axis
    b. are associated with preterm birth
    c. reflect maternal metabolic homeostasis
    d. are controlled by chorionic gonadotropin

20. Factors involving the control of human parturition include all of the following except:
    a. biomechanical changes in the myometrium and cervix
    b. altered expression of genes encoding contraction-associated factors in myometrial cells
    c. increased activity of the fetal hypothalamic-pituitary-adrenal axis
    d. tissue-level inflammation/immune cell activation in the myometrium, cervix, and decidua

8

Immunology of Pregnancy

GIL MOR | VIKKI M. ABRAHAMS

(see Creasy and Resnik's Maternal-Fetal Medicine, 9e: Ch 8)

Summary

This chapter provides a perspective on the role of the maternal innate immune system and its interactions with the trophoblast during pregnancy. The trophoblast and the maternal immune system act jointly to protect against infectious microorganisms. When the trophoblast identifies potentially dangerous molecular signatures, the maternal immune system responds with coordinate actions. Therefore pregnancy might resemble an orchestra in which the trophoblast serves as the conductor and each immune cell type represents a different musical instrument. The success of the pregnancy pivots on how well the trophoblast communicates and works together with each immune cell.

What was originally proposed to be only a graft-host interaction should now include a supportive regulatory interaction between the trophoblast and maternal immune system. As we learn more about the regulation of the expression and function of uterine immune cells and their regulatory molecules such as Toll-like receptors and nucleotide-binding oligomerization domain–like receptors during pregnancy, we will better understand the cellular cross-talk existing at the maternal-fetal interface.

QUESTIONS

1. During the COVID-19 pandemic, pregnant women were not included in the initial vaccine clinical trials because of the following concerns about the maternal immune system:
   a. Pregnant women are characterized by systemic immune suppression.
   b. The fetus suppresses the immune system of the mother, making her more susceptible to infections.
   c. Pregnant women lack an adequate T-cell response and cannot respond to viral infections.
   d. Hormonal changes during pregnancy make women less responsive to vaccines.

2. For many years the process of immune tolerance to paternal antigens has been associated with other immunologic processes. Which one of the following is most appropriate in view of advances in the field?
   a. The immunology of pregnancy is like a graft-versus-host condition, and success depends on a systemic immune suppression.
   b. The immunology of pregnancy is more like a tumor-immune response where small amounts of antigens induce tolerance to paternal antigens.
   c. During pregnancy, fetal-derived dendritic cells present paternal antigens to the maternal immune system, triggering a graft-versus-host response.
   d. Maternal immune cells are present in the uterus in response to paternal antigens.

3. Indicate in which of the following conditions rejection occurs and is similar to pregnancy (**Fig. 8.1**):

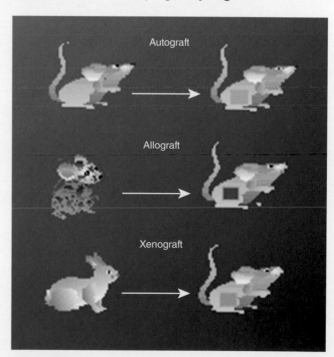

   a. Autograft
   b. Allograft
   c. Xenograft

4. Fetal cells have been shown to integrate into maternal tissue, and they play a role within the maternal physiology. In your opinion, which one describes the most advanced understanding of maternal chimerism?
   a. Fetal cells only are present in the maternal circulation.
   b. Fetal cells contribute to tissue renewal in maternal organs.
   c. There is no migration of fetal cells to maternal organs.

5. The inflammatory environment during pregnancy changes according development of the fetus. Which of the following best describes the dominant immunologic environment in a given trimester?
   a. The first trimester of pregnancy is an antiinflammatory condition.
   b. The second trimester of pregnancy is an inflammatory condition.
   c. The first trimester of pregnancy is an inflammatory condition.
   d. The third trimester of pregnancy is an antiinflammatory condition.

9

Maternal Cardiovascular, Respiratory, and Renal Adaptation to Pregnancy

MANJU MONGA | JOAN M. MASTROBATTISTA

(see Creasy and Resnik's Maternal-Fetal Medicine, 9e: Ch 9)

Summary

Profound physiologic changes occur in the cardiovascular, respiratory, and renal systems during pregnancy. An increase in plasma volume begins at 6 to 8 weeks' gestation, reaching a maximal volume of 4700 to 5200 mL at 32 weeks. Red blood cell mass increases by 250 to 450 mL, an increase of 20% to 30% by term compared with prepregnancy values. Because plasma volume increases disproportionately to the increase in red blood cell mass, physiologic hemodilution occurs, resulting in a mild decrease in maternal hematocrit. Cardiac output increases by 30% to 50% during pregnancy, and half of this increase occurs by 8 weeks' gestation. Stroke volume is primarily responsible for the early increase in cardiac output and declines toward term. Maternal heart rate increases from 5 weeks to a maximal increment of 15 to 20 beats/min by 32 weeks' gestation. Uterine blood flow increases 10-fold to between 500 and 800 mL/min, a shift from 2% of total cardiac output to 17% at term. Renal blood flow increases by 50% during pregnancy as does perfusion of the breasts and skin. Arterial blood pressure decreases in pregnancy beginning as early as the seventh week. Blood pressure nadir occurs at 24 to 32 weeks' gestation and is followed by a rise toward nonpregnant values at term. Late pregnancy is characterized by significant elevations in heart rate, stroke volume, and cardiac output, in concert with significant decreases in systemic and pulmonary vascular resistance and serum colloid osmotic pressure (COP). There is no significant alteration in pulmonary capillary wedge pressure, central venous pressure, or mean arterial blood pressure. Pregnant women are still at higher risk for pulmonary edema because of the significantly decreased gradient between COP and pulmonary capillary wedge pressure (gradient of 10.5 ± 2.7 mm Hg) compared with the nonpregnant state (gradient of 14.5 ± 2.5 mm Hg). The first stage of labor is associated with a 12% to 31% increase in cardiac output, primarily because of a 22% increase in stroke volume. The second stage of labor is associated with an even greater increase in cardiac output (49%). Pregnant women with cardiac disease are perhaps at greatest risk for pulmonary edema in the immediate postpartum period. Within 2 minutes of delivery, there is a 47% increase in cardiac index and a 39% decrease in systemic vascular index without appreciable change in mean arterial pressure. This immediate increase in cardiac output is caused by release of vena caval obstruction by the gravid uterus, autotransfusion of uteroplacental blood, and rapid mobilization of extravascular fluid. All these changes result in increased venous return to the heart and increased stroke volume. Cardiac output returns to prelabor values 1 hour after delivery.

There is a moderate decrease in functional residual capacity during pregnancy, attributed to a decrease in both expiratory reserve volume and residual volume. Maternal tidal volume increases by 40% in pregnancy, and this increase results in maternal hyperventilation and hypocapnia. Because maternal respiratory rate does not change during pregnancy, the 30% to 50% increase in minute ventilation that is noted as early as the first trimester is attributed to this increase in tidal volume alone. There is a decrease in the partial pressure of carbon dioxide from a prepregnancy level of 39 mm Hg to approximately 28 to 31 mm Hg at term. Serum bicarbonate decreases to 18−22 mEq/L. A mild respiratory alkalosis is therefore normal in pregnancy, with an arterial pH of 7.44 compared with 7.40 in the nonpregnant state.

Serum creatinine falls from prepregnancy values of 0.83 mg/dL to 0.7 mg/dL, 0.6 mg/dL, and 0.5 mg/dL in the first, second, and third trimesters. Blood urea nitrogen decreases from 12 mg/dL in the nonpregnant state to 11 mg/dL, 9 mg/dL, and 10 mg/dL in the first, second, and third trimesters. Colloids such as albumin, globulin, and fibrinogen are molecules that cannot pass through the cell membrane exert the force (COP) to maintain fluid within the capillary. Hemodilution of pregnancy is associated with a decrease in COP. This can be associated with an increased risk of pulmonary edema in patients with preeclampsia, sepsis, and hemorrhage.

QUESTIONS

1. When does an increase in maternal plasma volume begin?
   a. 6–8 weeks
   b. 12–14 weeks
   c. 20–22 weeks
   d. 30–32 weeks

2. In a singleton pregnancy, red blood cell mass
   a. increases by 1000 mL
   b. increases due to prolongation of red blood cell life
   c. increases by 20%–30%
   d. is associated with a decrease in maternal demand for iron

3. Physiologic hemodilution of pregnancy
   a. is due to disproportionate increase in plasma volume
   b. results in increase in maternal hematocrit
   c. increases blood viscosity
   d. is due to disproportionate increase in red blood cell mass

4. During pregnancy, cardiac output in a singleton gestation
   a. begins to increase at 18 weeks' gestation
   b. increases by 30%–50%
   c. is not affected by maternal posture
   d. increases by 60%–80%

5. Regional changes in distribution of blood flow in pregnancy include
   a. blood flow to the skin remains unchanged
   b. renal blood flow remains unchanged
   c. blood flow to the brain increases
   d. uterine blood flow increases

6. Pregnant women are at increased risk for pulmonary edema
   a. due to an increase in colloid osmotic pressure
   b. due to a decrease in colloid osmotic pressure
   c. due to an increase in pulmonary capillary wedge pressure
   d. due to a decrease in pulmonary capillary wedge pressure

7. During pregnancy
   a. diastolic murmurs develop in more than 95% of women
   b. systolic murmurs develop in more than 95% of women
   c. systolic murmurs louder than grade 2/4 are normal
   d. diastolic murmurs louder than grade 2/4 are normal

8. Postpartum hemodynamic changes
   a. increase the risk for pulmonary edema
   b. return to normal by 6 weeks' postpartum
   c. decrease the risk for pulmonary edema
   d. return to normal by one week postpartum

9. Which of the following is a normal respiratory change in pregnancy?
   a. Decrease in maternal respiratory rate
   b. Increase in maternal tidal volume
   c. Increase in maternal respiratory rate
   d. Decrease in maternal tidal volume

10. Which of the following changes in acid base status is normal in pregnancy?
    a. Mild respiratory alkalosis
    b. Mild respiratory acidosis
    c. Serum bicarbonate of 26–28 mEq/L
    d. Serum bicarbonate of 12–14 mEq/L

11. During normal pregnancy, sodium retention is promoted by
    a. progesterone
    b. vasodilatory prostaglandins
    c. atrial natriuretic factor
    d. aldosterone

12. In normal pregnancy,
    a. serum osmolality increases
    b. serum osmolality decreases
    c. osmotic threshold for thirst does not change
    d. osmotic threshold for thirst increases

13. Which of the following renal changes occur in a normal pregnancy?
    a. Renal plasma flow decreases.
    b. Glomerular filtration rate decreases.
    c. Uric acid increases.
    d. Serum creatinine decreases.

10

Endocrinology of Pregnancy

JAMES H. LIU | REBECCA K. CHUNG

(see Creasy and Resnik's Maternal-Fetal Medicine, 9e: Ch 10)

Summary

The endocrine changes of implantation, early and late pregnancy, and labor are complex. By understanding these processes, clinicians caring for obstetric and gynecologic patients can better recognize the management and treatment options for infertility and pregnancy complications.

Implantation is the initial step to establishing a pregnancy and involves many complex steps. A viable embryo implants into the endometrium about 8 to 10 days after ovulation. By day 10, the blastocyst is completely encased in uterine stromal tissue. Estradiol and progesterone and their receptors tightly regulate the remodeling and cellular differentiation of the endometrium to receive the blastocyst during the "receptive window." Many molecular pathways are needed to occur in synchrony for successful implantation including the localization of adhesive molecules, growth factors, cytokines, and proteinases. To add to the complexity of implantation, the concept of immunotolerance within the uterus to provide an immunologic barrier between the mother and fetus and post-translational gene expression through microRNA for implantation and endometrial receptivity have been described.

After implantation, the maintenance of early pregnancy is through human chorionic gonadotropin (hCG) and progesterone. hCG rescues the corpus luteum from early involution and allows for the continuation of progesterone production by the corpus luteum until the luteal-placental shift in progesterone synthesis occurs. When implantation does not occur, as in nonconception cycles, the corpus luteum will undergo luteolysis. In normal pregnancy, the luteal-placental shift occurs somewhere between the seventh and ninth week of gestation.

Throughout pregnancy, the major hormones are progesterone, estrogen, a number of growth factors, and many more that this chapter addresses. The main source of progesterone is from the placenta after the luteal-placental shift, which is synthesized from circulating maternal cholesterol. Estrogen is formed through placental aromatization of dehydroepiandrosterone, a major androgenic precursor from the fetal adrenal gland. Two genetic diseases that compromise placental estrogen synthesis are placental sulfatase deficiency and placental aromatase deficiency. Maintenance and growth of pregnancy is also regulated by multiple factors including growth factors (IGF, EGF, TGFα, VEGF, PGF), pregnancy-associated plasma protein−A, human chorionic somatomammotropin, human placental growth hormone, corticotropin-releasing hormone, and pregnancy-specific glycoproteins.

During pregnancy, a series of endocrine-metabolic changes are observed as the maternal metabolic demands alter with the development of the fetus. Hyperinsulinemia and insulin resistance associated with pregnancy are not fully understood but contribute to the development of gestational diabetes. They play a role in exaggerated hypoglycemia in prolonged fasting in pregnancy as gluconeogenesis is not increased as expected to compensate for low glucose levels during this state. Changes in lipid profile are also seen.

The onset of the labor process is thought to be largely regulated by progesterone. Progesterone is important for uterine quiescence, presumably through the inhibition of myometrial contractile protiens (e.g., gap junction connexins) and prostaglandin production and maintenance of cervical mucus barrier and collagenic structure. However, progesterone levels do not change at the onset of labor in humans. Rather it is decreased progetsreonc recpetor expression, a change in the ratio of the two progesterone receptor isoforms (A and B) or changes in progesterone receptor associated proteins that mediate and regulate uterine contractions. At the onset of labor, proinflammatory pathways are activated. Estrogen is also important for priming the uterus to be increasingly contractile during labor through multiple mechanisms including enhanced prostaglandin production, increasing formation of gap junction, modulation of adrenergic pathways, and increased uterine blood flow. Estrogen is also important for preparing the breast for lactation and increasing fetal lung surfactant production. Although oxytocin plays a role in labor, current data do not support oxytocin as the trigger for labor but rather as playing a role in the preparation of labor.

In summary, hormonal milieu and metabolic changes in pregnancy are complex, constantly changing throughout the gestational period. The key to understand complications of pregnancy is understanding these normal processes, which lead to further development of treatments for management of pregnancy complications.

QUESTIONS

1. A 28-year-old female, nulliparous woman presents with difficulty conceiving after 12 months of trying to do so. Her physical examination was within normal limits. She is doing timed intercourse with urine ovulation predictor kits and recently had a luteinizing hormone (LH) surge yesterday morning. How many days after ovulation does implantation occur?
   a. 2−4 days
   b. 4−6 days
   c. 6−8 days
   d. 8−10 days
   e. 10−12 days

2. A 32-year-old female with unexplained infertility and regular menses presents to the office for artificial insemination after ovulation induction. She feels bloated and has had mild pain in her left lower quadrant for the past day. She reported a urinary positive LH surge yesterday morning. After insemination, how early can hCG can be detected in the serum or urine before the next menses?
   a. 1−2 days
   b. 3−5 days
   c. 7−8 days
   d. 10−11 days
   e. 13−14 days

3. A 32-year-old female with worsening hirsutism, acne, and menstrual irregularity recently underwent an uncomplicated vaginal delivery of a term infant. On examination, the infant had ambiguous genitalia with urogenital sinus, posterior labial fusion, and clitoromegaly. Karyotype revealed 46XX and an elevated 17-hydroxyprogesterone level. Which of the following is the most likely cause?
   a. 21-Hydroxylase deficiency
   b. Maternal androgen-secreting tumor
   c. Polycystic ovarian syndrome
   d. Idiopathic hirsutism
   e. Theca lutein cyst

4. A 37-year-old female presented in active labor and delivered a term infant without complication. The infant presents with atypical genital appearance. Ultrasound revealed no uterus. Karyotype revealed 46XY, normal 17-hydroxyprogesterone, and a significantly elevated testosterone-to-dihydrotestosterone ratio >10:1. What is the likely phenotype of the infant?
   a. Hypovirilized external male genital structures
   b. Hypervirilized external male genital structures
   c. Hypovirilized external female genital structures
   d. Hypervirilized external female genital structures
   e. Gonads with both ovarian and testicular tissue

5. A 37-year-old female presented in active labor and delivered a term infant without complication. The infant presents with ambiguous genitalia. Ultrasound revealed no uterus with testes within the inguinal sac. Karyotype revealed 46XY, normal 17-hydroxyprogesterone, and

significantly elevated testosterone-to-dihydrotesterone ratio >10:1. What is the likely diagnosis of the infant?
   a. Androgen insensitivity syndrome
   b. Congenital adrenal hyperplasia
   c. Polycystic ovarian syndrome
   d. LH receptor deficiency
   e. 5-Alpha reductase deficiency

6. A 41-year-old female presents with recurrent pregnancy loss and recently underwent a frozen transfer of a euploid embryo. She had a serum hCG level of 17 mIU/mL on day 11 after her transfer with a repeat hCG 48 hours later of 10 mIU/mL. You counsel her regarding early pregnancy loss and state that the low hCG level is likely:
   a. a false-positive hCG and recommend a urine hCG test
   b. due to successful implantation but inadequate trophoblast invasion
   c. produced from the embryo but does not signify successful implantation
   d. pituitary hCG because she is perimenopausal
   e. from her hCG trigger for ovulation from her egg retrieval

7. A 24-year-old female who is 7 weeks' pregnant by last menstrual period presents to the emergency department with sudden left pelvic pain for 6 hours. She denies any vaginal bleeding. Her abdominal examination revealed tenderness in left lower quadrant and rebound tenderness but no guarding. Pelvic examination was unremarkable. She is afebrile, normotensive, mildly tachycardic, and oxygenating well at room air. Laboratory studies revealed a hemoglobin of 10.6 g/dL and platelets 251 × 109/L. Blood type is O positive. Transvaginal ultrasound confirmed an intrauterine pregnancy with fetal heartbeat and showed moderate fluid in the pelvis. You take her to the operating room due to concerns for a corpus luteum rupture with hemorrhage. You perform an uncomplicated surgery with removal of the corpus luteal cyst and evacuation of 300 mL of hemoperitoneum. She is stable postoperatively. What is the most appropriate next step in management?
   a. Recommend termination of the pregnancy
   b. Transfuse 2 units of packed red blood cells
   c. Administration of intramuscular Rhogam
   d. Obtain hCG level 24 hours after surgery
   e. Vaginal progesterone supplementation

8. A 35-year-old primigravid female at 28 weeks with gestational hypertension presents to labor and delivery with worsening headache. Blood pressure was 164/84 with repeat of 168/76. The urine protein creatinine ratio was 0.36. She was diagnosed with preeclampsia and her blood pressure was treated with antihypertensives. Preeclampsia is associated with which of the following?
   a. Placental sulfatase deficiency
   b. Reduced vascular endothelial growth factor activity
   c. Increased placental growth factor activity
   d. Low levels of maternal activin A
   e. Cigarette smoking

9. A 34-year-old primigravid female in the second trimester presents for routine obstetrics care. Her pregnancy is currently uncomplicated, except her prenatal genetic testing revealed an elevated risk for Down syndrome of 1 in 75. Results of which of the following laboratory findings would be most likely for this patient?
   a. Increased inhibin A
   b. Increased alpha-fetoprotein
   c. Increased unconjugated estriol
   d. Increased pregnancy-associated plasma protein−A
   e. Decreased hCG

10. A 40-year-old female, gravida 2 para 1 at 28 weeks' pregnant presents for routine obstetrics care. Her last delivery was an uncomplicated vaginal delivery of a 4400-g infant. At her visit, you discuss screening for gestational diabetes with a 50-g glucose tolerance test. She states that she was recently screened for diabetes at her annual exam before pregnancy and does not want to be screened again. Which of the following statements is true regarding screening?
   a. It is not recommended to be screened again because she was screened within 1 year.
   b. It is not recommended to be screened again because this is her second pregnancy.
   c. It is recommended that she is screened again because of her advanced maternal age.
   d. It is recommended that she is screened again because of her history of macrosomia.
   e. It is recommended that she is screened again due to insulin resistance in pregnancy.

11. A 25-year-old female, gravida 1 presents at 36 weeks' gestational age for routine obstetrics care. She is a surgical resident and states that during long operating room cases, she experiences lightheadedness, diaphoresis, pallor, and palpitations. She admits that she does not regularly eat breakfast. What metabolic changes are observed in gravid patients in late pregnancy?
   a. Increased gluconeogenesis
   b. Decreased insulin levels
   c. Decreased plasma lipids
   d. Decreased fasting glucose
   e. Decrease glucagon

12. A 19-year-old nulliparous female calls your office requesting a prescription for emergency contraception after unprotected intercourse. Ulipristal acetate was prescribed, and she was counseled regarding the side effects and efficacy of oral emergency contraceptive. What is the principal mechanism of action of ulipristal acetate?
   a. Decreases sperm viability and function
   b. Inhibits follicular rupture
   c. Prevents implantation
   d. Disrupts endometrial development
   e. Aborts existing pregnancy

13. A 25-year-old gravida 1 at 34 weeks presents with regular, painful contractions. Pelvic examination revealed a dilated cervix of 3 cm, 75% effaced, and −2 station. Membranes are intact. Fetal heart rate monitoring was category 1, and a course of antenatal corticosteroids was initiated. What occurs at the time of parturition?
   a. Increased progesterone receptor (PR)-A expression
   b. Increased PR-B expression
   c. Decrease in serum progesterone
   d. Increase in serum progesterone
   e. Expression of antiinflammatory genes

14. A 31-year-old female gravid 1 presents to labor and delivery at 41 weeks for induction of labor due to postdates. After a prolonged, failed induction, the patient underwent cesarean delivery of a male infant complicated by a postpartum hemorrhage with estimated blood loss of 1000 mL. After a few months, the male infant was noted to have dry, brown, scalelike skin on his back and legs. Which of the following is most likely underlying cause of the infant's condition?
   a. Seborrheic dermatitis
   b. Infantile acne
   c. Placental aromatase deficiency
   d. Steroid sulfatase deficiency
   e. Transient neonatal pustular melanosis

15. A 38-year-old female, gravida 2 para 1 at 39 weeks' pregnant presents to labor and delivery with regular painful contractions. Fetal heart tracing is category 1, and cervical examination revealed a dilated cervix of 6 cm, 90% effaced, and 0 station. What hormonal changes are observed during labor?
   a. Progesterone withdrawal
   b. Decline in corticotropin-releasing hormone
   c. Rise in circulating oxytocin
   d. Acute decrease of prostaglandins
   e. Reduced prolactin level

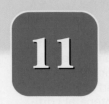

11

The Breast and Physiology of Lactation

RUTH A. LAWRENCE | ROBERT M. LAWRENCE | ADETOLA LOUIS-JACQUES

(see Creasy and Resnik's Maternal-Fetal Medicine, 9e: Ch 11)

Summary

The obstetrician serves an essential function in support of breastfeeding, beginning in the prenatal period and continuing throughout lactation. Expert knowledge of the anatomy and physiology of the human breast, an understanding of lactogenesis and all it entails, and experience in managing the challenges of breastfeeding are crucial prerequisites for successful support of the mother and infant through lactation. This chapter is an introduction to the majority of the essential topics for support of breastfeeding.

The conversation in support of breastfeeding begins with open-ended exploration of the mother's intentions for feeding her infant including the woman's knowledge concerning breastfeeding, previous experience with breastfeeding/lactation, her personal attitudes and those of her partner and extended family, and any questions, doubts, or concerns the woman may have about her ability to successfully breastfeed her infant. A balanced presentation of information about breastfeeding and lactation, including the benefits to the mother and infant compared with the potential risks of breastfeeding, is necessary to assist the mother in reaching an informed decision about feeding her infant. Respectful inclusivity and practiced equity will lead to "affirming health care" in support of the mother and her family's decision regarding infant feeding and practical nurturing.

The physician's expert knowledge and experience of breast anatomy, physiology, and development will additionally inform an assessment of the breast and "readiness" for lactation as the woman progresses through pregnancy, delivery, and postpartum periods. Potential problems with the breasts, lactation, and breastfeeding should be anticipated, discussed with the mother, and addressed with appropriately timed interventions. The numerous factors that can contribute to and facilitate the onset of normal successful lactation should be initiated and supported through the available health delivery services.

Initiation of lactation and breastfeeding begins at delivery within a breastfeeding-friendly environment, including skin-to-skin contact within the first "golden hour," limitation of the use of medications that could interfere with lactation or feeding, instruction and assistance to achieve an effective latch, observation of episodes of breastfeeding for the infant's suck–swallow–breath activity, and successful transfer of colostrum and mother's own milk. Early assessment of breastfeeding success should include continued direct observation of breastfeeding, discussing the mother's questions and concerns, documenting effective latch and milk transfer, instructing the mother regarding hand expression of milk and mechanical collection and storage of her own milk, the infant's frequency of feeding, urination and stooling along with the infant's weight maintenance and gain, and addressing any apparent difficulties with breastfeeding (inadequate latch, ineffective transfer of milk, nipple pain, engorgement, concerns regarding adequate milk productions, etc.).

Medical management of the challenges of breastfeeding is briefly addressed in this chapter, as the challenges are extensively addressed in other resources, including the American College of Obstetricians and Gynecologists, Committee on Obstetric Practice Breastfeeding Expert Work Group in Breastfeeding Challenges. *Obstet Gynecol.* 2021;137:e42-e54, Optimizing support for breastfeeding as part of obstetric practice. *Obstet Gynecol.* 2018;132:e187-e196, Barriers to breastfeeding: supporting initiation and continuation of breastfeeding. *Obstet Gynecol.* 2021;137:e54-e62, and the Academy of Breastfeeding Medicine (ABM) Protocols (https://www.bfmed.org/protocols). The important challenges addressed in this chapter will require ongoing study and clinical practice to master them, including breast engorgement, nipple tenderness/pain, failing milk supply, various breast masses, breastfeeding premature infants, and breastfeeding infants of multiple births.

Management of specific maternal infections during breastfeeding is also addressed in this chapter, including diphtheria; active pulmonary disease; brucellosis; cytomegalovirus; hemorrhagic fevers (Ebola, Marburg, or Lassa viruses); Dengue or other flaviviruses; human immunodeficiency viruses (HIV); human T-cell leukemia virus types I and II; hepatitis; and mastitis.

Contraception during lactation is another important issue necessitating the practice of "affirming health care" to support maternal and familial decision making about breastfeeding with sexuality, birth spacing, and contraception as important considerations. This vast topic is supported by recommendations from several organizations including the World Health Organization, American College of Obstetricians and Gynecologists, and ABM concerning contraception during lactation.

Medication use during lactation is common, leading to numerous questions on safety and management and informed decision making for medication use while breastfeeding. The basic pharmacophysiology of medication use during breastfeeding and the effect on breastmilk is discussed along with some recommendations for their safe use. In particular, analgesics, anesthetics, and radiopharmaceuticals are briefly discussed as there are again extensive resources available to the clinician regarding medication use during breastfeeding (Briggs et al: *Drugs in Pregnancy and Lactation*, 2021; Hale TW: *Hale's Medications & Mothers' Milk 2021: A Manual of Lactational Pharmacology,* 2021; American College of Radiology: *Manual on Contrast Media, v10.22016:* https://www.acr.org/Quality-Safety/Resources/Contrast-Manual; and ABM's various protocols (analgesia, anesthesia, antidepressants, contraception, substance use, and radiology, https://www.bfmed.org/protocols).

Ongoing breastfeeding support after delivery requires "breastfeeding-friendly" practices within the delivery facility and the clinic and office for appropriate supportive health care. Equally essential is addressing the many inequities in health care perpetuated by institutions and personal action related to race/ethnicity, socioeconomic status, gender, sexual orientation, and other social issues. Affirming health care in support of breastfeeding remains an important goal in support of breastfeeding, and use of human milk for all infants and the obstetrician will continue to play an essential role in offering affirming health care for the breastfeeding woman.

QUESTIONS

1. Breast milk is species specific, made uniquely for human infants. The components of human milk are present in specific amounts, readily digestible, and "bioavailable" to the human infant to optimize infant growth and development. Which of the following is not an example of the specificity of human milk?
   a. Human milk oligosaccharides
   b. Proteins and specific amino acids
   c. Lipids, especially cholesterol and docosahexanoic acid
   d. Lactose
   e. Immunoglobulins

2. A 36-year-old G1P0 patient presents for her second routine prenatal at 14 weeks' gestation. She wants to discuss the benefits of breastmilk against infection because her mother says breastmilk cannot prevent infection. What is the most appropriate next step for the obstetrician at this juncture?
   a. Tell her that her mother is wrong and convince the mother she should breastfeed.
   b. Provide her with lists of all the immunologically active components in breastmilk that protect against infection.
   c. Continue with open-ended questions about breast feeding regarding the mother's concerns about infection and breastfeeding, acknowledging her concerns and questions before providing specific information to answer her questions.
   d. Reassure the mother that breastmilk is the ultimate fluid in protecting against infection.
   e. Proceed with the rest of the history and physical examination needed for this visit.

3. As you continue the discussion of the benefits of breastfeeding with the same patient above, she asks about the benefits of breastfeeding for the mother. She has a history of breast surgery (reduction), hypertension, obesity, and polycystic ovary syndrome. She specifically asks about whether there is any benefit against ovarian cancer because her older sister was diagnosed with ovarian cancer. What is a reasonable next step to address the benefits of breastfeeding for the mother relative to the risk of cancer?
   a. Provide the mother with the list of all the benefits of breastfeeding for the mother (including decreasing the risk for ovarian cancer).
   b. Provide a balanced discussion of the various factors that relate to the risk of ovarian cancer (including family history, family genetics, number of pregnancies, duration of oral contraceptive use, and duration/intensity of lactation).
   c. Refer the mother to the American Cancer Society's information on ovarian cancer risk.
   d. Address the fact that obesity is a risk for ovarian cancer, and give the mother a plan for good weight loss during this pregnancy.
   e. Discuss the benefits of breastfeeding in protection against all types of cancer.

4. This same pregnant woman asks about the contraindications to breastfeeding. What is the most reasonable response to this mother's question about "contraindications"?
   a. Give this mother the list of contraindications against breastfeeding.
   b. Talk to the mother about HIV infection and counsel her about avoiding HIV infection.
   c. Discuss with the mother the various infections that can be transmitted via breastfeeding.
   d. Provide a balanced discussion of the potential risks of breastfeeding, and present examples when the potential risk of breastfeeding may outweigh the potential benefits of breastfeeding in a mother's decision making about infant feeding.

5. To continue to counsel this pregnant woman and promote breastfeeding, what counseling strategies are suggested by "Best Start"?
   a. Use open-ended questions of the mother about breastfeeding experience, knowledge, and attitudes (including her family's support).
   b. Acknowledge that every woman experiences some feelings of doubt about breastfeeding successfully—this is normal.
   c. Discuss how other women have dealt with various concerns and questions about breastfeeding at the same time as providing specific knowledge about breastfeeding.
   d. a and c
   e. a, b, and c

6. As you continue to explore this pregnant woman's attitudes, knowledge, and breast health history, she expresses concerns regarding whether she will produce sufficient milk for the infant. Along with discussing her personal risk factors for low milk supply, what else would you recommend to address these risk factors to successful breastfeeding?
   a. Treat the mother's hypertension and plan for serial blood pressure measurements.
   b. Give the mother a plan for effective weight loss during pregnancy.
   c. Refer the mother to a breast surgeon to discuss how surgery affects breastfeeding.

d. Discuss with the mother strategies to identify and address low milk supply, and provide additional breastfeeding support at delivery and through the course of lactation.

e. Treat her polycystic ovary syndrome aggressively.

7. Which one of the conditions in the patient history is not a risk factor for low milk supply?
   a. Hypertension
   b. Breast reduction surgery
   c. Obesity
   d. Polycystic ovarian syndrome

8. Milk synthesis is a complex process involving a number of important factors. Which hormones are essential to milk synthesis?
   a. Prolactin and progesterone
   b. Prolactin and oxytocin
   c. Prolactin, progesterone, and oxytocin
   d. Prolactin, insulin, and glucocorticoids
   e. Insulin, estrogen, and progesterone

9. What are the most important peripartum interventions to promote successful breastfeeding around the time of delivery?
   a. Immediate skin-to-skin contact between the mother and infant
   b. Facilitate the infant's first feeding at the breast within the first hour after delivery
   c. Encourage and facilitate "rooming in"
   d. Recommend feeding on demand and early breast-feeding support (including breastfeeding techniques) in the first 24–36 hours
   e. All of the above

10. You are rounding on a 28-year-old primiparous woman who underwent a spontaneous vaginal birth of a 37-week-old (2495 gm) male infant on postpartum day 2. The medical history, pregnancy, and birth were unremarkable. The infant is reported to have breastfed 2–3 times with difficulty since yesterday. What important steps should the obstetrical team complete before discharge of this mother/infant dyad?
   a. Inform the pediatrician.
   b. Observe a feeding session or have the bedside nurse observe a feeding session to confirm if there is effective transfer of milk.
   c. Document the number of feedings, voids, and stools per 24 hours.
   d. Initiate professional lactation assistance.
   e. All of the above

11. A 24-year-old, primiparous woman calls the obstetric service on postpartum day 4. She had no complications during pregnancy or vaginal delivery. The infant, a male born at 39 weeks' gestation (3425 gm), was discharged on hospital day 2 and reportedly breastfeeding well with insignificant weight loss before discharge. The mother reports some difficulty with latch, and she is concerned about engorgement (she has increasing nipple tenderness and her breasts remain full even

after feeding) and the infant being fussy and not feeding well. The baby appears well and has stooled once today and voided twice. What should you recommend at this time for suspected engorgement?
   a. Wear a well-fitting brassiere around the clock.
   b. Frequently feed the infant and gently massage to soften the areola before feeding to make the latch easier for the infant.
   c. If pain worsens, apply cold compresses after feeding and use ibuprofen or acetaminophen.
   d. a and b
   e. a, b, and c

12. The same 24-year-old mother reports recurrence of persistent nipple pain 3 weeks postpartum. At a recent visit to the pediatrician, the infant was thriving and the pediatrician ruled out various causes of nipple pain including ankyloglossia, incorrect latch, breast pump trauma, psoriasis, eczema, bacterial or fungal infection, HSV, or cracked/damaged nipples. You suspect a rarer cause of persistent nipple pain. What additional symptoms should you query the mother about?
   a. A history of varicella or zoster
   b. A history of recurrent genital herpes simplex virus
   c. An oversupply of milk
   d. A history of blocked ducts
   e. Shooting or burning breast pain with blanching or other color changes of the nipple with the pain

13. What is first step in the management of acute lactational infectious mastitis?
   a. Effective milk removal with supportive measures (rest, hydration, breast massage, and analgesia)
   b. Empiric antibiotics
   c. Breast ultrasound
   d. Aspiration or drainage

14. A new mother is referred to you regarding stopping breastfeeding because of concern of active pulmonary tuberculosis. The infant is continuing to breastfeed and is thriving. The mother reportedly has an abnormal chest roentgenogram consistent with tuberculosis but no symptoms of fevers, weight loss, fatigue, or a productive cough. The mother has had "sputum" cultures and smears done. Three smears are negative, and the cultures are negative to date. The mother is on isoniazid, rifampin, and pyrazinamide. What additional steps should be taken at this time for the mother to continue breastfeeding?
   a. Place the infant on preventive isoniazid for 3–6 months, with ongoing assessment of the infant's health.
   b. Follow up on the results of the mother's sputum cultures.
   c. Confirm the mother's compliance with her medications, and encourage continued compliance, explaining that these medications that can reach the breastmilk will not harm the infant.
   d. Document the absence of any nipple/breast lesions suggestive of extrapulmonary tuberculosis.
   e. All of the above

15. A patient at 32 weeks' gestational age is referred to you with questions about cytomegalovirus (CMV) and breastfeeding. She has worked in a daycare with infants younger than 2 years of age for the past 5 years. The mother has experienced no apparent infectious illness during this pregnancy, and CMV was noted at 26 weeks' gestation when there was a concern for fetal growth restriction. The mother's laboratory results show she is CMV IgG positive, CMV IgM negative. CMV IgG avidity testing was consistent with an old infection. Which of the following is reasonably true to discuss with this mother concerning CMV and breastfeeding her infant?
    a. Infants infected with CMV between 32 and 36 weeks are severely affected.
    b. Infants infected by their mothers with CMV via breastmilk will be deaf.
    c. CMV can be transmitted via breastmilk, but infants born after 36 weeks' gestational age are rarely, if ever, sick due to CMV infection.
    d. This infant should receive CMV negative donor human milk.
    e. This mother should pasteurize the breastmilk before giving it to the infant.

16. During the discussion with the pregnant woman above; the mother expresses concern about infections due to other viruses and breastfeeding. Which of the following viruses has not been associated with transmission via breastmilk?
    a. Human immunodeficiency virus
    b. Hepatitis C virus
    c. Human T-cell leukemia virus
    d. Epstein-Barr virus
    e. Dengue virus

12

Maternal Nutrition

LISA M. BODNAR | KATHERINE P. HIMES

(see *Creasy and Resnik's Maternal-Fetal Medicine, 9e*: Ch 12)

Summary

Sufficient intake of nutrients during pregnancy is essential to meet the demands of fetal growth and development, as well as maternal physiologic adaptations to pregnancy. Unfortunately, nutritional status is poor among pregnant women in the United States. Numerous poor pregnancy and birth outcomes have been associated with nutritional deficiencies, including preterm birth, fetal growth restriction, gestational diabetes mellitus, and preeclampsia. Maternal nutritional status may have a critical influence in the periconceptional period, when fetal growth trajectory, placental capacity to supply nutrients to the fetus, fetoplacental immunology and inflammation, and maternal hormonal and metabolic regulatory systems are established. A poor-quality diet during pregnancy also promotes excessive gestational weight gain and postpartum weight retention. Furthermore, poor maternal nutritional status has a powerful influence on the offspring's health and susceptibility to disease later in life. All clinicians caring for reproductive-age women should educate themselves and their patients about the importance of good nutritional health before, during, and after pregnancy.

Healthy eating during pregnancy follows the Dietary Guidelines for Americans. These national recommendations focus on eating patterns rather than intake of individual nutrients or foods because research shows that overall dietary patterns are most important in disease prevention. Pregnant women can put the Dietary Guidelines for Americans into practice using a tool called MyPlate (https://www.myplate.gov/widgets-sm/myplate-daily-checklist-input-start), an interactive resource for patients and providers to calculate what and how much to eat within the recommended calorie allowance. MyPlate encourages intake of 40% vegetables, 10% fruit, 20% protein, and 30% grains, along with a serving of dairy at each meal. Providers can also use an interactive tool (https://www.nal.usda.gov/human-nutrition-and-food-safety/dri-calculator) to calculate the Estimated Energy Requirement and recommend micronutrient and macronutrient intakes for patients.

Supplementation with 400 µg/day of folic acid starting before conception and 30 mg/day of iron from early pregnancy is recommended for all pregnant women. Maternal folic acid deficiency can cause neural tube defects in the fetus and other congenital anomalies. Iron deficiency has been associated with infant low birthweight, preterm birth, and other poor health outcomes. Universal multivitamin supplementation in the form of prenatal vitamins is routine and reasonable for pregnant women because detailed dietary assessments are burdensome.

Universal vitamin D deficiency screening or supplementation is not recommended during pregnancy. However, if deficiency is suspected and blood levels reveal deficiency, supplementation with 1000-2000 IU of vitamin D/day is safe. Calcium intakes are low in the United States, and supplementation may reduce risk of preeclampsia among women with low intake or among women at high risk of preeclampsia.

Docosahexaenoic acid and eicosatetraenoic acid are omega-3 polyunsaturated fatty acids that have roles in inflammatory pathways. Data suggest that omega-3 fatty acid supplementation may reduce risk of preterm birth and offspring neurologic development and asthma risk. Fish and seafood are the primary sources of these fatty acids. The U.S. Food and Drug Administration and American College of Obstetricians and Gynecologists (ACOG) recommend that pregnant women or women who want to become pregnant consume 8 to 12 oz of fish each week. Methylmercury accumulates in some seafood. The Environmental Protection Agency issued revised recommendations for fish consumption that highlight the best choices for fish consumption for pregnant and breastfeeding women.

Pregnant women should avoid or limit their intake of added sugars, solid fats, caffeine, and alcohol. They should be encouraged to avoid listeriosis and toxoplasmosis, the two foodborne illnesses more likely to affect pregnant women, and to follow food safety guidelines.

Gestational weight gain is a modifiable factor that is associated with adverse pregnancy outcomes. Current recommendations for how much weight women should gain during pregnancy were published in 2009 by the Institute of Medicine (IOM, now the National Academy of Medicine) and endorsed by the ACOG. The 2009 guidelines considered other short-term and long-term adverse outcomes for both mother and child with the goal of balancing these risks. The guidelines emphasize obesity prevention and reflect improved understanding of the developmental origins of disease in utero and the importance of considering a life course perspective in the relationship between pregnancy weight gain and health. The IOM guidelines for total pregnancy weight gain (and rate of weight gain in the second and third trimesters) for underweight, normal weight, overweight, and obese women are 28−40 lb (1−1.3 lb/week), 25−35 lb (0.8−1 lb/week), 15−25 lb (0.5-0.7 lb/week), and 11−20 lb (0.4−0.6 lb/week), respectively.

Helping women achieve optimal weight gain and learn healthy lifestyle habits during pregnancy is imperative. Overall, diet, exercise, and diet-plus-exercise interventions in pregnancy reduce total gestational weight by 20% on average and reduce the likelihood of postpartum weight retention at 6–12 months in the intervention compared with control groups.

The IOM guidelines advise that (1) women normalize their weight before pregnancy; (2) clinicians assess prepregnancy body mass index, recommend the appropriate target weight gain guideline, and track weight gain during pregnancy, ideally plotting on a graph to visualize progress; (3) individualized assessment and counseling be provided at the beginning of pregnancy and throughout pregnancy as needed to assist women in following dietary and physical activity patterns that support optimal weight gain; and (4) women be similarly assisted in returning to their prepregnancy body mass index after the birth.

Given the high prevalence of both prepregnancy obesity and excessive gestational weight gain and the possible long-term implications of weight and nutrition during pregnancy, helping women achieve optimal weight gain and learn healthy lifestyle habits during pregnancy is imperative.

QUESTIONS

1. A 28-year-old nulliparous woman presents for a preconception visit given her history of a laparoscopic Roux-en-Y gastric bypass procedure 2 years prior. Her weight has been stable for the past 13 months. She has not seen her surgeon or primary care physician in the past year because overall she has been doing well. She is at increased risk for which of the following during pregnancy?
   a. Miscarriage
   b. Micronutrient deficiencies
   c. Congenital anomalies
   d. Postpartum depression

2. A 19-year-old primigravid woman at 28 weeks has recently been diagnosed with iron deficiency anemia. She plans to start iron supplementation orally. What would be the best drink for her to have while she is taking her iron supplement?
   a. Orange juice
   b. Coffee
   c. Milk
   d. Water at the same time she takes her calcium supplement

3. A 43-year-old gravida 2, para 1 presents for a new obstetric visit at 7 weeks' gestation. Her previous pregnancy was 15 years ago, and she has several questions about healthy eating during pregnancy. She works long hours and frequently eats snack food or fast food. She rarely gets a prepared meal. Which of the following would you emphasize to her during the visit?
   a. She should not consume any caffeine during the pregnancy.
   b. Eat 16 to 20 oz of fish weekly.
   c. Limit foods with added sugars and solid fats.
   d. Energy needs increase by roughly 500 kcal during pregnancy, so she should increase her intake accordingly.

4. A 28-year-old gravida 3, para 2 presents for a new obstetric visit at 6 weeks' gestation. She read she should increase her intake of fish during pregnancy, as it is a high-protein food that provides fatty acids that help with fetal brain development. The only fish she eats is swordfish. Which of the following is a reasonable recommendation for her during pregnancy?
   a. She should aim to eat 8 to 12 ounces of swordfish weekly.
   b. She should consider supplements with docosahexaenoic acid.
   c. She should stop eating swordfish during pregnancy.
   d. She should stop eating swordfish during the rest of the first trimester.

5. A 41-year-old primigravid woman at 12 weeks presents for a return obstetric visit. She has heard that women older than the age of 40 have an increased risk of cesarean delivery. She is also concerned about postpartum weight retention. She wants to discuss all modifiable options for decreasing these risks. Which of the following could you address with her at this visit?
   a. Iron supplementation
   b. Fish oil supplementation
   c. Decreasing the consumption of fatty foods
   d. Gaining within the IOM guidelines for gestational weight gain

6. A 32-year-old gravida 3 para 3 presents for her postpartum visit. Her pregnancy was complicated by preeclampsia, as well as a fetus with an open neural tube defect confirmed on postnatal evaluation. She plans another pregnancy. She reports that she eats a well-balanced diet high in nutrient-dense food. What would you recommend to her?
   a. Take 4 mg of folic acid for at least a month before conception and continue it for the first trimester of pregnancy.
   b. Supplement with calcium in a future pregnancy.
   c. Take 4 mg of folic acid for at least a month before conception and continue it for the first trimester of pregnancy. Start a baby aspirin after the first trimester of pregnancy.
   d. Remain on a prenatal vitamin daily.

Fetal Cardiovascular Physiology

JEFFREY R. FINEMAN | EMIN MALTEPE

(see Creasy and Resnik's Maternal-Fetal Medicine, 9e: Ch 13)

Summary

Compared with its postnatal counterpart, the fetal cardiovascular system is characterized by marked differences in cardiac output and blood flow distribution, myocardial function, sympathetic and parasympathetic innervation, energy metabolism, and local and reflex control. In addition, the hypoxic environment that characterizes the fetus plays a critical role in cardiovascular development.

FETAL BLOOD FLOW PATTERNS

In the mammalian adult, oxygenation occurs in the lungs, and oxygenated blood returns via the pulmonary veins to the left side of the heart to be ejected by the left ventricle into the systemic circulation. In the fetus, gas exchange occurs in the placenta and the fetal lungs are nonfunctional as far as the transfer of oxygen and carbon dioxide is concerned. For oxygenated blood derived from the placenta to reach the systemic circulation, the fetal circulation is arranged so that several sites of intercommunication (shunts) are present, including the ductus arteriosus and foramen ovale. In addition, preferential flow and streaming occur to limit the disadvantages of intermixing the oxygenated and deoxygenated blood that returns to the heart. With fetal stress, these preferential streaming patterns may be modified even more to mitigate the adverse effects of disorders such as reduced umbilical blood flow and fetal hypoxemia.

VENOUS RETURN TO THE HEART

Approximately 40% of total fetal cardiac output (i.e., approximately 200 mL/kg of fetal body weight per minute) is distributed to the placental circulation; a similar amount returns to the heart via the umbilical venous system. Because umbilical venous blood is the most highly oxygen-saturated blood in the fetal circulation, distribution of umbilical venous return is most important in determining oxygen delivery to fetal tissues. After entering the intraabdominal portion of the umbilical vein, a portion of umbilical venous blood flow supplies the liver; the remainder passes through the ductus venosus, which directly connects the umbilical vein–portal sinus confluence to the inferior vena cava. In contrast to the umbilical and portal veins, the ductus venosus has no direct branches to the liver. Umbilical venous blood can enter the ductus venosus directly. However, portal venous return can reach the ductus venosus only through the portal sinus. Approximately 50% of umbilical blood flow passes through the ductus venosus; the remainder enters the hepatic-portal venous system and passes through the hepatic vasculature.

The fetal liver receives its blood supply from the umbilical vein (75%–80%), as well as the portal vein (15%) and hepatic artery (4%–5%). The blood from these sources is distributed differently to various parts of the liver. Hepatic arterial blood flow to the liver is equally distributed to the right and left lobes, but the left lobe is supplied almost exclusively (>95%) by umbilical venous blood. In contrast, the right lobe receives both umbilical venous blood (approximately 60%) and portal venous blood (approximately 30%). Because umbilical venous blood supplies a major portion of flow to the right liver lobe by traversing the portal sinus, little, if any, portal venous blood reaches the ductus venosus. Therefore the blood in the ductus venosus has pH, blood gas, and hemoglobin oxygen saturation values similar to those of umbilical venous blood. The portion of umbilical venous blood flow that passes via the ductus venosus directly into the inferior vena cava meets the systemic venous drainage from the lower body.

CARDIAC OUTPUT AND ITS DISTRIBUTION

In the fetus, because of the blood flow across the ductus arteriosus into the descending aorta, lower body organs are perfused by both the right and the left ventricles (across the aortic isthmus). For this reason and because of intracardiac shunting, it is customary to consider fetal cardiac output as being the total output of the heart, or the combined ventricular output (~450 mL/kg/min). In contrast to adults, and because of the various sites of intracardiac and extracardiac shunting, the left and right ventricles in the fetus do not eject in series and therefore do not need to have the same stroke volume. In fact, the right ventricle ejects approximately two-thirds of total fetal cardiac output (approximately 300 mL/kg/min), whereas the left ventricle ejects only a little more than one-third (approximately 150 mL/kg/min).

MYOCARDIAL FUNCTION

Studies of fetal myocardium show immaturity of structure, function, and sympathetic innervation relative to the adult myocardium. At all muscle lengths along the curve of length versus tension, the active tension generated by fetal myocardium is lower than that generated by adult myocardium. In addition, resting, or passive, tension is higher in fetuses than in adults, suggesting lower compliance of fetal myocardium. Importantly, the right ventricle is unable to increase stroke work or output to the same extent as in the adult. This is particularly true in less mature fetuses, in whom right ventricular end-diastolic pressure is markedly elevated without any obvious change in right ventricular stroke work. Fetal and adult sarcomeres have equivalent lengths, but there are major ultrastructural differences between fetal myocardium and adult myocardium. The diameter of the fetal cells is smaller, and, perhaps more importantly, the proportion of noncontractile mass (i.e., of nuclei, mitochondria, and surface membranes) to the number of myofibrils is significantly greater than in the adult. In the fetal myocardium, only about 30% of the muscle mass consists of contractile elements; in the adult, the proportion is about 60%. These ultrastructural differences are probably responsible for the age-dependent differences in performance.

SYMPATHETIC AND PARASYMPATHETIC INNERVATION AND ENERGY METABOLISM

In addition, there are marked differences in the sympathetic and parasympathetic innervation and energy metabolism between fetal and adult myocardium. For example, isolated fetal cardiac tissue has a lower threshold of response to the inotropic effects of norepinephrine than adult cardiac tissue and is more sensitive to norepinephrine throughout the dose-response curves. This supersensitivity of fetal myocardium to norepinephrine is probably the result of incomplete development of sympathetic innervation in fetal myocardium. In addition, in the normal unstressed fetus, myocardial blood flow is approximately 180 mL/min/100 gm tissue, approximately 80% greater than in the adult. Fetal myocardial oxygen consumption is similar to that in the adult. Free fatty acids provide the major source of energy for the adult myocardium, and carbohydrate accounts for only about 40% of myocardial oxygen consumption. However, in the fetus, free fatty acid concentrations are extremely low under normal conditions, and almost all the oxygen consumed by the left ventricular wall can be accounted for by carbohydrate metabolism: 33% by glucose, 6% by pyruvate, and 58% by lactate metabolism.

HYPOXIA AND ORGAN DEVELOPMENT

Fetal tissues in all mammals are exposed to a hypoxic environment compared with neonates and adults, and oxygen entry from the vasculature into cells is entirely driven by diffusion. The partial pressure of oxygen in the fetal circulation is typically approximately 25 to 35 mm Hg compared with 75 to 100 mm Hg in adults. Cellular responses to hypoxia are complex and profound. The most widely studied response is mediated by a family of hypoxia-inducible factor (HIF) transcription factors. HIF family members form heterodimeric complexes that bind DNA to regulate the expression of hundreds of genes in response to decreases in oxygen tension. Interestingly, HIF transcription regulation of cardiovascular development is well documented, suggesting that the fetal hypoxic environment is a significant driver of fetal development.

REGULATION OF FETAL CIRCULATION

Maintenance of normal cardiovascular function, blood pressure, heart rate, and distribution of blood flow represents a complex interrelationship among local vascular and reflex effects. Regulation includes local organ regulation, baroreflex and chemoreflex regulators, and autonomic control. In addition, several vasoactive substances have been identified as important regulators of fetal circulation. These include products of the reninangiotensin system, vasopressin, natriuretic peptides, arachidonic acid metabolites, and endothelial-derived vasoactive factors such as nitric oxide and endothelin-1.

QUESTIONS

1. Intracardiac fetal communications include:
   a. ductus arteriosus
   b. ductus venosus
   c. foramen ovale
   d. a and c
   e. all of the above

2. The most highly oxygen-saturated blood in fetal circulation is:
   a. umbilical arterial blood
   b. umbilical venous blood
   c. ductus venosus blood
   d. portal venous blood
   e. blood in the ductus arteriosus

3. The fetal liver receives its blood supply from the:
   a. ductus venosus
   b. hepatic artery
   c. umbilical vein
   d. portal vein
   e. b, c, and d

4. Regulators of fetal circulation include:
   a. autonomic nervous system
   b. baroreflex
   c. chemoreflex
   d. nitric oxide
   e. all of the above

5. The partial pressure of oxygen in fetal circulation is:
   a. 75−85 mm Hg
   b. 25−35 mm Hg
   c. 10−20 mm Hg
   d. 50−65 mm Hg
   e. none of the above

6. The major regulator of the fetal hypoxic environment is:
   a. TGF transcription factor family
   b. nitric oxide
   c. HIF transcription factor family
   d. endothelin 1
   e. arachidonic acid

7. All of the following induce fetal vascular relaxation EXCEPT:
   a. nitric oxide
   b. prostacyclin
   c. natriuretic peptides
   d. thromboxane
   e. prostaglandin E2

8. Which of the following is FALSE regarding endothelin−1?
   a. It always induces pulmonary vasoconstriction.
   b. Its vasoactive effects are mediated by two different receptors.
   c. It always induces systemic vasoconstriction.
   d. It is a 21-amino acid polypeptide.
   e. ETb receptor activation can result in nitric oxide stimulation.

9. Which of the following is true regarding the fetal myocardium?
   a. Fetal myocardium generates greater active tension than adult myocardium.
   b. Fetal myocardium generates lower passive tension that adult myocardium.
   c. Fetal sarcomeres are longer than adult sarcomeres.
   d. The fetal right ventricle is able to increase stroke work as well as the adult right ventricle.
   e. The fetal myocardium demonstrates similar maturity of the structure, function, and sympathetic innervation compared with the adult.

10. Which of the following is TRUE regarding energy metabolism?
    a. Fetal myocardial oxygen consumption is greater than the adult.
    b. Fetal myocardial blood flow is greater than the adult.
    c. Free fatty acids are the major source of energy for the fetal myocardium.
    d. ATP activity is greater in the fetal myocardium.
    e. None of the above

14

Placental Respiratory Gas Exchange and Fetal Oxygenation

GIACOMO MESCHIA | RANDALL WILKENING

(see Creasy and Resnik's Maternal-Fetal Medicine, 9e: Ch 14)

Summary

The understanding of placental gas exchange and fetal oxygenation must be grounded in the basic principles of diffusion gradients across membranes, carrying capacity, substrate delivery, the oxyhemoglobin dissociation curve, and the Fick Principle. Once oxygen has been taken up by blood in the pulmonary capillaries, the transport of oxygen to the fetal tissues is a sequence of four steps alternating bulk transport with transport by diffusion. Blood transports oxygen in two forms: free oxygen dissolved in the water of the blood and oxygen bound to hemoglobin. There is a reversible equilibrium between these two forms defined by the binding characteristics of the specific hemoglobin present in the blood.

Oxygen diffuses from the water of the blood across membranes by passive diffusion and is therefore dependent on a concentration gradient across the membrane. In the case of oxygen diffusion across the placental membrane, the gradient from mother to fetus is maintained by the higher oxygen affinity of fetal hemoglobin compared with maternal hemoglobin.

The Fick Principle allows the calculation of a substrate uptake of a tissue or a collection of tissues by determining the arteriovenous concentration difference and multiplying that concentration difference by the blood flow to the tissue or tissues involved. Applying this principle to the pregnant uterus allows for the determination of a substrate uptake across the entire uterus, placenta, and conceptus. Similarly, application of this principle to the umbilical circulation allows for the calculation of a substrate uptake by the fetus. For oxygen these uptake calculations are a direct measurement of oxygen consumption by the tissue or tissues involved.

Placental vascular architecture and placental tissue structure also impact placental gas exchange and fetal oxygenation. The importance of placental vascular architecture, specifically the direction of blood flow across the placental membrane, determines whether fetal blood has the potential of equilibrating with maternal venous or arterial blood. Countercurrent and concurrent flow patterns represent two opposite possibilities of blood flow separated by a diffusion membrane. A concurrent pattern of blood is one of several blood flow patterns, which are termed *venous equilibrators*. The ovine placenta and the human placenta have characteristics observed in venous equilibrators. Mammalian placentas with a countercurrent vascular architecture (rabbits, rodents) make these placentas effective in extracting oxygen from uterine circulation.

The changes in placental tissue structure between midgestation and late gestation highlight the impact that the placenta has on both respiratory gas exchange and fetal oxygenation. Early in gestation, both human and ovine placentas are relatively poor (ineffective) respiratory organs, which are compensated for by relatively high uterine blood flow. However, with the formation of terminal villa, the effectiveness of gas exchange improves dramatically and allows umbilical blood flow to grow in synchrony with the growth in fetal oxygen demand.

An understanding of homeostatic control of fetal oxygenation was based initially on detailed study of the normal ovine late gestation fetus. In the second half of gestation, uterine and umbilical oxygen uptakes increase exponentially. Constancy of fetal oxygenation in the face of such changes implies homeostatic control of fetal oxygenation. The function of this control is to equalize the growth rates of oxygen supply and demand and to prevent a decline of fetal oxygenation to the point of severe hypoxia.

One line evidence of the homeostatic control of fetal oxygenation can be developed by comparison of placental respiratory gas exchange and fetal oxygenation in two groups of sheep under normal conditions. One group of ewes was homozygous for hemoglobin B, and the other group was homozygous for hemoglobin A. Hemoglobin A has a higher affinity for oxygen than does hemoglobin B. Fetal oxygenation, consumption, and growth were identical between the two groups; the fetus was unaware that the maternal hemoglobin types were quite different. This was the result of two compensatory mechanisms impacting placental respiratory gas exchange. First was an increase in uterine blood flow in the hemoglobin A ewes, and second was a decrease in the uterine vein to umbilical vein PO_2 gradient.

A second line of evidence can be developed by examining the normal variability around umbilical venous oxygen saturations and PO_2 and its relationship to norepinephrine concentrations and cardiac output. This evidence points to the conclusion that the homeostatic control of fetal oxygenation depends on a negative feedback mechanism and suggests that there is some degree of fetal growth restriction (FGR) as a part of what is normally considered statistically normal.

The recognition that cyclic thermal stress is associated with ovine FGR has led to one the few natural animal models of FGR. This model exhibits characteristics virtually identical to human FGR and allows for additional evidence for the homeostatic control of fetal oxygenation over an extended range of fetal growth. Further, the permeability to the transplacental diffusion of maternal glucose into fetal blood is also reduced. Interdependence of fetal oxygen and glucose homeostasis explains why chronic infusion of glucose into the circulation of growth-restricted fetal lambs aggravates fetal hypoxia.

Insights into fetal oxygen homeostasis can also be developed from the fetal response to acute hypoxia, the metabolic adaptations occurring from the transition from acute to chronic hypoxia and the effect of maternal oxygen administration on fetal PO_2. A basic understanding of fetal respiratory gas exchange and fetal oxygenation is a necessary foundation for the study of the role of hormonal regulation of fetal growth and metabolism.

QUESTIONS

1. The amount of oxygen carried in the blood is determined primarily by which of the following?
   a. Concentration of hemoglobin
   b. Oxygen saturation of hemoglobin
   c. pO_2

2. There is a difference in the amount of oxygen carried by maternal blood compared with the amount of oxygen carried by fetal blood. This is because:
   a. the fetal hemoglobin concentration is lower than the maternal hemoglobin concentration.
   b. fetal hemoglobin can carry more oxygen molecules than maternal hemoglobin.
   c. the fetal hemoglobin dissociation curve is shifted to the left of the maternal hemoglobin dissociation curve.

3. Compared with maternal hemoglobin, at the same pO_2, fetal hemoglobin binds oxygen less avidly.
   a. True
   b. False

4. The solubility of oxygen in the water of the blood is the same for mother and fetus. Nevertheless, at the same pO_2, maternal whole blood carries less oxygen than fetal whole blood.
   a. True
   b. False

5. In a normal late-gestation human pregnancy, the oxygen consumption of the fetus on a per-weight basis is:
   a. higher than that of the mother.
   b. lower than that of the mother.
   c. the same as that of the mother.

6. Oxygen dissolved in the water of the blood diffuses from uterine circulation across the placenta into fetal circulation. Which of the following statement(s) is correct?
   a. The pO_2 in the umbilical vein is lower than the pO_2 in the uterine artery but equal to the PO_2 in the intervillous space of the placenta.
   b. The pO_2 in the umbilical vein is equal to both the pO_2 in the uterine vein and the pO_2 in the intervillous space of the placenta.
   c. The pO_2 in the umbilical vein is lower than the pO_2 in the uterine vein and lower than the pO_2 in the intervillous space of the placenta.
   d. The pO_2 in the umbilical vein is lower than the pO_2 in the umbilical artery.
   e. The pO_2 in the umbilical vein is lower than the pO_2 in the intervillous space of the placenta.

7. The umbilical vein supplies nutrients and oxygen to the fetus. Which of the following statement(s) is correct?
   a. Fetal arterial blood is formed by mixing umbilical venous blood with venous blood from fetal tissues.
   b. The arterial oxygen saturation is higher in the ascending fetal aorta than the descending fetal aorta.
   c. The fetal arterial oxygen saturation is highest in the blood perfusing the fetal heart and brain.

8. The uptake of oxygen by the pregnant uterus can be determined by multiplying uterine blood flow by the difference in oxygen content between the uterine arterial blood and uterine venous blood (Fick Principle). The oxygen uptake measured in this manner is the amount of oxygen consumed by the:
   a. fetus.
   b. fetus and placenta.
   c. fetus, placenta, myometrium, and endometrial glands.

9. The uptake of oxygen by the fetus can also be determined by applying the Fick Principle to umbilical circulation. In absolute terms, the oxygen consumption of the fetus is:
   a. higher than that of the mother.
   b. lower than that of the mother.
   c. the same as that of the mother.

10. The slope of the maternal oxyhemoglobin dissociation curve defines an increase in maternal arterial pO_2 from 90 torr in room air to a maximum of 410 torr when breathing 100% oxygen. Is the following statement true or false?
    Under normal conditions of uterine perfusion and oxygen uptake by the conceptus, such an increase in maternal arterial pO_2 results in a similar increase in a fetal arterial pO_2.
    a. True
    b. False

11. The diffusion of carbon dioxide follows a concentration gradient exactly opposite that of oxygen from the fetus to the mother. Which of the following statements is correct?
    a. The pCO_2 in the umbilical vein is higher than the pCO_2 in the umbilical artery.
    b. The pCO_2 in the umbilical vein is lower than the pCO_2 in the uterine vein.
    c. The pCO_2 in the umbilical vein is lower than the pCO_2 in the uterine artery.
    d. The pCO_2 in the umbilical vein is higher than the pCO_2 in the uterine vein.

12. Diffusion of oxygen from uterine circulation to umbilical circulation depends on the PO_2 gradient between the mother and fetus. Which of the following statement(s) are true?
    a. The uterine vein PO_2 and the PO_2 in the intervillous space of the placenta are the same.
    b. The uterine vein PO_2 and PO_2 in the intervillous space of the placenta are higher than the PO_2 in the umbilical vein.
    c. The PO_2 in the intervillous space of the placenta is lower than the PO_2 in the umbilical vein.

13. Diffusion of oxygen from uterine circulation to umbilical circulation depends on the PO_2 gradient between the mother and fetus. Which of the following statement(s) is/are true?
    a. Maternal oxygen consumption determines the PO_2 gradient.
    b. Placental oxygen consumption determines the PO_2 gradient.
    c. Fetal oxygen consumption determines the PO_2 gradient.

14. In the third trimester, the normal PO_2 in the umbilical vein is 35 torr and in the umbilical artery is 21 torr. In the growth-restricted fetus, the difference between these two values is:
    a. the same.
    b. decreased.
    c. increased.

15. Placental oxygen consumption is one of the factors that prevents equilibration of umbilical venous PO_2 with intervillous PO_2.
    a. True
    b. False

16. Compared with the normal adult, the cardiac output of the fetus on a per-weight basis is:
    a. higher.
    b. the same.
    c. lower.

17. As uterine blood flow decreases, the PO_2 difference between the mother and the fetus:
    a. increases.
    b. stays the same.
    c. decreases.

18. In the growth-restricted fetus, there is reduction in growth of the placenta, especially in the growth of terminal villi. As a result, the umbilical blood flow per kg fetus is:
    a. the same.
    b. decreased.
    c. increased.

19. Fetal cardiac output is normally near its maximum. In this situation, negative changes in fetal oxygenation can result in which of the following?
    a. Redistribution of fetal cardiac output, increased oxygen extraction, decrease in fetal growth rate
    b. Increased oxygen extraction, redistribution of fetal cardiac output, decrease in fetal growth rate
    c. Decrease in fetal growth rate, redistribution of fetal cardiac output, increased oxygen extraction

20. The hyperbolic relationship between oxygen content and percentage of cardiac output directed to the heart and central nervous system suggests that the physiologic difference between an APGAR score of 1 and 4 is less than the physiologic difference of an APGAR score of 6 and 9:
    a. True
    b. False

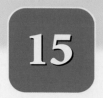

15

Evidence-Based Practice in Perinatal Medicine

GEORGE MACONES | METHODIUS TUULI

(see Creasy and Resnik's Maternal-Fetal Medicine, 9e: Ch 15)

Summary

Several study designs are reported in medical literature.

DESCRIPTIVE STUDIES

Case reports and case series are descriptions of either a single case or several cases and, thus, are termed *descriptive studies.* They often focus on an unusual disease, an unusual presentation of a disease, or an unusual treatment for a disease. In case reports and case series, there is no control group. Therefore, drawing any inference on causality is impossible.

OBSERVATIONAL STUDIES

The two main types of observational studies are case-control studies and cohort studies. These study designs attempt to assess the relationship between an exposure and an outcome. In case-control studies, subjects are identified on the basis of disease rather than exposure. Cohort studies identify subjects on the basis of exposure and assess the relationship between the exposure and the clinical outcome of interest. Cohort studies can be either retrospective or prospective.

RANDOMIZED CLINICAL TRIAL

The *randomized clinical trial* is the gold standard of clinical research design. In this type of clinical trial, eligible consenting participants are randomly allocated to receive different therapies. Differences in clinical outcomes are then compared on the basis of treatment assignment. Clinical trials are powerful because the likelihood that confounding and bias will influence the results is minimized.

SYSTEMATIC REVIEWS AND META-ANALYSIS

Systematic review and *meta-analysis* are two related but different terms, and they are often confused. A *systematic review* is a scientific investigation that focuses on a specific question and uses explicit, planned methods to identify, select, assess, and summarize the findings of similar but separate studies. It may or may not include a quantitative synthesis of the results from separate studies. A *meta-analysis* is the process of using statistical methods to quantitatively combine the results of similar studies identified in a systematic review to allow inferences to be made from the sample of studies.

SOURCES OF ERROR IN CLINICAL RESEARCH

Broadly speaking, two types of error can occur in clinical research studies: systematic error and random error. Random error, which is due to chance, is assessed using various methods for hypothesis testing, as described in the textbook chapter in detail. Systematic error is generally introduced into the study design by the investigator. Sources of systematic error include confounding and bias. As consumers of clinical research, our goals are to understand and try to interpret the role of these errors in the studies we read.

SAMPLE SIZE AND POWER

Type II (or β) error is defined as the probability of accepting the null hypothesis when, in fact, it is false. In a study with type II error, results are falsely reported as negative, and thus a true difference is missed. This typically occurs when the sample size is insufficient. Sample size estimates should be performed before any observational or interventional study.

SCREENING AND DIAGNOSIS

It is critical to understand the characteristics of both screening and diagnostic tests. Sensitivity and specificity are characteristics inherent in the test and are independent of the prevalence of the disease. *Sensitivity* is the probability, expressed as a percentage, that if the disease is present, the test is positive. *Specificity* is the probability, expressed as a percentage, that if the disease is absent, the test is negative. A *positive predictive value* is the probability that if the test is positive, the subject has the disease. A *negative predictive value* is the probability that if the test is negative, the subject does not have the disease.

QUESTIONS

1. Which of the following is an advantage of a case-control study over a cohort study?
   a. Direct calculation of relative risk
   b. Less prone to bias
   c. Less prone to confounding
   d. Lower expense

2. Which of the following is true of randomized controlled trials?
   a. Limited concern about confounding
   b. Easy logistically
   c. Highly generalizable
   d. Must be multicenter

3. Which of the following is true about subgroup analyses in randomized controlled trials?
   a. Generally, are well powered to detect important differences
   b. Should be planned a priori
   c. Are subject to type I error

4. You are interested in studying the association between first-trimester exposure to azithromycin and fetal hydranencephaly. Which would be the most appropriate study design to assess this association?
   a. Randomized controlled trial
   b. Prospective cohort study
   c. Decision analysis
   d. Case-control study

5. You are studying the association between maternal fever in the first trimester and fetal cleft palate, using a case-control study design. Which of the following is a likely source of error for this study design?
   a. Selection bias
   b. Type II error
   c. Confounding
   d. Recall bias

6. Which of the following measures of effect can be reliably calculated in a case-control study?
   a. Odds ratio
   b. Risk difference
   c. Relative risk
   d. None of the above

7. Which of the following is not an approach to the assessment and control of confounding in an observational study?
   a. Multivariable modeling (such as logistic regression)
   b. Stratified analysis
   c. Bayesian analysis

8. Which of the following is not an element in a sample size calculation for a randomized clinical trial?
   a. Type I error
   b. Type II error
   c. Incidence of disease in control arm
   d. Minimum detectable odds ratio

9. Which of the following terms does the following describe? The probability that if the test is positive, the disease is present.
   a. Sensitivity
   b. Positive likelihood ratio
   c. Positive predictive value
   d. Specificity

10. Which of the following is a graphical way of representing the trade-off between sensitivity and false-positive rate for a screening test?
    a. Likelihood ratio
    b. Funnel plot
    c. Receiver operating characteristic curve
    d. None of the above

Obstetric Imaging

Performing and Documenting the Fetal Anatomy Ultrasound Examination

JOSHUA A. COPEL | THOMAS R. MOORE

(see *Creasy and Resnik's Maternal-Fetal Medicine, 9e: Ch 16*)

Summary

The midtrimester fetal ultrasound examination ("anatomy scan") is important for obstetric dating, identifying fetal anatomic defects, and evaluating maternal conditions such as uterine fibroids and placental abnormalities (previa, accreta).

Most series suggest 50%−60% of major birth defects are detected with typical ultrasound anatomy surveys, especially with recent efforts to push the examination into the late first and early second trimesters.

Examinations are typically characterized as basic (standard, Current Procedural Terminology [CPT] 76805) and detailed (targeted, CPT 76811) depending on the level of risk of birth defects.

CPT codes are submitted for insurance reimbursement paired with codes from the International Statistical Classification of Diseases and Related Health Problems, 10th Revision (ICD-10), which describe the medical justification for the visit or procedure. Codes for obstetric ultrasound are found in Chapter 15 ("Pregnancy, Childbirth, and the Puerperium") and all begin with the letter "O."

All ultrasound examinations require a report to be placed in the patient's medical record, including the indication for the study, relevant findings, and their interpretation. The content of the report depends on the indication for the ultrasound study and should include enough information for clinicians to incorporate the findings into the patient's care.

CPT guidelines for each examination type provide specific elements that must be evaluated and reported in the fetus, placenta, and uterus. The images required for the specific level of the examination should be obtained, labeled appropriately, and stored. Images should remain available as long as required by local statutory regulations, which vary from state to state.

The detailed obstetric examination (76811) should be performed only once per pregnancy by any practice. After a detailed fetal anatomic examination and maternal risk assessment are completed, all subsequent procedures should be considered "follow-up" and coded as CPT 76816.

QUESTIONS

1. You are counseling a couple about the results of their midtrimester anatomy examination. What proportion of fetal anomalies should they expect to be detected?
   a. 20%−30%
   b. 40%−50%
   c. 50%−60%
   d. Well over 95%

2. When coding a fetal ultrasound examination in which a fetal neurologic anomaly is found, which of the following is the appropriate area of the CPT book to use to find the correct code?
   a. The chapter on diseases of the nervous system
   b. The chapter on obstetrics
   c. The chapter on conditions originating in the perinatal period
   d. The chapter on congenital malformations

3. For what period of time should images and reports be retained by a practice?
   a. For 7 years
   b. Until the baby is 21 years old
   c. Per local regulations
   d. Indefinitely

4. Which of the following best describes how to decide whether to use the 76811 versus 76805 CPT code?
   a. The indication for the scan
   b. What the insurance company will reimburse
   c. Whether all the anatomy is seen
   d. If the practice is accredited or not

5. When doing a routine anatomy scan, you identify a mass consistent with dermoid cyst of the ovary. Which of the following is the best way to handle this finding?
   a. No need to report when documenting a fetal scan.
   b. Call the managing medical doctor or certified nurse midwife but do not put it in the report.
   c. Bring the patient back at another date for a pelvic scan.
   d. Report all pelvic findings with interpretation of significance.

Doppler Ultrasound: Select Fetal and Maternal Applications

MERT OZAN BAHTIYAR | JOSHUA A. COPEL

(see *Creasy and Resnik's Maternal-Fetal Medicine, 9e: Ch 17*)

Summary

1. Umbilical Artery (UA): The number of umbilical arteries should be documented routinely during ultrasound examination, commonly by documenting two UAs traveling around the fetal bladder with color Doppler. Alternatively, one can identify a cross section of a freely floating loop of cord. Most UA Doppler indices are calculated ratios (e.g., S/D, RI, PI) and do not require measurement of absolute flow velocities. Attention should be paid to avoid compression of the umbilical cord. There is a progressive reduction in UA diastolic flow velocity from increasing placental impedance in growth-restricted pregnancies, with risk of stillbirth and asphyxia. Use of UA Doppler studies in small-for-gestational-age fetuses have been associated with reduction in perinatal mortality. These changes in Doppler waveforms should be seen as a marker of high-risk conditions and an indication for further surveillance and should not be used in isolation as an indication for delivery. Routine use of UA Doppler ultrasound in low-risk or unselected populations does not improve neonatal or maternal outcomes. Ultrasound-based twin-twin transfusion syndrome and twin anemia polycythemia staging systems that incorporate umbilical artery, umbilical vein, ductus venosus (DV), and middle cerebral artery (MCA) Doppler flow patterns are used in clinical practice. UA Doppler is also used to determine selective fetal growth restriction associated with monochorionic twin gestations. UA Doppler should not be measured during fetal breathing.

2. Middle Cerebral Artery (MCA): Correct technique is critical in determining the MCA peak systolic velocity (PSV). The peak velocity and shape of the peak velocity waveform become highly variable during episodes of fetal breathing. Excessive pressure on the fetal head should be avoided. The MCA is commonly used to assess suspected fetal anemia. Moderate or severe anemia is predicted by values of PSV in the fetal MCA greater than 1.5 times the median for gestational age, with a sensitivity of 100% and a false-positive rate of 12% in fetuses with red blood cell alloimmunization. Increased MCA PSV can also reliably predict anemia in fetuses with parvovirus B19 infection and twin anemia polycythemia sequence.

3. Ductus Venosus: The DV may be identified in sagittal, oblique parasagittal, or cross-sectional abdominal planes. The DV flow pattern directly reflects pressure changes within the right heart. The DV signal should be obtained during fetal rest and in the absence of fetal breathing. Growth-restricted fetuses with absent or reverse DV flow during atrial systole have worse perinatal outcomes. Absent or reverse flow during atrial systole in the DV is a strong indication of a pending fetal demise within 1 week. In most intrauterine growth-restricted fetuses, sequential deterioration of venous flow precedes biophysical profile score deterioration.

4. Doppler ultrasound assessment of the DV in the first trimester, between 10 and 14 weeks of gestation, has been suggested as a tool to identify fetuses at increased risk for chromosomal anomalies. In approximately 90% of fetuses with chromosomal anomalies, reversed or absent flow during atrial contraction has been reported. A similar blood flow pattern is seen in only 3.1% of chromosomally normal fetuses.

QUESTIONS

1. Which of the following fetal vessels provides the most information about fetal anemia?
   a. Umbilical artery
   b. Umbilical vein
   c. Middle cerebral artery
   d. Uterine artery
   e. Ductus venosus

2. Which of the following Doppler indices is used to assess for fetal anemia?
   a. Umbilical artery S/D ratio
   b. Middle cerebral artery S/D ratio
   c. Cerebroplacental ratio
   d. Middle cerebral artery peak systolic velocity
   e. Umbilical artery peak systolic velocity

3. Middle cerebral artery peak systolic velocity can be used to assess fetal polycythemia.
   a. True
   b. False

4. Doppler in which of the following fetal vessels is used for clinical diagnosis of twin anemia polycythemia sequence?
   a. Umbilical artery
   b. Umbilical vein
   c. Middle cerebral artery
   d. Ductus venosus
   e. Twin anemia polycythemia sequence cannot be diagnosed prenatally

5. Doppler in which of the following fetal vessels is used to determine the type of selective fetal growth restriction (sFGR) in monochorionic twin gestations?
   a. Umbilical artery
   b. Umbilical vein
   c. Middle cerebral artery
   d. Ductus venosus
   e. Doppler ultrasound does not have clinical utility in sFGR

6. Which of the following is the most helpful Doppler ultrasound finding in type 3 selective fetal growth restriction in monochorionic twin gestation?
   a. Intermittently elevated peak systolic velocity in middle cerebral artery
   b. Intermittently abnormal (absent or reverse end diastolic flow) in umbilical artery
   c. Pulsatile umbilical vein Doppler flow pattern
   d. Absent end diastolic flow in ductus venosus

7. Which of the following is the expected worsening sequence in umbilical artery Doppler findings in fetal growth restriction?
   a. Decreased end diastolic flow, absent end diastolic flow, reverse end diastolic flow
   b. Reverse end diastolic flow, absent end diastolic flow, decreased end diastolic flow
   c. Absent end diastolic flow, decrease diastolic flow, reverse end diastolic flow
   d. Decreased end diastolic flow, reverse end diastolic flow, absent end diastolic flow

8. Which Doppler finding indicates the worst perinatal outcome in growth-restricted fetuses?
   a. Decreased end diastolic flow in umbilical artery
   b. Reverse end diastolic flow in ductus venosus
   c. Elevated peak systolic velocity in middle cerebral artery
   d. Notching in the uterine artery

9. Abnormal ductus venosus Doppler in the first trimester has been suggested to indicate chromosomal abnormality.
   a. True
   b. False

10. DV blood flow pattern is identical to that of the inferior vena cava.
    a. True
    b. False

18

Clinical Applications of Three-Dimensional Sonography in Obstetrics

REEM S. ABU-RUSTUM | LAURA A. MONTANEY | DOLORES H. PRETORIUS | LAURYN C. GABBY | DORA J. MELBER

(see *Creasy and Resnik's Maternal-Fetal Medicine, 9e: Ch 18*)

Summary

Three-dimensional (3D) and four-dimensional (4D) ultrasonography (US), also referred to as volume sonography, has developed significantly in recent years. Two-dimensional US remains the backbone of sonographic imaging, to which 3D and 4D US has contributed an additional layer of problem-solving tools. This chapter addresses the obstetric applications of 3D US.

Volume data sets are typically obtained with a 3D mechanical probe by performing an automated volume sweep, of a certain size and quality, at a constant speed. This volume information may be displayed on the 2D screen in various types of display. Oftentimes, 3D US is routinely used as an adjunct to 2D US of the fetus. A significant advantage of 3D over 2D US is that once data are acquired, the image can be reviewed and manipulated in different planes for diagnostic clarification, even after the patient has left the US examination suite.

3D US and its clinical application are limited by various factors, including gestational age, maternal obesity, fetal motion, and imaging technique. With increasing experience among sonographers and sonologists, as well as more user-friendly 3D and 4D software programs, 3D US is expected to provide important additional information. The type of 3D US imaging tools used depends on the specific clinical question. For example, when evaluating bony abnormalities, use of maximum intensity projection would be appropriate. Conversely, surface rendering would be most helpful in assessment of soft tissue pathology, such as cleft lip, and minimum mode for the study of vasculature.

In the first trimester, key advantages of 3D imaging are primarily related to the size of the fetus and the ability to obtain a single volume of the entire fetus that contains all the anatomic and biometric planes needed for a complete assessment. In addition, 3D imaging is of critical value in the evaluation of ectopic pregnancies.

In the second and third trimesters, 3D is most useful in the evaluation of midline brain anatomy and the posterior fossa. It is also a valuable adjunct to 2D US imaging in the evaluation of neural tube defects: It allows more accurate determination of the exact level of the lesion. In the fetal face, various 3D techniques have been described to help evaluate the palate where they have been shown to improve diagnostic accuracy. In addition, it helps in the diagnoses of abnormal sutures.

Perhaps one of the most powerful applications of 3D imaging is in the evaluation of the fetal cardiovascular system. From the various modes that allow the interrogation of vascular abnormalities, to spatiotemporal image correlation, which is a method allowing acquisition of a fetal heart volume and its visualization as a 4D cine sequence, the applications are particularly useful. In addition, using automation, from a standardized acquisition of the plane of the four-chamber view, software has been developed to retrieve the plane of the abdominal circumference, four-chamber view, outflow tracts, three-vessel view, sagittal arches, and bicaval views automatically.

With respect to the fetal chest, abdomen, and pelvis, 3D is most helpful in volume calculation of various organs and abnormal masses that aid in prognostication and counseling of families. 3D US has also proved to be the adjunctive imaging modality of choice in evaluation of fetal skeletal anomalies detected on 2D US.

A unique attribute of 3D ultrasound is that 3D rendering of the fetal face has added another dimension to parental bonding, and facial expressions and fetal behavior have also been studied with 3D and 4D ultrasound.

As with any new technology, care must be exercised with respect to both false-positive and false-negative results. This is particularly applicable to 3D ultrasound, where the third dimension may allow better visualization of certain structures but introduces a third dimension of potential errors with it.

As an increasing number of sonographers use 3D US with greater confidence, application of 3D US to solve specific diagnostic issues will lead to improved diagnostic accuracy and clinical management.

QUESTIONS

1. **BASICS OF VOLUME SONOGRAPHY**
   A 26-year-old woman, gravida 1, para 0, is referred for ultrasound at 22 weeks of gestation due to concern for cleft lip. A 3D US study of the face and palate is considered. Which of the following is an advantage of 3D over 2D imaging?
   a. 3D imaging can be manipulated in different planes, even after the patient has left the US examination suite.
   b. 3D imaging is not affected by fetal motion or position.
   c. 3D imaging can be easily optimized even if the quality of the 2D image from which it is acquired is poor.
   d. 3D imaging is not limited by imaging technique or maternal body habitus.

2. **ECTOPIC PREGNANCY**
   A 30-year-old woman, gravida 2, para 0, is referred for ultrasound at 6 weeks of gestation due to concern for abnormal position of the gestational sac. A transvaginal 3D US study is performed, and a hyperechoic line is visualized, extending from the lateral aspect of the uterine cavity into the midsection of the gestational sac along with a thin mantle of myometrium surrounding the gestational sac. Which of the following is the most likely diagnosis?
   a. Septate uterus with intrauterine pregnancy
   b. Interstitial ectopic pregnancy
   c. Angular pregnancy
   d. Ovarian ectopic pregnancy

3. **ECTOPIC PREGNANCY**
   A 23-year-old woman, gravida 1, para 0, is referred for ultrasound at 6 weeks of gestation due to concern for a pregnancy of unknown location. A transvaginal 3D US study shows no intrauterine gestational sac. However, a gestational sac is seen in the fallopian tube. What unique feature on 3D ultrasound best allows visualization of the fallopian tube during evaluation of pregnancy of unknown location?
   a. Fallopian tube surrounded by a fine hypoechoic border
   b. Hyperechoic line extending from the uterine cavity into the midsection of the gestational sac
   c. Gestational sac visualized in the adnexa
   d. Dilation of the fallopian tube

4. **SONOEMBRYOLOGY AND SONOAUTOPSY**
   A 41-year-old woman, gravida 1, para 0, is referred for ultrasound at 14 weeks of gestation with a suspected missed abortion. Her physician suspected a fetal anomaly on an earlier ultrasound. Which anomaly would most likely be detected by a 3D ultrasound at this time?
   a. Absent cavum septum pellucidum
   b. Absent bladder
   c. Neural tube defect
   d. Hypoplastic left cardiac ventricle

5. **CENTRAL NERVOUS SYSTEM**
   A 25-year-old woman, gravida 2, para 0, is referred for a first-trimester ultrasound at 10 weeks of gestation. Her previous pregnancy was affected by anencephaly. How early can anencephaly be detected using 3D ultrasonography?
   a. 11 weeks
   b. 12 weeks
   c. 13 weeks
   d. 14 weeks

6. **CENTRAL NERVOUS SYSTEM**
   A 30-year-old woman, gravida 1, para 0, is referred for ultrasound at 20 weeks of gestation. A previous ultrasound suggested agenesis of the corpus collosum (ACC). 3D ultrasound may aid in the diagnosis through visualization of the corpus callosum, as well as which of the following structures that is used as an indirect finding of ACC?
   a. Cavum septi pellucidi
   b. Cisterna magna
   c. Cerebellum
   d. Vermis

7. **FETAL FACE (first trimester)**
   A 30-year-old woman, gravida 3, para 2, is referred for ultrasound at 12 weeks of gestation. A 3D US study is performed, and the retronasal triangle view is obtained. You notice that the normal gap in the midaspect of the mandible (mandibular gap) is absent. Which of the following is the most likely diagnosis?
   a. Cleft lip
   b. Cleft palate
   c. Micrognathia
   d. Absent nasal bone

8. **CENTRAL NERVOUS SYSTEM—Vermis**
   A 32-year-old woman, gravida 3, para 2, is referred for ultrasound at 21 weeks of gestation due to difficulty in evaluating the cerebellar vermis on 2D imaging. A 3D US study of the posterior fossa shows a vermis of normal length and a brainstem-vermis (BV) angle >45 degrees. Which of the following is the most likely diagnosis?
   a. Vermian hypoplasia
   b. Blake pouch cyst
   c. Dandy-Walker malformation
   d. Mega cisterna magna

9. CENTRAL NERVOUS SYSTEM

A 27-year-old, gravida 1, para 0, is referred for a routine anatomy ultrasound at 19 weeks of gestation. 2D ultrasound imaging of the cisterna magna was limited. Which of the following is a true statement?

a. 3D ultrasound is more accurate than 2D ultrasound in assessment of the cisterna magna.

b. In some cases, 3D ultrasound may aid in measuring the cisterna magna.

c. 3D ultrasound should always be applied in cisterna magna evaluations.

d. No reference ranges have been presented to describe 3D evaluation of the cisterna magna.

10. CENTRAL NERVOUS SYSTEM—Neural Tube Defect

A 32-year-old woman, gravida 3, para 2, is referred for ultrasound at 23 weeks of gestation given concern for neural tube defect on anatomy survey. Which of the following is an advantage of 3D imaging in this clinical scenario?

a. 3D imaging allows for optimized imaging regardless of fetal position or movement.

b. 3D imaging allows for more accurate determination of the vertebral level of defect.

c. 3D imaging can be obtained faster than 2D imaging.

d. 3D imaging can improve detection of neural tube defects on routine screening.

11. FETAL FACE, HEAD, AND NECK—Cleft Palate

A 26-year-old, gravida 4, para 3, is referred for anatomy ultrasound at 18 weeks of gestation. One of her previous children has a cleft palate. 2D ultrasound demonstrates a normal-appearing coronal view of the face, and the palate appears normal in the midsagittal plane. How could 3D ultrasound help in your evaluation?

a. 3D ultrasound improves diagnostic sensitivity for cleft palate in low-risk pregnancies.

b. Diagnostic accuracy for cleft palate is greatly improved with surface rendering on 3D ultrasound.

c. Multiplanar views on 3D ultrasound can help detect isolated cleft palate.

d. 3D volume acquisition can best be performed in an oblique plane.

12. FETAL MANDIBLE

A 21-year-old woman, gravida 1, para 0, is referred for anatomy ultrasound at 20 weeks of gestation. The facial profile in 2D imaging appears abnormal, so you perform a 3D ultrasound to investigate a potential mandible abnormality. What is an advantage of 3D ultrasound in this scenario?

a. 3D ultrasound allows all three planes to be manipulated for a perfectly symmetrically positioned face and assessment in the true midline.

b. Unlike with 2D imaging, 3D ultrasound will avoid misdiagnosis of micrognathia even when only the sagittal view is obtained.

c. 3D is the only modality that can distinguish micrognathia from retrognathia.

d. Surface rendering is more accurate than multiplanar imaging for fetal jaw evaluation.

13. FETAL NECK

A 30-year-old woman, gravida 1, para 0 is referred for ultrasound at 24 weeks of gestation. A recent ultrasound showed a suspected upper airway abnormality. The earliest age at which 3D ultrasound is most sensitive for detecting abnormalities of the pharynx and larynx is at what gestational age?

a. 15—19 weeks

b. 20—24 weeks

c. 25—29 weeks

d. 30—34 weeks

14. FETAL HEART AND VASCULAR SYSTEM

A 23-year-old woman, gravida 2, para 1, is referred for detailed anatomy ultrasound at 19 weeks of gestation. You decide to obtain views of the heart using 3D ultrasound using a method that allows for simultaneous display of multiple sequential cardiac images that can be rotated in any plane. This technology is called:

a. Surface rendering

b. Tomographic ultrasound imaging

c. Volume contrast imaging

d. B-Flow imaging

15. THORAX

A 31-year-old woman, gravida 1, is referred for follow-up ultrasound for suspected diaphragmatic hernia involving the liver at 29 weeks of gestation. What 3D ultrasound mode would be most useful for diagnosis?

a. Surface rendering

b. Tomographic ultrasound imaging

c. Volume contrast imaging

d. B-Flow imaging

16. FETAL EXTREMITIES AND SKELETON

A 27-year-old, gravida 1, para 0, is referred for detailed anatomy ultrasound at 18 weeks of gestation. An abnormally short limb is suspected on 2D ultrasound. Which 3D ultrasound technique has been shown to detect limb shortening and may aid in diagnosis?

a. Volume-rendering with maximum-intensity projection

b. Surfacing rendering

c. Tomographic ultrasound imaging

d. Multiplanar views

17. PARENTAL BONDING AND FETAL BEHAVIOR

A 32-year-old woman, gravida 1, para 0, is referred for anatomy ultrasound at 19 weeks of gestation. She asks you to perform a 3D ultrasound so that she can "see the baby's face." Which of the following statements are true regarding 3D imaging and fetal bonding?

a. 3D ultrasound has been shown to improve a patient's ability to form a mental picture of the baby.

b. 3D ultrasound for the purpose of parental bonding is not medically indicated and therefore should not be done.

c. 3D ultrasound can upset parents if there is a visible anomaly and therefore should be avoided.

d. 3D ultrasound used in excess has been shown to cause fetal harm, especially during the second trimester.

18. FUTURE OF VOLUME SONOGRAPHY IN OBSTETRICS
Regarding 3D ultrasound, which of the following is most likely to become common practice in the near future?
a. Enhanced surface rendering with true color depiction that more accurately depicts fetal skin tones
b. Sound wave acquisition that allows perception of fetal noises
c. Replacement of 2D with 3D ultrasound as the primary fetal imaging modality
d. Enhanced image manipulation that automatically acquires key images from volume sweeps using artificial intelligence

19

Role of Magnetic Resonance Imaging in Obstetric Imaging

ANNE KENNEDY | PAULA WOODWARD

(see Creasy and Resnik's Maternal-Fetal Medicine, 9e: Ch 19)

Summary

Magnetic resonance imaging (MRI) has a well-established role in evaluation of fetal anomalies, as its superior contrast resolution complements the superior spatial resolution of ultrasound (US). It is most useful for evaluation of the central nervous system and complex body malformations. It is, however, a highly technical and expensive examination that must be performed by technologists with dedicated training and be monitored by radiologists with expertise in fetal imaging so that the examination is tailored to answer specific clinical questions.

ADVANTAGES OF MRI OVER ULTRASOUND

MRI has superb contrast resolution, allowing delineation of anatomic structures that appear similar on US. It is less compromised by maternal obesity and oligohydramnios than is US. Acoustic shadowing from overlying bone, extremities, or parts of another fetus in multiple gestations is not an issue. Orthogonal planes are easy to set up, and the large field of view is often helpful when counseling parents or planning interventions, both fetal and neonatal.

The studies are fast in experienced hands, with a targeted study taking approximately 20 minutes. No sedation is required in the majority of cases. There is no exposure to ionizing radiation, and the studies are safe with no demonstrated adverse impact on maternal or fetal health.

DISADVANTAGES OF MRI OVER ULTRASOUND

While cine images can be obtained (e.g., for evaluation of fetal swallowing), MRI does not allow for real-time assessment of the fetus, nor can scan planes be continuously adjusted to compensate for fetal movement. The equipment is expensive and neither universally available nor portable, unlike US.

Maternal discomfort can be an issue, particularly in the third trimester, but this can be overcome by scanning in the lateral decubitus position. Maternal claustrophobia can be eased with the use of feet-first positioning, use of headphones, short examination times, and, occasionally, administration of oral anxiolytics before the examination. In cases of extreme obesity, table weight limits and gantry diameter may preclude performance of MRI in pregnancy.

BASICS OF IMAGE INTERPRETATION

Most magnetic resonance sequences are either T1 or T2 weighted. T2-weighted imaging (T2WI) is the mainstay of fetal MRI, whereas T1-weighted imaging (T1WI) is used for problem solving. Also, to compensate for fetal movement, only fast, single-slice techniques are used.

T2WI shows fluid as high signal or white. Solid organs are intermediate in signal or various shades of gray. Gas-filled and calcified structures are low signal and appear black. Flowing blood also appears black on T2WI due to the "flow void" created by lack of signal from moving objects in the scan plane.

On T1WI, fluid is low signal (dark gray), as are most of the soft tissues. However, meconium, fat, and blood products are high signal (white); this allows for specific problem solving such as mapping the colon in complex genitourinary malformations and confirming that a low-signal area on T2WI represents clotted blood.

Diffusion-weighted imaging and apparent diffusion coefficient mapping are more advanced techniques that may be used in fetal brain imaging. Restricted diffusion is seen in the setting of hypoxic-ischemic injury and in some congenital brain malformations. The demonstration of ischemic injury can be important in countries where termination is legal at any gestational age. In countries where late-pregnancy termination is not allowed, detection of severe brain injury or malformation is still useful for delivery planning and provides proof that the insult did not occur during labor or delivery.

ANOMALIES/ANATOMIC AREAS IN WHICH MRI IS MOST USEFUL

Brain: MRI can show additional findings even after dedicated neurosonography in the setting of ventriculomegaly or absent cavum septi pellucidi. Ischemic injury in association with vascular malformations and fetal intervention or following maternal trauma is reliably demonstrated by MRI. The vermis and brainstem are challenging to assess with US even when transvaginal imaging can be performed. MRI allows rapid evaluation in orthogonal planes, making it easy to differentiate between Dandy-Walker malformation and the less severe posterior fossa malformations.

Abdomen: MRI can delineate the course of the colon and rectum and demonstrate anal position in urogenital septum anomalies and complex abdominal wall malformations such as bladder and cloacal exstrophy. It also helps determine the organ of origin of an abdominal mass, narrowing the differential diagnosis. The internal extent of a sacrococcygeal tumor is easily demonstrated on MRI, whereas it can be quite difficult on US.

Chest: Measurement of lung volume and demonstration of liver position in fetuses with congenital diaphragmatic hernia is simple with MRI. Lung volume measurement may also be used for prognostication in fetuses with large or multiple chest masses, or with giant omphalocele.

Head and neck: MRI is used to assess the extent of masses and to evaluate airway patency for delivery planning, especially when an EXIT (ex utero intrapartum treatment) procedure may be appropriate. In fetuses with CHAOS (congenital high airway obstruction syndrome), MRI may be used in an effort to determine the level of obstruction.

Fetal tumors: Fetal tumors are uncommon but may be life-threatening. MRI is used to fully characterize these masses, as well as to determine extent and plan intervention.

ANOMALIES/ANATOMIC AREAS IN WHICH MRI IS LEAST USEFUL

Vertebral/bone detail: Fetal motion and the types of sequences available limit bone evaluation. With three-dimensional (3D) reconstruction, vertebral segmentation anomalies and the level of open neural tube defects can be reliably demonstrated on US, as can the presence of a tethered cord.

Cardiac imaging: Cardiac gating is not possible for the fetal heart. The small size and rapid rate limit the applications of MRI in fetal cardiac abnormalities.

Facial and extremity malformations: The real-time assessment of the face and extremities possible with ultrasound and the use of 3D and four-dimensional imaging makes US far superior to MRI.

Conclusion

Fetal MRI is additive to US; it is not a substitute for a poorly performed study. MRI should never be performed in a vacuum; knowledge of the clinical history and review of the sonographic findings are essential before performing the examination. When appropriately performed and interpreted, MRI is an extremely useful adjunct to US in providing precise and comprehensive information on fetal diagnosis. The additional information often has a direct impact on patient management.

QUESTIONS

1. An obese patient at 20 weeks' gestation is referred for evaluation of "abnormal ultrasound findings, concern for absent cavum septi pellucidi." On review of the 18-week office scan, fetal size was concordant with dates but views of the head were in nonstandard projections. What is the appropriate next step in imaging?
   a. Detailed anatomic ultrasound
   b. Contrast-enhanced ultrasound
   c. Fetal MRI
   d. Fetal MRI with contrast

2. A 20-week scan of twins shows absent cavum septi pellucidi in twin B with atrial diameters of the lateral ventricles measuring 10.2 mm and 11 mm. The family would not terminate an abnormal pregnancy but would consider comfort care for an infant with a significant brain abnormality. Which of the following studies would provide most information for delivery planning?
   a. Fetal MRI at 22 weeks
   b. Fetal MRI at 32 weeks
   c. Transvaginal ultrasound
   d. 3D ultrasound

3. In which of the following clinical situations is fetal MRI considered "usually appropriate" by the American College of Radiology Appropriateness Criteria Second and Third Trimester Screening for Fetal Anomaly? The term usually appropriate is defined as "imaging procedure or treatment is indicated in the specified clinical scenarios at a favorable risk-benefit ratio for patients."
   a. Increased nuchal translucency
   b. Abnormal cell free DNA screen
   c. Echogenic bowel
   d. Diaphragmatic hernia

4. A pregnant patient is in a high-speed motor vehicle collision with multiple injuries at 30 weeks. To look for which of the following complications would an MRI 10−14 days later be indicated?
   a. Fetal skull fracture
   b. Fetal ischemic brain injury
   c. Maternal liver laceration
   d. Maternal pelvic fracture

5. In a 32-week fetus with newly diagnosed hydrocephalus, which of the following diagnoses would have the most impact on method and timing of delivery?
   a. Dandy-Walker malformation
   b. Interhemispheric cyst
   c. Hydranencephaly
   d. Aqueductal stenosis

6. Which of the following is the most likely diagnosis if fetal MRI shows elevation of the torcular, vermian rotation with tegmentovermian angle of 72 degrees, large posterior fossa cyst, and severe ventriculomegaly with lateral ventricular diameters of 17 and 20 mm?
   a. Mega cisterna magna
   b. Blake pouch cyst
   c. Vermian dysgenesis
   d. Dandy-Walker malformation

7. Which of the following signs that may be demonstrated on MRI is considered diagnostic of Joubert syndrome?
   a. Molar tooth sign
   b. Lemon sign
   c. Steer horn sign
   d. Bat wing sign

8. What information does MRI provide that is critical in determining the need for an EXIT (ex utero intrapartum treatment) procedure in a fetus with a solid neck mass most consistent with a cervical teratoma?
   a. Composition of mass
   b. Extent of mass
   c. Tracheal compression
   d. Choanal atresia

9. Which of the following pieces of information obtained at fetal MRI is important in fetal prognosis with a left-sided congenital diaphragmatic hernia?
   a. Lung volume
   b. Liver volume
   c. Lung displacement
   d. Liver displacement

10. Which of the following findings on fetal MRI has a high positive predictive value for the diagnosis of esophageal atresia?
    a. Vertebral segmentation anomaly
    b. Ureteropelvic junction obstruction
    c. Esophageal pouch
    d. Unilateral renal agenesis

Fetal Central Nervous System Imaging

ANA MONTEAGUDO | ILAN E. TIMOR-TRITSCH

(see *Creasy and Resnik's Maternal-Fetal Medicine,* 9e: Ch 20)

Summary

Encephaloceles are cranial defects through which there is a herniation of the brain and/or meninges. They can occur anywhere in the skull, although the majority in the Western Hemisphere are occipital or posterior. The exact pathogenesis is unclear. Cephaloceles are classified as neural tube defects. Prenatal diagnosis at 11 $^{0/7}$–13 $^{6/7}$ weeks is possible, and the sonographic appearance is similar to that described during the second trimester. The important sonographic clues are a saclike structure adjacent or posterior to the fetal head containing brain tissue, meninges, and/or cerebrospinal fluid protruding through a skull defect. The herniated sac may be covered by skin. Hydrocephaly is commonly present.

Choroid plexus cysts are well-demarcated, anechoic, fluid-filled structures within the choroid plexus of the lateral ventricles of the brain. In the past they have been referred to as "soft sonographic markers of aneuploidy." However, when isolated, and in the presence of low-risk noninvasive testing, they are considered a benign normal "variant."

Alobar holoprosencephaly is the most severe of the spectrum of holoprosencephalies, which are characterized by failure of the forebrain to properly divide along the midline. The three classic forms are alobar, semilobar, and lobar. The sonographic features include a monoventricle; absence of the interhemispheric fissure, falx cerebri, corpus callosum, and *cavum septi pellucidi;* fusion of the thalami and cerebral hemispheres; and possibly various facial anomalies (e.g., cyclopia, proboscis, median clefts). Nonvisualization of the "butterfly sign" in an axial section or the midline falx flanked by the choroid plexus of the brain between 11 $^{0/7}$ and 13 $^{6/7}$ weeks is a reliable diagnostic clue to the presence of alobar holoprosencephaly.

Porencephaly refers to a pathologic brain cavity or cyst filled by cerebrospinal fluid, typically seen late in gestation. The cyst is the result of a vascular insult occurring between the second trimester of pregnancy and early postnatal period. Areas affected by the insult undergo tissue necrosis and resorption, leaving behind a cavity in the brain (porencephalic cavity). Sonographic diagnosis is made when there is a cyst or cavity within the brain parenchyma that communicates with the ventricles and/or subarachnoid space; there is ventriculomegaly on the same side as the cyst; no mass effect is present; and the cyst is seen along the distribution of the middle cerebral artery or other arteries.

Ventriculomegaly is defined as dilation of the lateral ventricle measuring ≥10 mm. It can be further divided into mild, moderate, and severe when the ventricles measure 10–12 mm; 13–15 mm, and >15 mm, respectively. Ventriculomegaly is a sign, not a diagnosis; therefore once the diagnosis is made, a search for possible etiologies must be undertaken. Evaluation of the fetus diagnosed with ventriculomegaly includes detailed anatomic survey including fetal echocardiography and brain scan, infection workup (cytomegalovirus and toxoplasmosis), genetic counseling and testing, and often fetal brain magnetic resonance imaging (MRI).

Arnold Chiari malformation refers to a constellation of findings resulting from a complex congenital anomaly resulting from the presence of an open spinal defect (myelomeningocele or myeloschisis) with subsequent herniation of the cerebellar vermis and brainstem through the foramen magnum. It is associated with elevated maternal serum alpha fetoprotein (MSAFP). The sonographic features include change in the head contour ("lemon" sign) and flattening of the cerebellar hemispheres ("banana sign"), both seen best in an axial plane of the head, as well as ventriculomegaly or hydrocephaly. Direct visualization of the spine in sagittal section in cases of myelomeningocele reveals a cystic bulging mass and in myeloschisis is a flat defect with no bulging mass, while in the transverse section the bony spine has a U shape due to the missing spinal processes.

Dandy-Walker spectrum refers to a spectrum of malformations that include enlargement of the posterior fossa with an elevated cerebellar tentorium and torcular, dilation of the fourth ventricle, and small, malformed, or entirely missing cerebellar vermis. In the majority of cases, some degree of ventriculomegaly or hydrocephaly is present. Sonographic clues to the diagnosis include a large cisterna magna that communicates with the fourth ventricle, absent or hypoplastic vermis, cerebellar hemispheres splayed apart with varying degrees of dysplasia, elevated tentorium and torcular Herophili, and ventriculomegaly.

Agenesis of the corpus callosum is diagnosed when colpocephaly (ventriculomegaly) with teardrop-shaped, parallel lateral ventricles are imaged on the axial section of the fetal brain. In addition, there is an absent *cavum septi pellucidi,* absent corpus callosum, and absent or abnormal pericallosal artery with color/power Doppler. During the third trimester the gyri and sulci result in the "sunburst" sign—on the median surface of the brain. On the coronal plane the anterior horns of the lateral ventricle are widely spaced and upward pointing, resembling the shape of a "Viking helmet." Approximately 30%–45% of the cases have an identifiable cause, of which 10%–17% have chromosomal anomalies, such as deletions, trisomies, and duplications. Furthermore, another 20%–35% have recognizable genetic syndromes. The prognosis ranges from normal to severe psychomotor delay; however, in the presence of other brain findings or associated anomalies, the prognosis is more guarded. Outcome is not clearly worse for individuals with isolated complete agenesis compared with individuals with partial agenesis.

Arachnoid cysts are collections of cerebrospinal fluid on the brain surface. These cysts are usually benign, congenital, space-occupying lesions. Cysts occur in Sylvian fissure, brain convexity, or interhemispheric spaces. Approximately 25%–30% of cysts occur in posterior fossa. The cyst is well demarcated, with smooth borders. It does not communicate with the ventricular system or subarachnoid space. Color Doppler reveals no blood flow in the walls. Ventriculomegaly or hydrocephaly is secondary to pressure effects.

Exencephaly-anencephaly sequence is one of the most common neural tube defect. Sonographic findings include the absence of cranium beyond the area of the forehead with exposed brain tissue, prominent orbits with preservation of the base of the skull and facial features, and echogenic amniotic fluid. It can be reliably diagnosed during the first trimester at the time of the nuchal translucency scan or even before. In the second trimester, it is associated with elevated MSAFP.

Microcephaly is a condition in which the head circumference is two to three standard deviations below the mean for gestational age on standardized charts. The pathogenesis is multifactorial and is the common end point of a group of heterogeneous conditions that interfere with growth of the brain. The condition results from abnormal cell division and

proliferation. Microcephaly has been associated with genetic conditions, infections, maternal conditions, as well as alcohol and illicit drug usage.

Vein of Galen malformation (VGAM) is a rare type of arteriovenous malformation involving the predecessor of the vein of Galen, which typically results in high-output congestive heart failure. It may lead to developmental delay, hydrocephaly, and seizures in the neonate. Typically, it is first seen in the late second or third trimester. Sonographic findings on an axial section of the brain show VGAMs as tubular structures located superior to the thalamus; they are contiguous with the dilated sagittal sinus, giving it the appearance of a "comet tail" or "keyhole" shape. Color/power Doppler imaging demonstrates high-velocity turbulent flow within the structure, which is the most helpful method differentiating VGAM from other pathologies.

Hydranencephaly is a rare brain malformation that results from a destructive process in which both cerebral hemispheres may be entirely, or almost entirely, absent, with cerebrospinal fluid filling the space. The falx cerebri, cerebellum and brainstem are usually intact. The head size may be normal or large (macrocephaly). Polyhydramnios is usually present.

QUESTIONS

1. A 31-year-old woman gravida 4 para 3 is referred for a first-trimester scan at 13 1/7 weeks. The ultrasound reveals a saclike structure on the back of the head with a cranial defect. Which of the following is the most likely diagnosis?
   a. Cystic hygroma
   b. Amniotic band syndrome
   c. Posterior encephalocele
   d. Nuchal tumor

2. A 22-year-old woman gravida 1 para 0 had a detailed anatomic survey performed at 20 5/7 weeks after normal cfDNA testing. The scan was significant for large bilateral choroid plexus cysts, but otherwise the scan was within the normal limits for the gestational age. Which of the following is the most appropriate next step in management?
   a. Reassure the patient, given low-risk noninvasive prenatal testing
   b. Recommend amniocentesis for karyotype
   c. Fetal echo due to the association with congenital heart defects
   d. Fetal brain MRI

3. A 28-year-old woman gravida 4 para 1 with a history of prior pregnancy complicated by alobar holoprosencephaly diagnosed at 22 6/7 weeks presents at 12 6/7 weeks for a nuchal translucency scan; she is anxious to find out if this fetus also has alobar holoprosencephaly. Which of the following is the most appropriate step in the management?
   a. Chorionic villous sampling for karyotype
   b. MRI of the fetus
   c. Detailed anatomic survey at 20–22 weeks
   d. Evaluate brain for the "butterfly" sign

4. A 32-year-old woman gravida 3 para 2 at 34 5/7 weeks has an ultrasound that revealed a cyst in the fetal brain that freely communicates with the ventricular system. There is ventriculomegaly in the same side as the cyst, with no mass effect. Which of the following is the most likely diagnosis?
   a. Arachnoid cyst
   b. Porencephaly
   c. Brain tumor

5. You inform a 27-year-old woman gravida 1 para 0 having an anatomic survey at 20 3/7 weeks that the fetal lateral brain ventricles measured 13 mm. Which of the following is the most appropriate step in the management?
   a. Evaluate for the presence of extracardiac anomalies
   b. A detailed fetal neuroscan
   c. Infection workup
   d. Genetic counseling and amniocentesis
   e. All of the above

6. A 33-year-old gravida 2 para 1, with a body mass index of 40, presents for an anatomic survey at 20 1/7 weeks. The scan is significant for spine in contact with the posterior uterine wall, normal *cavum septi pellucidi*, cerebellum poorly seen, cisterna magna not seen, and lateral ventricles measuring 10.4 mm. The head has a bilateral frontal indentation; the kidneys, abdominal wall, and hands appeared normal; the heart and legs are poorly seen; and amniotic fluid was normal. Which of the following is the most likely diagnosis?
   a. Borderline ventriculomegaly
   b. Reassurance that this is normal
   c. Arnold-Chiari II malformation
   d. Brachycephaly

7. A 37-year-old gravida 1 para 0 conceived via in vitro fertilization, with low-risk preimplantation genetic testing, was diagnosed with borderline ventriculomegaly at 20 1/7 weeks of gestation. Which of the following is the most appropriate next step in the management?
   a. Fetal echocardiogram
   b. Infection workup
   c. Amniocentesis for karyotype and microarray
   d. Repeat ultrasound to monitor progression
   e. All of the above

8. A 25-year-old gravida 3 para 2 at 20 2/7 weeks was diagnosed with cisterna magna measuring 14 mm on the transcerebellar view; the vermis was not seen, and a wide communication with the fourth ventricle was apparent. Which of the following is the most likely diagnosis?
   a. Persistent Blake pouch cyst
   b. Dandy-Walker spectrum
   c. Posterior fossa arachnoid cyst
   d. Megacisterna magna

9. A 33-year-old gravida 2 para 1 was diagnosed with agenesis of the corpus callosum during the detailed anatomic survey; confirmed by fetal MRI; fetal echocardiogram was unremarkable. The couple reports a normal nuchal translucency scan and a low-risk noninvasive prenatal screen. Which of the following is the most appropriate next step in the management?
   a. Amniocentesis for karyotype and microarray
   b. Repeat noninvasive prenatal screen with a different lab
   c. Blood work for MSAFP
   d. Schedule for cesarean delivery at 39 weeks

10. A 36-year-old primigravida comes to the office for counseling due to the diagnosis of partial agenesis of the corpus callosum confirmed by MRI; otherwise, her detailed anatomic survey is normal. She reports a normal fetal echocardiogram, karyotype, microarray, and infection workup. Which of the following advice should be given to this patient?
    a. This condition is always associated with severe neurologic outcomes.
    b. Outcomes are comparable with complete agenesis of the corpus callosum.
    c. Autism is not associated with this condition.
    d. Fine motor control is never a problem with this condition.

11. A 22-year-old gravida 2 para 1 had a detailed anatomic survey at 22 weeks, which was significant for the cerebral lateral ventricles measuring 10.5 mm. The cavum septi pellucidi was not seen, and the anterior horns were widely spaced and upwardly pointing. There was also a ventricular septal defect and urinary tract dilatation. Which of the following is the most likely diagnosis?
    a. Agenesis of the corpus callosum
    b. Arnold-Chiari type II malformation
    c. Alobar holoprosencephaly
    d. Persistent Blake pouch

12. A 42-year-old primigravida during a routine growth scan at 28 weeks' gestation is diagnosed with a well-defined cystic fetal brain structure near the interhemispheric fissure measuring 1.8 cm. It does not communication with the ventricles, and color Doppler reveals no blood flow. Which of the following is the most likely diagnosis?
    a. Cavum veli interpositi cyst
    b. Persistent Blake pouch cyst
    c. Arachnoid cyst
    d. Choroid plexus cyst

13. An 18-year-old primigravida with known LMP presents for a transabdominal dating scan at 11 6/7 weeks. The scan reveals size dates discrepancy and speckled amniotic fluid. The cranial vault is poorly visualized with an irregular appearance. Which of the following is the most likely diagnosis?
    a. Wrong dates, redate the pregnancy
    b. Subchorionic hematoma
    c. Posterior encephalocele
    d. Exencephaly-anencephaly sequence

14. A 29-year-old gravida 4 para 3 veterinarian had a growth scan at 32 weeks, which reveals the head circumference at <3 standard deviations below the mean. She has not traveled out of the country, no history of febrile illness, no history of substance abuse, no history of diabetes, and no family history of microcephaly. Which of the following is the most appropriate next step in the management?
    a. Refer for fetal MRI
    b. Genetic counseling
    c. Reassure the patient that this is likely normal
    d. Repeat scan in 2 weeks
    e. Infection workup (TORCH titers)

15. A-30-year-old gravida 2 para 1 during a routine growth scan was diagnosed with a tubular structure superior to the fetal thalamus and extending to the sagittal sinus. It was reported that it looks like a comet's tail. The office ultrasound machine does not have color Doppler, but pulsed Doppler revealed high-velocity turbulent flow. Which of the following is the most likely diagnosis?
    a. Vein of Galen malformation
    b. Teratoma of the brain
    c. Intracranial hemorrhage
    d. Cerebral venous thrombosis

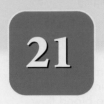

21

Imaging of the Face and Neck

KATHERINE H. CAMPBELL | CHRISTINA S. HAN | SONYA S. ABDEL-RAZEQ

(see *Creasy and Resnik's Maternal-Fetal Medicine, 9e: Ch 21*)

Summary

CLEFT LIP AND PALATE

Cleft lip or palate, or both, are conditions that result in a broad spectrum of potential implications for the health and well-being of the affected fetus/neonate. The cleft may be an isolated defect or present as part of a more global syndrome that may involve additional structural and genetic anomalies. The most common presentation is unilateral cleft lip with cleft palate. However, other combinations and cleft type can occur including isolated unilateral cleft lip, bilateral cleft lip and palate, midline cleft lip and palate, and isolated cleft palate. The structural anomaly occurs during fetal embryogenesis between weeks 7 and 12. In addition to genetic associations, environmental and pharmacologic exposure can increase the risk of clefting. Ultrasound imaging may allow visualization as early as 13—14 weeks' gestation; however, the sensitivity is low at early gestational ages and repeat ultrasound assessment should be performed at the time of the anatomy ultrasound at 18—20 weeks' gestation. If a cleft is identified on ultrasound, further assessment should be undertaken to look for the presence of any other birth defects. Lumbar and cervical spine anomalies are the most common type of associated anomalies, followed by cardiac defects. If a cleft is diagnosed, multidisciplinary management should be pursued including involvement with maternal fetal medicine, prenatal genetics, and the appropriate pediatric specialists. Postnatal management should be planned in advance and include the physician specialists, as well as any required supporting services that will be required in the early neonatal period including feeding evaluation and support.

CYSTIC HYGROMA

Cystic hygromas are congenital thin-walled cysts that contain lymphatic fluid, arising from failure of the primitive lymphatic tree to connect to the venous system. Key diagnostic features include anechoic fluid-filled cavities that are encircled by soft tissue, most commonly located in the posterior region of the neck. These structures may also extend cephalad to engulf the fetal head or caudad to cover the dorsum of the fetus. Cystic hygromas occur in 1 in 100 pregnancies in the first trimester. Differential diagnoses include thickened nuchal translucency, neural tube defects, cystic teratoma, hemangioma, fetal hydrops, and residual developmental cysts. A finding of cystic hygroma should prompt evaluation for associated structural anomalies and genetic etiologies. Prognosis and management of pregnancies with cystic hygroma are individualized on the basis of the underlying diagnosis and associated anomalies and may require a multidisciplinary approach with genetics, pediatric cardiology, pediatric surgery, and neonatology involvement. Fetal magnetic resonance imaging may also be used to distinguish between differential diagnoses.

MICROGNATHIA

Micrognathia is characterized by the presence of a hypoplastic mandible and receding chin with a wide spectrum of severity. The tongue is displaced posteriorly and superiorly, resulting in a clefted or high-arched palate and glossoptosis. Though it may be the sole ultrasound finding, it is seen in association with a heterogeneous group of conditions, ranging from autosomal dominant transmission in Treacher-Collins syndrome to autosomal recessive in Smith-Lemli-Opitz syndrome. The defect originates in the first and second branchial arches and involves abnormal migration and proliferation of neural crest cells. Mandibular hypoplasia results from superior displacement of the tongue and failure of palate fusion. Ultrasound findings allow for calculation of the jaw index (anteroposterior diameter mandible/biparietal diameter mandible) $\times$ 100, with value <21 carrying 100% PPV. Three-dimensional imaging may provide additional information regarding severity. Associated anomalies often involve limbs and teratogen exposure. Genetic counseling, as well as multidisciplinary management involving neonatology, otolaryngology, and perinatology experts, should be undertaken. Approximately two-thirds of affected fetuses will have abnormal karyotypes. A detailed fetal survey looking for other structural anomalies and a fetal echocardiogram should be performed. Delivery should take place in a tertiary referral center given the possibility of severe respiratory complications and difficult airway management. Prognosis depends on final diagnosis and etiology of micrognathia.

ABNORMAL ORBITS

The diagnosis of abnormal orbits includes hypertelorism, hypotelorism, and microphthalmia. Hypertelorism and hypotelorism involve an increase and a decrease in the interorbital distance, respectively. The size of the eyeball is decreased in microphthalmia. Hypotelorism and microphthalmia are usually found in conjunction with other severe anomalies and genetic syndromes. Genetic counseling and a detailed fetal survey are indicated in evaluation of abnormal orbits. Fetal magnetic resonance imaging may be considered to assess for brain anomalies not detected on ultrasound. Prognosis is grim if other severe anomalies are present.

QUESTIONS

1. What is the most common type of cleft?
   a. Isolated cleft lip
   b. Combined bilateral cleft lip and palate
   c. Isolated cleft palate
   d. Combined unilateral cleft lip and palate

2. Differential diagnosis of suspected facial cleft should include all of the following conditions EXCEPT:
   a. amniotic band syndrome
   b. macroglossia
   c. posterior encephalocele
   d. premaxillary agenesis
   e. anterior meningocele

3. Which aneuploidy is most strongly associated with midline cleft lip and/or palate?
   a. Trisomy 13
   b. Trisomy 16
   c. Trisomy 18
   d. Trisomy 21

4. Three-dimensional ultrasound may enhance the visualization of both the primary and secondary fetal palate (True/False).
   a. True
   b. False

5. Which of the following is the most common defect associated with cleft lip/palate?
   a. Lumbar and cervical spine
   b. Cardiac
   c. Genetic
   d. Micrognathia

6. Which micronutrient, taken before a subsequent pregnancy, can provide risk reduction for the recurrence of cleft lip or palate, or both?
   a. Iron sulfate
   b. Vitamin B$_{12}$
   c. Dehydroepiandrosterone
   d. Folic acid

7. Which clinical scenario below would prompt delivery at a facility with expertise in management of a potential difficult airway in the newborn?
   a. Isolated unilateral cleft lip and palate in a fetus with first-trimester exposure to phenytoin
   b. Unilateral cleft lip and palate in a fetus with severe polyhydramnios in the third trimester
   c. Midline cleft lip and palate in a fetus with a membranous ventricular septal defect
   d. a, b, and c
   e. b and c

8. Cystic hygroma develops from:
   a. abnormal vasculature
   b. residual branchial cleft cysts
   c. abnormal lymphatics
   d. residual thyroglossal duct cysts
   e. swallowed fluid from a tracheoesophageal fistula

9. Which of these are NOT a potential location for cystic hygroma involvement?
   a. Forehead
   b. Axilla
   c. Scalp
   d. Mediastinum
   e. Hands

10. What is the frequency of cystic hygroma in the first trimester?
    a. 1:100
    b. 1:250
    c. 1:400
    d. 1:1000
    e. 1:5000

11. Which of the following is not a described genetic etiology of cystic hygroma?
    a. Turner syndrome
    b. Trisomy 21
    c. Triploidy
    d. Delta-F508 mutation
    e. Mosaic deletions of chromosomes

12. Which of these syndromes is not associated with cystic hygroma?
    a. Noonan syndrome
    b. Potter syndrome
    c. Thanatophoric dysplasia
    d. Costello syndrome
    e. Diamond-Blackfan anemia

13. Antenatal monitoring modalities that are appropriate for a fetal diagnosis of cystic hygroma include:
    a. a detailed fetal anatomic survey
    b. a fetal echocardiogram
    c. serial fetal ultrasounds
    d. nonstress tests
    e. all of the above

14. Of all associated structural abnormalities associated with cystic hygroma, cardiac abnormalities account for what percentage of findings?
    a. 5−10
    b. 25−30
    c. 45−50
    d. 70−75
    e. 85−90

15. The yield of karyotype, microarray, and whole exome sequencing in evaluation of cystic hygroma are (respectively):
    a. 75%, 5%, and 3%
    b. 50%, 5%, and 24%
    c. 25%, 40%, and 62%
    d. 10%, 8%, and 11%
    e. 5%, 3%, and 8%

16. Which of the following are potential outcomes in pregnancies with cystic hygromas?
    a. Spontaneous resolution
    b. Intrauterine fetal demise
    c. Neonatal demise
    d. Normal outcomes
    e. All of the above

17. Micrognathia is:
    a. a posteriorly displaced mandible
    b. a hypoplastic mandible
    c. a receding chin
    d. b and c
    e. all of the above

18. Which of these has NOT been associated with increased risk for micrognathia?
    a. Isotretinoin
    b. Ciprofloxacin
    c. Penicillamine
    d. Valproate
    e. Maternal diabetes

19. The differential diagnosis for micrognathia includes:
    a. skeletal dysplasia
    b. incorrect imaging plane
    c. amniotic band sequence
    d. a and b
    e. a, b, and c

20. Genetic etiologies of micrognathia include:
    a. aneuploidy
    b. sporadic new mutation
    c. autosomal dominant
    d. autosomal recessive
    e. all of the above

21. Anomalies associated with hypertelorism include:
    a. facial clefting
    b. craniosynostosis
    c. skeletal dysplasia
    d. polydactyly
    e. a, b, and c

22. The chromosome abnormality most often associated with abnormal orbits is:
    a. chromosome 5p deletion syndrome (Cri du chat syndrome)
    b. XXY syndrome (Klinefelter syndrome)
    c. 21q11.2 deletion syndrome (DiGeorge syndrome)
    d. trisomy 13
    e. none of the above

23. Which of these should most often prompt referral to a tertiary center for delivery?
    a. Hypertelorism
    b. Hypotelorism
    c. Microphthalmia
    d. Micrognathia
    e. Ankyloglossia

22

Fetal Thoracic Imaging

ANNA KATERINA SFAKIANAKI | KATHERINE H. CAMPBELL

(see *Creasy and Resnik's Maternal-Fetal Medicine, 9e*: Ch 22)

Summary

CONGENITAL DIAPHRAGMATIC HERNIA

Congenital diaphragmatic hernia (CDH) refers to an embryologic defect in the diaphragm resulting in variable degrees of herniation of abdominal contents into the thoracic cavity. It results from abnormal diaphragm development at 6–10 weeks with incomplete closure of the pleuroperitoneal folds. Herniated viscera cause decreased bronchial branching, alveolar number, and pulmonary vascularization and overmuscularization of pulmonary arterial tree, leading to pulmonary hypoplasia and pulmonary hypertension. The majority of CDHs are left sided. The major ultrasound finding is a thoracic mass accompanied by mediastinal shift. Associated anomalies are common. Evaluation includes genetic testing, fetal echocardiography, serial ultrasound, and, increasingly, magnetic resonance imaging (MRI). In utero therapy using fetal endoscopic tracheal occlusion, or FETO, is becoming more common. An ongoing US trial is under way. Referral to a tertiary care facility is suggested.

CYSTIC LUNG LESIONS, CONGENITAL PULMONARY MALFORMATION, AND BRONCHOPULMONARY SEQUESTRATION

The most common cystic lung lesions include congenital pulmonary airway malformation (CPAM) and bronchopulmonary sequestration (BPS). CPAMs are hamartomatous lesions composed of the different elements of the respiratory tract and are connected to that tract. BPS is composed of nonfunctioning respiratory tract tissue that does not connect with the respiratory tract. Both develop during the pseudoglandular phase of lung development (7–17 weeks' gestation); they may have common origin. Both lesions are noted on prenatal ultrasound as masses within or associated with the fetal lungs. They differ from the (normal) surrounding lung by their echogenicity, cystic components, and/or position with respect to the diaphragm.

CPAM is classified histologically, by the degree of microcystic versus macrocystic composition. BPS is classified as intralobar sequestration (ILS) or extralobar sequestration (ELS). CPAM is usually isolated and sporadic; other anomalies (in 15%–20%) are most commonly cardiac and renal. BPS is more commonly associated with other anomalies than is CPAM. Antenatal management involves serial assessment of lesion stability, prediction of adverse outcome using the CPAM volume ratio (CVR), and referral to a tertiary care facility as indicated. Many lesions regress; however, the potential for malignant transformation dictates that neonates be followed by a specialist. Hydrops is a poor prognostic indicator.

CONGENITAL HIGH AIRWAY OBSTRUCTION

Congenital high airway obstruction syndrome (CHAOS) refers to a constellation of findings on prenatal ultrasound resulting from an intrinsic obstruction in the upper airway of the fetus, most often from laryngeal atresia; other causes include tracheal atresia or stenosis, subglottic stenosis, obstructing web, or cyst. Different etiologies can lead to the same clinical findings. It is rare and the true incidence is not known. Obstruction of the egress of fluid from the lungs leads to accumulation of secretions, with massive overexpansion of the lungs. Ultrasound findings include large echogenic lungs, a flattened or inverted diaphragm, and compressed mediastinal structures. Hydrops is common, and polyhydramnios results from esophageal compression by the lungs. CHAOS may be syndromic and has been associated with aneuploidies. Fetal demise is common. The EXIT (ex utero intrapartum treatment) procedure may result in newborn survival; therefore, if pregnancy termination is not pursued, referral should be made to a tertiary care facility. Long-term outcome is unknown.

PLEURAL EFFUSION

Fetal pleural effusion is a nonspecific fluid collection located in the pleural space. It is noted to be primary (direct result of lymphatic leakage into the pleural space and a diagnosis of exclusion) or secondary (as a result of a wide array of conditions—structural, infectious metabolic, or chromosomal, which may cause an effusion to develop). Pleural effusions are uncommon (1 in 10,000 to 1 in 15,000 pregnancies), and they develop when there is any disruption along the lymphatic drainage pathway from the pleura to the mediastinal lymph nodes. The effusions are usually easily seen on ultrasound imaging and, once visualized, should prompt development of a broad differential diagnosis and thorough ultrasound assessment of the fetus including structural defects, stigmata of infection, presence of fetal anemia, and consideration for genetic testing. Prenatal diagnosis, when possible, will provide opportunity for thorough patient counseling, consideration for intervention including thoracentesis or thoracoamniotic shunt placement, delivery planning, and preparation for care of the neonate. Overall prognosis is directly related to any underlying etiology of the pleural effusion, as well as presence of any subsequent pulmonary hypoplasia as a result of long-standing lung compression from the effusion.

QUESTIONS

1. Prognosis for CDH is associated with all of the following except
   a. Presence of other anomalies
   b. Liver herniation
   c. Lung area to head circumference ratio
   d. Maternal age

2. Workup for the CDH should include all of the following except
   a. Offer genetic testing
   b. Thorough evaluation with a detailed ultrasound and echocardiogram to assess for other structural defects
   c. Umbilical artery Doppler to assess for anemia
   d. MRI to evaluate liver herniation

3. The most common anomalies associated with CDH occur in the cardiac system.
   a. True
   b. False

4. A CDH is more commonly left sided.
   a. True
   b. False

5. Workup for cystic lung lesions should include the following except
   a. Offer genetic testing
   b. Thorough evaluation with a detailed ultrasound and echocardiogram to assess for other structural defects
   c. Umbilical artery Doppler to assess for anemia
   d. Serial ultrasound to assess for stability of lesion and for hydrops

6. Which of the following best describes the blood supply to a CPAM?
   a. Systemic
   b. Pulmonary

7. Which of the following best describes the blood supply to a BPS?
   a. Systemic
   b. Pulmonary

8. Hydrops is most common in which of the following?
   a. BPS
   b. Type 1 CPAM
   c. Type 2 CPAM
   d. Type 3 CPAM

9. Which is the most common pathologic feature of CHAOS?
   a. Laryngeal atresia
   b. Tracheal atresia
   c. Subglottic stenosis
   d. Obstructing web/cyst

10. Workup for CHAOS should include the following except
    a. Offer genetic testing
    b. Thorough evaluation with a detailed ultrasound and echocardiogram to assess for other structural defects
    c. MRI to distinguish from CCAM
    d. Thoracentesis to obtain fluid for analysis

11. Differential diagnoses for secondary causes for fetal pleural effusion include all of the following except
    a. Metabolic storage disease
    b. Turner syndrome
    c. Fetal anemia
    d. Pericardial effusion

12. Workup for the fetal pleural effusion should include the following except
    a. Offer genetic testing
    b. Consideration for maternal serologies for TORCH infections
    c. Thorough evaluation with a detailed ultrasound and echocardiogram to assess for other structural defects
    d. Umbilical artery Doppler to assess for anemia

13. Early elective delivery is indicated so that a large isolated effusion can be drained.
    a. True
    b. False

14. Pleural effusions without clear etiology tend to be stable not to progress, so close fetal surveillance is not indicated.
    a. True
    b. False

15. Drainage of a pleural effusion can be considered for the following scenarios:
    a. Large effusion with mass effect
    b. Rapidly enlarging effusions
    c. To aid with ventilation after delivery
    d. To aid in visualization of the cardiac anatomy
    e. All of the above

23

Fetal Cardiac Malformations and Arrhythmias: Questions and Answers

KOYELLE PAPNEJA | MARK STEVEN SKLANSKY

(see *Creasy and Resnik's Maternal-Fetal Medicine, 9e: Ch 23*)

Summary

Congenital heart disease (CHD) represents the most common form of birth defect around the globe (roughly 1% of newborns) and accounts for a vastly disproportionate share of neonatal mortality related to congenital malformations. Much of the substantial neonatal/childhood morbidity and mortality related to CHD stems from delays in detection, diagnosis, and management. Outcomes for infants and children with major forms of CHD can be improved with prenatal detection and diagnosis, followed by perinatal management by a collaborative, multidisciplinary team of fetal, neonatal, and pediatric subspecialists—obstetricians, maternal-fetal medicine practitioners, radiologists, pediatric cardiologists, neonatologists, congenital cardiac and general pediatric surgeons, anesthesiologists, intensive care subspecialists, nurses, social workers, and others. The practice of fetal cardiology represents a "team sport," wherein optimal outcomes derive from a collaborative, multidisciplinary team approach at every point in time, from early prenatal detection/diagnosis, through delivery, the neonatal period, and infancy. It is for this team of subspecialists that this chapter is dedicated.

Fetal, maternal, and familial risk factors for CHD have been identified, but most cases of CHD still occur in pregnancies not identified as high risk. Positive predictive value appears greatest when a cardiac abnormality is suspected on routine fetal cardiac screening. Most of the world focuses on the midgestation anatomic survey as the primary opportunity to detect cardiac abnormalities. Second-trimester fetal cardiac screening typically involves the use of two-dimensional (2D) imaging to evaluate the position of the heart and stomach, the four-chamber view, the left- and right-ventricular outflow tracts, and, increasingly, the three-vessel view(s). Many practices incorporate color Doppler into fetal cardiac screening. The acquisition and storage of cine or video clips, with subsequent review in real time or slowed down and reviewed back and forth, has also become widely recognized to help improve detection. In many regions of the world, efforts to screen for fetal heart disease are being incorporated into late first-trimester examinations. Most importantly, efforts must be made to optimize both the image and the angle of acquisition; the ventricular septum should be evaluated using a perpendicular angle to optimize detection of septal defects and aortic/pulmonary override. Efforts have been made to apply three-dimensional/four-dimensional technology to enhance both the detection and evaluation of fetal heart disease; results have been mixed.

Pregnancies identified to be at risk for fetal heart disease, or who are suspected or confirmed to have structural/functional heart disease or arrhythmia, generally undergo detailed fetal echocardiographic evaluation, typically during the second trimester. In experienced hands, fetal echocardiography has been found to be far more sensitive than fetal cardiac screening for detection of CHD. Fetal echocardiography provides a more detailed evaluation of the fetal heart, including acquisition of cine clips, the use of color Doppler, and detailed evaluation of cardiac anatomy and function. While fetal cardiac screening generally focuses on views, fetal echocardiography includes a comprehensive evaluation of cardiac anatomy and function, with specific focus on structures rather than views. Fetal echocardiographic evaluation also includes an assessment of fetal cardiac rhythm. Fetal cardiac function may be evaluated with a variety of qualitative and quantitative tools. In comparison with fetal cardiac screening, fetal echocardiography often includes multiple quantitative measurements to help assess suspected abnormalities. Such quantitative measurements may include assessment of not only ventricular function but also flow, such as quantitative evaluation of flow through the ductus arteriosus (pulsatility index).

Fetal cardiac malformations can be classified according to the component of the fetal heart involved with the defect. In some cases, particularly in the setting of heterotaxy, abnormalities of the fetal heart may be first identified/suspected with abdominal imaging, which focuses on the position of the descending aorta, inferior vena cava, stomach, and size/position of the azygous vein. Abnormalities of the systemic and pulmonary venous returns can be challenging but important, particularly in the case of total anomalous pulmonary venous return. Multiple forms of abnormalities may be identified with evaluation of the mitral and tricuspid valves and their respective ventricles. Outflow tract abnormalities, although typically more challenging to evaluate than abnormalities of the four-chamber view, are also more likely to represent ductal dependent cardiac malformations in need of neonatal intervention. Fetal echocardiography may be performed most commonly at midgestation but also as early as 10–13 weeks, for at-risk pregnancies, or later in the third trimester.

Fetal arrhythmias can be classified as premature atrial or ventricular contractions, bradycardia, or tachycardia. The diagnosis of fetal arrhythmias may use multiple different approaches, always beginning with optimization of the 2D image and angle of acquisition to allow evaluation of atrial and ventricular activity. Multiple modalities may be used including 2D imaging; 2D with color Doppler; pulsed Doppler (most commonly within the left ventricular inflow and outflow, or within the superior vena cava and aorta); m-mode; or m-mode with color Doppler. Fetal magnetocardiography can provide detailed diagnostic information, but this technique requires highly specialized equipment and expertise not widely available. Increasingly, efforts are being made to extract the fetal from the maternal electrocardiogram; such an approach may facilitate evaluation of fetal arrhythmias in the future. Fetal bradyarrhythmias may be related to structural CHD (commonly with polysplenia/left-sided isomerism phenotype) or congenital (i.e., long QT syndrome) or acquired (i.e., anti-Sjögren-syndrome-related antigen A

[SSA] antibodies or viral processes) pathology. Fetal tachyarrhythmias may be related to structural CHD (such as Ebstein anomaly) or fetal exposure to stimulants. Most fetal arrhythmias, like most CHD, occur without a clear etiology. Treatment of fetal arrhythmias is usually approached conservatively, given the generally benign natural history of most cases of fetal arrhythmias and the potential for maternal/fetal toxicity with pharmacologic management. When pharmacologic therapy appears indicated, ideally patients are managed by a multidisciplinary group with experience in the treatment of fetal arrhythmias. Under such settings, the vast majority of fetal arrhythmias requiring treatment may have favorable outcomes.

QUESTIONS

1. At 12 weeks' gestation, which of the following factors most increases the risk of congenital heart disease in the fetus?
   a. Fetal left ventricular echogenic focus
   b. Increased nuchal translucency thickness
   c. Group B streptococcus in a prior pregnancy
   d. Family history of stroke

2. Which of the following signs on an anatomy scan is most indicative of the need for further specialized fetal cardiac evaluation?
   a. The heart and stomach are both on the fetal left.
   b. The circumference of the fetal heart is approximately half of the circumference of the thorax.
   c. The flap of the foramen ovale is visualized in the left atrium.
   d. The left side of the fetal heart appears larger than the right side of the heart.

3. A vascular structure between the descending aorta and left atrium ("twig sign") raises suspicion for which of the following abnormalities?
   a. Total anomalous pulmonary venous return
   b. Tetralogy of Fallot
   c. Truncus arteriosus
   d. Atrial septal defect

4. Which of the following fetal cardiac conditions is most likely to cause fetal congestive heart failure?
   a. Supraventricular tachycardia
   b. Hypoplastic left heart syndrome (HLHS)
   c. Transposition of the great arteries
   d. Tetralogy of Fallot with pulmonary atresia

5. If a left superior vena cava is seen, careful evaluation for which of the following associated fetal cardiac lesions is warranted?
   a. Pulmonary stenosis
   b. Ventricular septal defect
   c. Coarctation of the aorta
   d. Complete heart block

6. Which of the following conditions is most likely to be readily detected with a routine four-chamber view?
   a. Coarctation of the aorta
   b. Small membranous ventricular septal defect
   c. Tetralogy of Fallot
   d. Complete atrioventricular canal defect

7. Tricuspid valve regurgitation, pulmonary hypoplasia, supraventricular tachycardia, and hydrops are associated with a severe form of which of the following conditions?
   a. Ebstein anomaly
   b. Coarctation of the aorta
   c. Tricuspid atresia
   d. Partial atrioventricular canal defect

8. Which of the following is the most appropriate delivery plan for a fetus with HLHS at 29 weeks' gestation?
   a. Delivery at a local community hospital with planned outpatient pediatric cardiology follow-up 2 weeks after discharge home
   b. Home birth, if this is the patient's preference
   c. Delivery at a tertiary care center with pediatric cardiology and cardiac surgical expertise
   d. Emergent delivery by caesarean section

9. Which of the following lesions detected at 19 weeks' gestation requires ongoing prenatal follow-up to evaluate for the potential development of HLHS?
   a. Valvar aortic stenosis
   b. Transposition of the great arteries
   c. Large apical muscular ventricular septal defect
   d. Truncus arteriosus

10. Which of the following associated findings will most likely be seen with a fetal diagnosis of tetralogy of Fallot with absent pulmonary valve?
    a. Mitral valve regurgitation
    b. Dilated branch pulmonary arteries
    c. Aneurysmal flap of the foramen ovale
    d. Patent ductus arteriosus

11. Which of the following is most appropriate to convey in counseling about a fetus with dextro-transposition of the great arteries (D-TGA) and intact ventricular septum?
    a. The newborn is expected to be clinically well at birth and likely will not require surgery until early adolescence.
    b. The newborn will likely not require any immediate specialized cardiac care after birth but may require surgery within the first month of life.
    c. The newborn will likely require a prostaglandin infusion and may potentially require an emergent balloon atrial septostomy within hours after delivery.
    d. Fetal demise before term is highly likely.

12. Which of the following syndromes is most closely associated with truncus arteriosus?
    a. Down syndrome (Trisomy 21)
    b. DiGeorge syndrome
    c. Noonan syndrome
    d. Turner syndrome

13. Which of the following conditions is most associated with multiple echogenic, homogenous, well-circumscribed masses in the ventricular septum and right ventricular free wall?
    a. Tuberous sclerosis
    b. Trisomy 18
    c. Neurofibromatosis
    d. Alpha-thalassemia

14. Which of the following is true regarding premature atrial contractions in a pattern of bigeminy?
    a. There is a high risk of development of hydrops.
    b. There is a high risk of development of ventricular tachycardia.
    c. There is a high risk of development of complete heart block.
    d. There is a low risk of development of associated cardiac problems, and no treatment is required.

15. Treatment with which of the following medications may be indicated in a mother with anti-SSA antibodies, a prior child with congenital complete heart block, and a mechanical PR interval of 160 msec?
    a. Sotalol
    b. Dexamethasone
    c. Indomethacin
    d. Insulin

16. Which of the following is the most likely associated abnormality in a fetus with heart rate of 65 beats per minute, a right-sided inferior vena cava, moderate tricuspid regurgitation, a large ventricular septal defect, transposition of the great arteries and pulmonary stenosis?
    a. Trisomy 21
    b. Omphalocele
    c. L-looped ventricles or ventricular inversion
    d. Coarctation of the aorta

17. Which of the following findings would be LEAST likely in a fetus with left-sided obstructive disease?
    a. Predominantly left-to-right flow through the foramen ovale
    b. Predominantly left-to-right flow through the ductus arteriosus
    c. Increased pulsatility index in the ductus arteriosus
    d. Dilated right ventricle

18. Which of the following is the most likely finding in a fetus with a dilated right atrium, right ventricle, and pulmonary artery, as well as an increased velocity with an elevated pulsatility index in the ductus arteriosus?
    a. Atrial septal defect
    b. Mitral atresia
    c. Ductal constriction
    d. Ventricular septal defect

19. Which of the following is most likely with fetal cardiomegaly, pericardial effusion, ascites, and a normal karyotype and microarray?
    a. Atrial bigeminy
    b. Ventricular septal defect
    c. Tetralogy of Fallot with absent pulmonary valve
    d. Transposition of the great arteries

20. Which of the following is the most likely chromosomal finding in a fetus with an enlarged right ventricle, 2 m/second flow velocity in the ascending aorta, and a pleural effusion?
    a. 47, XXX
    b. 47, XX + 18 (trisomy 18)
    c. 46 XX (del22q11) 22q11 microdeletion
    d. 46, X (Monosomy X)

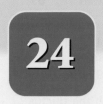

24

Fetal Abdominal Imaging

RICHARD B. WOLF

(see *Creasy and Resnik's Maternal-Fetal Medicine, 9e*: Ch 24)

Summary

The fetal abdomen contains primarily isoechoic structures (bowel, liver, and kidneys). Physiologic echolucent structures include the stomach; bladder; the renal pelvis of each kidney; larger blood vessels (e.g., umbilical vein, aorta); and, variably, the gallbladder. Nonphysiologic fluid collections include abdominal cysts and dilated intestines due to obstruction, or fluid can fill the abdomen as ascites. The abdominal contents can become herniated during early embryologic development (e.g., gastroschisis, omphalocele, limb–body stalk) or fail to develop properly (e.g., esophageal atresia). Unusually echodense (bright) areas can involve any fetal abdominal organ. A thorough assessment is needed if suspecting sonographic abnormalities.

Ascites is an abnormal fluid collection within the fetal peritoneal cavity and often the first finding in hydrops fetalis. Ascites is present in 85% of cases of nonimmune hydrops fetalis; the incidence of *isolated* ascites is quite low. When ascites is present, free fluid outlines the fetal liver, loops of bowel, stomach, and bladder. Free abdominal fluid can represent a *transudate, exudate, leaked urine, meconium* from a perforated bowel, or *chylous fluid*. If ascites is visualized sonographically, a systematic assessment of fetal anatomy should be undertaken to rule out hydrops fetalis or other anomalies.

Intestinal *atresia* indicates *complete* absence of the lumen in a portion of the bowel; *stenosis* is a *narrowing* of the lumen. Atresia or stenosis can occur at any level in the gastrointestinal tract (esophagus to anus) and should be suspected if dilated bowel is seen, due to distention of the proximal gastrointestinal tract, particularly in the third trimester. Duodenal atresia produces the classic "double bubble" sign of collected fluid below the stomach and above the area of atresia. In contradistinction, esophageal atresia (with or without tracheoesophageal fistula) presents with a small or absent stomach. Polyhydramnios is typical with esophageal or proximal small bowel atresia. Duodenal and esophageal atresia carry a high risk of trisomy 21.

Ventral wall defects, not to be confused with *physiologic* gut herniation at the 6th to 10th week of embryonic development, include gastroschisis, omphalocele, and limb–body stalk anomaly. Gastroschisis is a *paraumbilical* ventral defect through which bowel herniates, with *free-floating* bowel loops observed in the amniotic fluid, giving a typical "cauliflower" appearance. Omphalocele is a *midline* ventral wall defect with bowel and/or liver herniating through the base of the umbilicus, with bowel covered by a membrane. With gastroschisis, the defect is typically to the right of abdominal cord insertion (though it can, less commonly, be to the left), while with omphalocele, the umbilical cord passes *through* the mass and inserts on the membranes. This can be a key feature to distinguish gastroschisis from omphalocele with a ruptured sac. Maternal serum alpha fetoprotein is usually elevated with gastroschisis but not uniformly with omphalocele. About 40% of omphalocele cases are associated with aneuploidy (e.g., trisomy 18), particularly if the omphalocele sac contains *only* bowel loops, without liver; fetuses with gastroschisis are usually euploid. Fetal growth restriction is common but may be overestimated, as herniated abdominal contents result in an undersized abdominal circumference. Prolonged stays in the neonatal intensive care unit are typical for newborns with gastroschisis and omphalocele. Limb–body stalk anomaly is a significantly larger ventral defect, often adherent to the placenta and/or with a short umbilical cord, and is considered a lethal birth defect.

Cystic or echogenic abdominal lesions can arise in any abdominal organ. In female fetuses, abdominal cysts most frequently represent *ovarian cysts*, particularly in the third trimester. The organ system of cysts or echogenic lesions may be identified on the basis of their size and location; most resolve spontaneously. Color flow Doppler imaging can help distinguish cysts from vascular structures (e.g., umbilical vein varix, which, as an *isolated* finding, usually has a favorable outcome). Echogenic abdominal lesions should be "bright as bone" and persist with lowered gain and harmonic-enhanced imaging disabled. Echogenic abdominal lesions can indicate infection, inflammation, thrombosis, tumor, or thickened meconium.

QUESTIONS

1. Which underlying condition associated with fetal ascites carries the best prognosis for survival?
   a. Chylous ascites
   b. Early hydrops fetalis
   c. Inherited metabolic storage disease
   d. Urinary ascites

2. Finding of a "double bubble" on abdominal imaging is suggestive of which of the following?
   a. Esophageal atresia
   b. Duodenal atresia
   c. Jejunal atresia
   d. Imperforate anus

3. Where is the gastroschisis mass most commonly located relative to the umbilicus?
   a. Superior to the umbilicus
   b. Central to the umbilicus (i.e., the cord passes through the gastroschisis mass)
   c. To the left of the umbilicus
   d. Io the right of the umbilicus

4. Which condition associated with omphalocele has the highest risk of aneuploidy?
   a. Intracorporeal liver (i.e., omphalocele sac contains only bowel loops)
   b. Extracorporeal liver (i.e., omphalocele contains bowel and liver)
   c. Giant omphalocele (greater than 5 cm diameter)
   d. Finding of fluid (ascites) within the omphalocele sac

5. Which is the most common cystic abdominal fetal mass?
   a. Renal cyst
   b. Choledochal cyst
   c. Ovarian cyst
   d. Splenic cyst

6. Which imaging technique tends to make fetal bowel appear falsely more echogenic (bright)?
   a. Low gain settings
   b. Low-frequency transducer
   c. Harmonic-enhanced imaging
   d. Full maternal bladder (i.e., through transmission acoustic enhancement)

7. What is the most common abnormality associated with esophageal atresia with tracheoesophageal (TE) fistula?
   a. Central nervous system abnormalities
   b. Polyhydramnios
   c. Oligohydramnios
   d. Duodenal atresia

8. Which of the following is most likely to be associated with isolated ascites?
   a. Gastroschisis
   b. Esophageal atresia with TE fistula
   c. Bladder outlet obstruction
   d. Diaphragmatic hernia

9. Which of the following carries the highest association with aneuploidy?
   a. Duodenal atresia
   b. Omphalocele
   c. Gastroschisis
   d. Esophageal atresia with TE fistula

10. The finding of ectopia cordis is most likely associated with which condition?
    a. Tetralogy of Fallot
    b. CHARGE syndrome
    c. VATER or VACTERL association
    d. Pentalogy of Cantrell

11. Which of the following ratios is used to predict short-term neonatal outcomes with omphalocele?
    a. Omphalocele circumference-to-head circumference ratio
    b. Omphalocele diameter-to-chest circumference ratio
    c. Omphalocele circumference-to-abdominal circumference ratio
    d. Omphalocele diameter-to-abdominal circumference ratio

12. What is most predictive of perinatal mortality with umbilical vein varix?
    a. Concomitant abnormalities
    b. Turbulent flow on color Doppler imaging
    c. Fetal growth restriction
    d. Preterm delivery

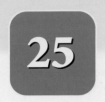

25

Fetal Urogenital Imaging

RICHARD B. WOLF

(see Creasy and Resnik's Maternal-Fetal Medicine, 9e: Ch 25)

Summary

Most congenital anomalies of the kidney and urinary tract can be identified during routine fetal imaging. Excess fluid within the kidneys, ureters, or bladder can indicate urinary obstruction, renal duplication, or renal parenchymal cysts. Unusually echodense kidneys indicate inherited polycystic kidney disease or obstructive cystic dysplasia. Failure to identify kidneys bilaterally may be due to unilateral or bilateral renal agenesis, or the kidney(s) may occupy an ectopic location (e.g., pelvic kidney). A persistently absent bladder can be due to bladder exstrophy, while cyst(s) identified within the bladder are typically ureteroceles, prompting evaluation for renal duplication. Atypical or ambiguous genitalia may be part of a larger syndrome.

Pyelectasis is a common sonographic finding, with urine dilating the fetal renal pelvis, often due to ureteropelvic junction obstruction or vesicoureteral reflux (VUR), particularly in males. Clinically significant pyelectasis is defined as renal pelvic diameter ≥4 mm at 16–27 weeks or ≥7 mm at 28–40 weeks. *Hydronephrosis* is diagnosed when pyelectasis is accompanied by *caliectasis* (distended renal calyces). *Ureterovesical junction* obstruction can cause pyelectasis, and is distinguished from ureteropelvic junction obstruction by a dilated ureter (ureters usually *not visible* on ultrasound).

Echogenic kidneys indicate abnormal renal parenchyma, suggesting abnormal function, likely needing postnatal dialysis and/or transplantation. This can be inherited as *autosomal dominant polycystic kidney disease*, also known as "adult" PKD, or *autosomal recessive polycystic kidney disease*, or "infantile" PKD, or it can be due to *obstructive cystic dysplasia*, resulting from chronic first- or second-trimester urinary tract obstruction or persistent vesicoureteral reflux. Autosomal dominant PKD produces moderately enlarged echogenic kidneys with *increased* corticomedullary differentiation, while autosomal recessive PKD yields massively enlarged echogenic kidneys with *loss* of corticomedullary differentiation. Small echogenic kidneys are typically seen with obstructive cystic dysplasia. Enlarged echogenic kidneys can also be part of a syndrome (e.g., Beckwith-Wiedemann).

Multicystic dysplastic kidney (MCDK) disease is a nonhereditary renal disease with multiple irregular noncommunicating echolucent cysts seen within the kidney and an irregular reniform but normal-appearing bladder and ureters. Bilateral MCDK or unilateral MCDK with contralateral renal agenesis can result in lethal pulmonary hypoplasia.

Posterior urethral valves (PUVs) are membranes within the posterior urethra causing lower urinary tract obstruction, producing hydronephrosis and pressure-induced renal dysplasia. A dilated posterior urethra *("keyhole" sign)* is virtually pathognomonic for PUV, which occurs almost exclusively in *males*; in females, *urethral atresia* may present similarly with complete bladder outlet obstruction. In utero therapy to prevent pulmonary hypoplasia and preserve renal function is variably successful; if antenatal intervention is considered, vesicocentesis should be used to assess fetal renal function before proceeding.

Renal duplication occurs when the kidney divides during embryogenesis into separate upper and lower pole sections (moieties) with separate duplicated ureters. The upper pole ureter often ends in an obstructed *ureterocele* (cystic dilation of the ureter within the fetal bladder), while the lower pole ureter develops reflux, resulting in two separate and dilated renal pelves. Lower urinary tract obstruction can result if the ureterocele is large enough to obstruct the urethra.

Renal agenesis is the congenital absence of one or both kidneys; bilateral renal agenesis is incompatible with extrauterine life and associated with virtual anhydramnios, with resultant Potters sequence and pulmonary hypoplasia. Renal agenesis should be suspected with severe oligohydramnios and an absent bladder. Normal amniotic fluid volume with a persistently absent bladder yet normal-appearing kidneys likely indicates *bladder exstrophy*.

Ambiguous genitalia can be a component of many syndromes, including bladder exstrophy, and merits careful assessment of the fetal anatomy. Suspected congenital adrenal hyperplasia, which is the most common cause of ambiguous genitalia, merits immediate evaluation and treatment.

QUESTIONS

1. In the 2014 Multidisciplinary Consensus Statement, what renal dilation would be considered abnormal in the third trimester (>28 weeks)?
   a. >4 mm
   b. >5 mm
   c. >6 mm
   d. >7 mm

2. Which of the following abnormally echogenic kidneys have increased cortical medullary differentiation?
   a. Autosomal dominant polycystic kidney disease
   b. Autosomal recessive polycystic kidney disease
   c. Meckel-Gruber syndrome
   d. Obstructive cystic dysplasia

3. Which of the following abnormally echogenic kidneys would typically be smaller than expected?
   a. Autosomal dominant polycystic kidney disease
   b. Autosomal recessive polycystic kidney disease
   c. Meckel-Gruber syndrome
   d. Obstructive cystic dysplasia

4. Which of the following is a feature of unilateral MCDKs?
   a. Noncommunicating echolucencies
   b. Renal length decreased
   c. Polyhydramnios
   d. Decreased echogenicity of surrounding renal parenchyma

5. How can you distinguish PUV from megacystis-microcolon-intestinal hypoperistalsis syndrome (MMIHS)?
   a. Polyhydramnios
   b. Echogenic bowel
   c. Megacystis
   d. Sonographically evident microcolon

6. Which of the following is associated with ureteroceles?
   a. Megacystis
   b. Renal duplication
   c. PUVs
   d. Pelvic kidney

7. Which of the following is not associated with fetal bladder exstrophy?
   a. Persistently absent bladder visualization
   b. Ambiguous genitalia
   c. VUR
   d. Isoechoic mass inferior to abdominal cord insertion

8. What is the most common cause of 46,XX disorder of sexual development (ambiguous genitalia)?
   a. Placental aromatase deficiency
   b. Congenital adrenal hyperplasia
   c. Testosterone insensitivity
   d. Maternal Sertoli-Leydig tumor

9. Which abdominal magnetic resonance imaging or ultrasound finding would likely assign a baby with ambiguous genitalia as being female gender?
   a. Ovaries
   b. Uterus
   c. Small phallus/clitoris
   d. Pubic ramus angle ≥90 degrees

10. Which of the following is true regarding renal duplication?
    a. The upper pole ureter is typically affected with VUR.
    b. The lower pole moiety often undergoes cystic dysplastic changes.
    c. The upper pole ureter is often obstructed with an ureterocele.
    d. The lower pole moiety is more likely to be seen dilated than the upper pole moiety.

11. Which of the following sonographic findings confirms bilateral renal agenesis?
    a. Persistent nonvisualization of fetal bladder
    b. Empty renal fossa bilaterally
    c. Anhydramnios
    d. Absent renal arteries on color Doppler imaging

12. Which of the following regarding the fetal ureters is true?
    a. Fetal ureters normally measure 3-4 mm in diameter in the third trimester (>28 weeks).
    b. Fetal ureters can be identified using color Doppler imaging.
    c. Fetal ureters are usually not sonographically visualized, unless dilated.
    d. Fetal ureters are sonographically visualized only during fetal micturition.

26

Fetal Skeletal Imaging

RICHARD B. WOLF

(see *Creasy and Resnik's Maternal-Fetal Medicine, 9e: Ch 26*)

Summary

The fetal skeletal system should be assessed during routine anatomy sonographic imaging. Abnormalities of the skeletal system can be due to malformation, disruption, or deformation from intrinsic or extrinsic factors. The skull can be misshaped (e.g., craniosynostosis) as an isolated abnormality or as part of a broader syndrome involving the entire skeletal system (i.e., skeletal dysplasia). Abnormal development of the fetal spine can lead to scoliosis, lordosis, or kyphosis; cause foreshortening (e.g., sacral agenesis); or result in open neural tube defects (e.g., meningomyelocele, meningocele, myeloschisis) and closed neural tube defects (e.g., sacrococcygeal teratoma). Bony abnormalities in the extremities can cause anomalous shapes or positions (e.g., arthrogryposis or clubfoot), or portions of limbs may be missing entirely due to amniotic band syndrome.

Skeletal dysplasia is a genetically diverse group of disorders of the skeleton causing abnormal bone length, shape, and density, with varying degrees of disability. The most common *lethal* skeletal dysplasia is thanatophoric dysplasia, followed by osteogenesis imperfecta type II and achondrogenesis. The most common *nonlethal* skeletal dysplasia is achondroplasia. Systematic assessment for skeletal dysplasia is indicated if the femur length is >2 standard deviations below mean, any long bones appear angulated or bowed, or limbs subjectively appear short. The term *rhizomelia* indicates shortened proximal bones (humerus, femur); *mesomelia* indicates short intermediate bones (radius, ulna, tibia, fibula); *acromelia* affects the distal limbs (hands, feet); and with *micromelia* the entire limb is short. *Craniosynostosis* is a malformed calvarium due to premature closure of single or multiple calvarial suture(s). Although craniosynostosis can be associated with skeletal dysplasia (e.g., thanatophoric dysplasia), it can also be an isolated finding. Accurate prediction of lethality is an important goal of prenatal diagnosis if skeletal dysplasia is suspected.

Limb abnormalities can result from *malformation* due to embryonic teratogen exposure (e.g., viral infection, radiation, medications, diabetes), *disruption* with breakdown of normal tissue (e.g., *amniotic band sequence*), or *deformation* with distortion of normal tissue (e.g., *clubfoot*). Limb abnormalities also include *arthrogryposis* (fixed joint contractures) and *polydactyly* (supernumerary digits present in the hand and/or foot). Arthrogryposis and "clubfoot" are caused by lack of fetal movement (akinesia) resulting from intrinsic factors (neuromuscular disorders, skeletal dysplasia, aneuploidy); extrinsic factors (compression from oligohydramnios, malpresentation, uterine abnormalities); or environmental factors (infection, teratogen exposure), with resultant exaggerated posturing of the limb(s). Postaxial (ulnar) polydactyly is common, more prevalent in fetuses with African American ancestry. Polydactyly is an isolated finding in the majority of cases (85%). *Amniotic band syndrome*, an atypical nonembryonic pattern of fetal malformations, arises from amniotic membrane disruption early in gestation, typically causing extensive craniofacial or visceral defects (similar to limb−body stalk), whereas later disruption involves distal extremities (hands, feet).

Neural tube defects observed with ultrasound can be closed (e.g., *sacrococcygeal teratoma*, *sacral agenesis*) or open to the amniotic space (e.g., meningomyelocele, myeloschisis). Sacrococcygeal teratoma (SCT) is a mixed echogenic mass extending from the coccyx to beyond the skin, though 10% of SCT cases are confined internally to the presacral area. Sacral agenesis arises from abnormal embryonic development of the sacrum and lower spine. Both SCT and sacral agenesis are examples of *closed* spinal dysraphism. *Open neural tube defect* (ONTD) is a defect in the formation of the posterior vertebral arches of the spine. ONTD appears as a cystic mass overlying a defect in the posterior aspect of the spine, with or without neural elements extending into the cyst (*myelomeningocele* or *meningocele*), or as a soft tissue defect with neural elements exposed (*myeloschisis*). Most (>80%) ONTD defects are located in the lumbosacral region of the spine. *Hemivertebrae* are incomplete vertebral bodies that act as a wedge against adjacent normal vertebrae, causing scoliosis, lordosis, or kyphosis.

QUESTIONS

1. What is the most common cause of lethal skeletal dysplasia?
   a. Osteogenesis imperfecta, type II
   b. Homozygous Achondroplasia
   c. Achondrogenesis
   d. Thanataphoric dysplasia

2. What is the most common cause of nonlethal skeletal dysplasia?
   a. Rhizomelic dysplasia
   b. Heterozygous achondrogenesis
   c. Homozygous achondroplasia
   d. Heterozygous achondroplasia

3. Shortened proximal bones are classified as:
   a. rhizomelia
   b. micromelia
   c. acromelia
   d. mesomelia

4. The most common form of polydactyly is which with the following?
   a. Preaxial
   b. Postaxial
   c. Mesoaxial
   d. Subaxial

5. Initial treatment of clubfoot is most often by which of the following?
   a. Casting followed by foot abduction bracing (Ponseti method)
   b. Splinting and taping, followed by tendon reimplantation (French physiotherapy)
   c. Initial tendon release surgery, followed by physical therapy (surgical release method)
   d. Early ambulation with crutches or walker (physiologic therapy)

6. According to the American Academy of Pediatrics—Surgical Section, a sacrococcygeal teratoma that is entirely internal without external components is classified as which of the following?
   a. Type I
   b. Type II
   c. Type III
   d. Type IV

7. Sacral agenesis is most commonly associated with which of the following underlying factors?
   a. Maternal diabetes
   b. Maternal seizure disorder (regardless of antiepileptic medications)
   c. Maternal teratogen exposure (e.g., tetracycline in first trimester)
   d. Maternal pelvic radiation exposure in early pregnancy

8. What is the term for an open neural tube defect characterized by a bony spinal defect without an overlying sac?
   a. Myelomeningocele
   b. Meningocele
   c. Myeloschisis
   d. Myelodysplasia

9. Which of the following central nervous system findings on first trimester nuchal translucency screening (11–14 weeks) raises suspicion for fetal open spina bifida?
   a. Bifrontal retraction or scalloping of the frontal bone ("lemon sign")
   b. Qualitative nonvisualization of the brainstem, fourth ventricle, or cisterna magna
   c. Brainstem-to–brainstem-to-occipital bone ratio <1
   d. Cerebral ventriculomegaly

10. Which of the following is associated with a "strawberry-shaped" fetal calvarium?
    a. Trisomy 8 (Warkany syndrome)
    b. Trisomy 13 (Patau syndrome)
    c. Trisomy 18 (Edwards syndrome)
    d. Trisomy 21 (Down syndrome)

11. Which of the following diagnoses is unlikely to cause abnormal curvature of the spine?
    a. Open neural tube defect
    b. Limb—body stalk abnormality
    c. Amniotic band sequence
    d. Sacrococcygeal teratoma

12. Which of the following abnormalities associated with amniotic band syndrome is most likely to result in perinatal mortality?
    a. Visceral abdominal wall defects
    b. Umbilical cord involvement
    c. Caudad neural tube defects
    d. Facial involvement

27

Placenta and Umbilical Cord Imaging

THOMAS R. MOORE

(see Creasy and Resnik's Maternal-Fetal Medicine, 9e: Ch 27)

Summary

Recently, obtaining "critical images" during pregnancy ultrasound examinations, which can provide significant prognostic information about fetal and newborn downstream risk, has received increased emphasis. Details of fetal anatomy (especially brain and cardiac) and lists of "must have" measurements (e.g., nasal bone length and posterior fossa dimensions) are considered essential in anatomic fetal assessment. To some, this may appear to leave placental and umbilical imaging in the category of secondary interest. However, abnormalities of placental and cord anatomy can not only draw attention to associated anatomic abnormalities in the fetus but also lead to significant fetal morbidity and mortality in addition to significant maternal risk. Thus, placental and umbilical cord imaging must be performed meticulously in order to assure accurate assessment of pregnancy prognosis.

PLACENTA

Location. The location of the placenta should be documented in every obstetric ultrasound examination (e.g., fundal, right fundal, anterior, low-lying, marginal previa). While there are no commonly used standards for sonographic placental dimensions (e.g., thickness, length/width) at various gestational ages, the distance from the inferior placental margin to the endocervical os is a critical measurement, as placenta previa is associated with significant maternal and neonatal morbidity. Because the placenta expands during gestation, documentation of the lower extent of placentation is essential with most ultrasound examinations.

Placenta Previa. Previa is identified when the inferior placental edge covers the internal cervical os. Low-lying placenta, which can have significant associated obstetric morbidity, has its inferior margin <2 cm from the endocervix but not covering the os. In patients with prior cesarean delivery or myomectomy, the presence of placental tissue overlying the cesarean scar should be noted and assessed with color Doppler imaging. Because delivery planning is dependent on placental position, low-lying or previa placentas noted in the second trimester should be reassessed at 32–34 weeks of gestation.

Succenturiate Lobe. Also termed a *bilobed placenta*, two placental masses are linked by connecting intramembranous blood vessels, with the umbilical cord usually originating from one of the placental lobes, although it can also originate from the connecting vessels in the membranes (membranous cord insertion). Succenturiate placenta has an increased risk of "vasa previa" in which the connecting vessels pass over the endocervical os.

Placenta Accreta. Occurring in ~1/500 deliveries, the accreta spectrum is associated with placental invasion into the adjacent myometrium, especially where a cesarean or prior myomectomy scar is present. Patients with three or more cesareans have accreta risk ~40% if the placenta is implanted in the lower uterine segment but only 0.1% if the implantation is fundal. Anterior location of placenta accreta in the lower uterine segment is associated with significantly higher blood loss than if attachment is predominantly posterior. Accreta markers on sonography or magnetic resonance imaging include loss of the normal hypoechoic boundary between placental and myometrial tissues, bright color-Doppler vascular lacunae in the placental-myometrial bed, and bulging of the placenta into the muscular wall of the uterus or bladder.

Molar Gestation. Complete and partial hydatidiform moles are genetically aberrant conceptuses. Typically, complete moles, comprising ~85% of molar gestations, have 46 chromosomes (diploidy), all of paternal origin. Partial moles usually have 69 chromosomes (triploidy), with 23 chromosomes of maternal and 46 chromosomes of paternal origin. Molar pregnancy occurs in 1/1000 pregnancies in the United States, whereas in Asia the frequency is as high as 1/100.

UMBILICAL CORD

Appearance and Structure. The human umbilical cord typically has two arteries carrying fetal blood to the placenta and a single vein returning to the fetus surrounded by Wharton jelly and a covering of amnion.

Single Umbilical Artery (SUA). In 1/200 singletons and 5% of twins, a single umbilical artery and vein are present. With SUA, coexistent structural anomalies are found in up to 30% of affected fetuses, typically involving cardiac, gastrointestinal, and renal defects. In fetuses with SUA and anatomic anomalies, aneuploidy is present in 5%–50%, with elevated rates of fetal growth restriction (odds ratio [OR] 2.75), preterm birth (OR 2.10), neonatal intensive care unit admission (OR 2.06), and perinatal mortality (OR 2.29).

Cord Insertion Site Into the Placenta. Marginal and velamentous cord insertions are distinguished by insertion within 2 cm of the placental edge (marginal) and ≥2 cm distant from the placental edge (velamentous). Marginal cord insertions are diagnosed in ~8% of singleton pregnancies, and velamentous insertion occurs in 1%. Vasa previa is diagnosed when the umbilical vessels pass within 2 cm of the cervical os.

QUESTIONS

1. A velamentous umbilical cord insertion into the placenta is defined as at least _____ mm of umbilical vessels traveling in the amniotic membranes beyond the placental edge.
   a. 5
   b. 10
   c. 15
   d. 20

2. What percentage of singleton gestations have a marginal umbilical cord insertion?
   a. 4%
   b. 8%
   c. 12%
   d. 18%

3. Vasa previa is defined when membranous umbilical vessels travel within what distance from the internal cervical os?
   a. 20 mm
   b. 15 mm
   c. 10 mm
   d. 5 mm

4. Which of the following statements about molar gestation is NOT true?
   a. The molar gestation genotype is typically 46,XX (diploid), with both X chromosomes of paternal origin.
   b. A complete mole is caused when a single (90%) or two (10%) sperm combine with an egg that lacks nuclear DNA.
   c. In partial moles, it is common to have a fetus with normal development and genotype.
   d. In Asia, the frequency of molar gestation is as high as 1% of pregnancies.

5. Although clinical judgment should be applied, the typical recommended timing of delivery for placenta accreta is
   a. 39–40 weeks of gestation
   b. 37–38 weeks of gestation
   c. 35–36 weeks of gestation
   d. 32–34 weeks of gestation

6. The frequency of placenta accreta is rising and currently occurs in 1 of every _____ pregnancies.
   a. 100
   b. 200
   c. 500
   d. 1000

7. Which of the following facts about placental lakes is NOT true?
   a. Placental lakes are enlarged intervillous vascular spaces containing maternal blood.
   b. Placental lakes are diagnosed in 1%–2% of second-trimester ultrasound examinations.
   c. Color Doppler shows no arterial flow within placental lakes.
   d. The majority of placental lakes resolve or decrease in size with advancing gestation.

8. During a midtrimester ultrasound examination, the lowest edge of the posterior placenta is 2.9 cm from the internal cervical os. Which of the following is the best way to describe the placental position in the ultrasound report?
   a. Normal
   b. Low-lying
   c. Marginal previa
   d. Previa

9. During sonographic examination at 18 weeks of gestation, the anterior placenta is noted to be 4 mm from the internal cervical os and reported as "placenta previa." Which of the following best represents the likelihood of this still being placenta previa at 37 weeks?
   a. ~5%
   b. ~10%
   c. ~30%
   d. ~40%

10. During an ultrasound examination, a single umbilical artery (SUA) is documented. Which of the following are associated with SUA?
    a. More than half of fetuses with SUA have major structural anomalies.
    b. With SUA and omphalocele present on ultrasound, abnormal karyotype occurs in more than 80%.
    c. With isolated SUA, fetal growth restriction is uncommon.
    d. If SUA is present on anatomy scan but no structural anomalies are noted, chromosome anomalies are uncommon.

11. Which of the following is true about subchorionic hemorrhage (SCH) found at 12 weeks' gestation?
    a. SCH occurs in 20%–30% of pregnancies.
    b. SCH always has associated vaginal bleeding.
    c. Most SCHs resolve over the subsequent 6–8 weeks.
    d. SCH is associated with third-trimester growth restriction.

12. At 12 weeks' gestation, uterine ultrasound demonstrates no fetus or placenta but a uterus of 16 weeks' size with a mass of multiple small cysts within the cavity. What should be the next step in care?
    a. Obtain quantitative human chorionic gonadotropin and thyroid function tests.
    b. Schedule dilatation and curettage.
    c. Reassess with ultrasound in 1–2 weeks.
    d. Perform an endometrial biopsy.

Uterus and Adnexae Imaging

THOMAS R. MOORE | ALESSANDRO GHIDINI

(see Creasy and Resnik's Maternal-Fetal Medicine, 9e: Ch 28)

Summary

Adnexal Masses. The majority of these masses are detected incidentally during obstetric ultrasound examinations; however, some masses are diagnosed due to symptoms related to their size or complications. Adnexal masses are detected in 1%–4% of pregnant women. Among cystic lesions, those smaller than 3 cm with no internal echoes are typically follicular cysts; corpus luteum cysts are 3–6 cm, with a color Doppler circumferential "ring of fire"; theca lutein cysts are multiloculated; and cystadenomas are predominantly cystic but may have internal excrescences. The most common solid masses are fibromas, which should be distinguished from pedunculated uterine myomas. Mixed cystic and solid components can be found in hemorrhagic cysts (with internal echoes), endometriomas, and teratomas (which have multiple echogenic and cystic components and may have shadowing due to calcifications). Differential diagnosis includes paraovarian cysts, hydrosalpinx, and leiomyomas. Resolution occurs in 80%–90% of adnexal masses, and it is more common to occur in simple cysts <6 cm in diameter and those diagnosed before 16 weeks of gestation. Persistent and large masses are more likely to result in torsion (up to 25%, typically in the first trimester), rupture (0%–9%), or obstruction of labor (2%–17%). Malignancy (usually of low malignant potential) occurs in 1%–3% of lesions overall. Magnetic resonance imaging may help differentiate dermoid tumors from other neoplasms. Surgery is commonly recommended in the presence of persistent and large masses, which are at risk for torsion or rupture, or when the morphologic pattern suggests malignancy. Surgery, if performed, has the least fetal morbidity in the early second trimester. Laparoscopy has a similar risk of fetal loss as open surgery but lower risk of preterm labor and lower blood loss. Routine obstetric management is recommended for stable cystic lesions <6 cm. If cesarean delivery is performed, appropriate surgical management, including staging if indicated, should be performed on all adnexal masses. Planned cesarean delivery should be reserved for complex lesions that are strongly suspected to be malignant or likely to obstruct labor.

Uterine Anomalies. Congenital uterine anomalies are rare (4%) in the general population, but they may have significant effects on fertility and risk of pregnancy complications (miscarriage, fetal growth restriction, premature birth, and malpresentation). They arise from abnormal fusion or canalization of müllerian ducts during embryonic development and may be complete, yielding two uteri and two cervices (Didelphys), or with varying degrees of incompleteness, including arcuate (a single, shallowly indented, heart-shaped uterine fundus), bicornuate, and unicornuate uteri. In bicornuate uteri, the second horn adjacent to the gravid horn may appear to be a uterine or adnexal mass but will have an echogenic endometrial "stripe." A septate uterus has a single uterine horn but with two cavities divided by a septum of varying length. It can be distinguished from bicornuate uterus because the latter has a fundal cleft in the outer contour of the uterus (due to the presence of two horns), whereas the former is without a fundal cleft. Differential diagnosis includes adnexal masses, uterine fibroids, gastrointestinal tumors, and localized fundal uterine contraction (for arcuate uterus). Three-dimensional ultrasound before pregnancy or in the first trimester can often aid with diagnosis. Associated maternal anomalies can be found in the kidneys (absent kidney in 30% of anomalies) and vagina (septate vagina in 5%, typically in uterus didelphys); thus, evaluation for coexisting maternal renal anomalies is recommended. Uterine anomalies are associated with increased risks of fetal malpresentation in labor (adjusted odds ratio [OR] = 9), preterm birth <34 weeks of gestation (adjusted OR = 7), placental abruption (adjusted OR = 3), fetal growth restriction (adjusted OR = 2.0), cervical incompetence, and second-trimester loss. Incidence of preterm birth is not increased in women with arcuate uteri. Risk of miscarriage is highest in septate uteri (44%). Cerclage placement may be considered in the presence of history of preterm delivery and cervical shortening. Fetal growth should be checked serially in the third trimester, and fetal position should be assessed near term for delivery planning.

Uterine Myomas. Also known as fibroids or leiomyomas, uterine myomas are the most common uterine tumors; they are benign monoclonal smooth muscle tumors originating from the myometrial layer of the uterus. They are detected in 3%–4% of midtrimester ultrasound evaluations. Fibroid growth is stimulated by estrogen and progesterone. However, most fibroids typically do not grow during pregnancy. Ultrasound appearance is generally that of a spherical, well-defined, largely hypoechoic mass located anywhere in the uterus (including the lower uterine segment or cervix). Myomas can be submucosal, intramural, subserosal, or pedunculated. Degeneration/internal infarction may occur during pregnancy, resulting in pain and, rarely, uterine contractions. On ultrasonography, degenerated fibroids have heterogeneous internal echoes and may have internal liquefaction. Differential diagnosis includes localized contractions (for intramural fibroids), ovarian tumors or duplicate uterine horn (for pedunculated fibroids), placental abruption or chorioangiomas (for intramural or submucosal fibroids located below the placental plate), and uterine sarcomas (particularly for degenerated fibroids). Fibroids are associated with increased risks of placenta previa (OR: 2.2) and placenta abruption (OR: 2.6), as well as preterm delivery, malpresentation, cesarean delivery, and postpartum hemorrhage. In case of fibroid degeneration, a cyclooxygenase inhibitor (nonsteroidal antiinflammatory drugs) can provide optimal analgesia; however, it must be used with caution in the third trimester due to risk of narrowing of the fetal ductus arteriosus. Cervical or lower uterine segment fibroids may obstruct delivery. A trial of labor is not contraindicated after myomectomy provided the cavity was not entered during the myomectomy.

QUESTIONS

1. A 23-year-old primigravida at 18 weeks' gestation comes for routine ultrasound survey of fetal anatomy. The pregnancy has been uncomplicated and she is asymptomatic for abdominal pain or vaginal bleeding. A 5-cm unilocular left ovarian cyst is noted at the scan, without internal echoes, septations, or increased vascularity on color Doppler. Which one is the most likely diagnosis?
   a. Follicular cyst
   b. Benign cystoadenoma
   c. Corpus luteum cyst
   d. Ovarian fibroma
   e. Ovarian endometrioma

2. In the case described above, which of the following is the most appropriate next step in diagnosis and management?
   a. Request magnetic resonance imaging.
   b. Laparoscopically remove the cyst before 24 weeks' gestation.
   c. Aspirate the cyst for cytology assessment.
   d. Request maternal serum markers for ovarian cancer: cancer antigen 125, human epididymis protein 4, carcinoembryonic antigen.
   e. Repeat the ultrasound scan in a few weeks to document resolution of the cyst or changes in the findings.

3. At a 12-week gestation scan, an intrauterine pregnancy is identified with fetal size appropriate for gestational age, and a solid, pear-shaped mass 10 cm in length is seen at the left side of the uterus. Differential diagnoses should include:
   a. pedunculated uterine fibroid
   b. ovarian fibroid
   c. uterus didelphys
   d. rectal tumor
   e. all of the above

4. In the case described above, documentation of an endometrial stripe at the center of the mass and presence of two cervices at vaginal speculum examination establish the diagnosis of uterus didelphys. Which obstetric complication has the highest relative risk in the presence of uterus didelphys?
   a. Preterm birth <34 weeks
   b. Cervical incompetence
   c. Fetal growth restriction
   d. Fetal malpresentation in labor
   e. Placental abruption

5. In the case described above, which of the following is the most appropriate step in diagnosis and management?
   a. Schedule a follow-up scan in the third trimester to monitor fetal growth and presentation.
   b. Request a computed tomography scan of the pelvis to confirm the diagnosis.
   c. Schedule a fetal echocardiogram at 24 weeks.
   d. Monitor cervical length with transvaginal scans every 2 weeks.
   e. Place a prophylactic cervical cerclage.

6. During a 24-week ultrasound scan, fetal biometry appears appropriate for gestational age and a 10-cm spherical mass is visible at the right lower uterine segment between the myometrium and placental plate. The differential diagnosis includes:
   a. localized uterine contraction
   b. occult placental abruption
   c. intramural uterine fibroid
   d. duplicate uterine horn in a bicornuate uterus
   e. all of the above

7. In the case described above, the patient mentions that a small fibroid had been diagnosed years prior during a gynecologic visit. The patient should be informed that a large uterine fibroid is associated with increased risks of the following complications EXCEPT:
   a. fetal growth restriction
   b. preterm delivery
   c. malpresentation
   d. cesarean delivery
   e. postpartum hemorrhage

8. In the case described above, what is an appropriate step in diagnosis and management?
   a. Schedule an elective cesarean delivery before labor.
   b. Schedule a follow-up ultrasound scan in the third trimester to check fetal presentation and growth.
   c. Plan for fibroid removal at the time of cesarean delivery.
   d. Schedule a magnetic resonance imaging scan.

9. In the case described above, the patient presents at 30 weeks with severe right lower abdominal pain. At physical examination, the pain is exquisite and located in the area of the fibroid. At tocographic monitoring, regular uterine contractions are detected every 3 minutes. At ultrasound scan, the fibroid has changed in echotexture, now an inhomogeneous structure, with heterogeneous internal echoes and signs of liquefaction. All of the following management steps may be appropriate EXCEPT:
   a. Perform serial vaginal examinations to document changes in cervical status.
   b. Obtain a transvaginal scan to assess cervical length.
   c. Explain to the patient that the findings and symptoms are consistent with sarcomatous degeneration of the fibroid so that a consultation with a gynecologic oncologist is indicated to plan hysterectomy.
   d. Administer a brief (<2-day) course of an oral or intravenous nonsteroidal antiinflammatory drug.
   e. Explain to the patient that the symptoms are due to degeneration of the fibroid, which does not have long-term adverse maternal effects.

10. In the case described above, the pregnancy continues until 39 weeks, when she presents in early labor. Clinical and vaginal examination suggests fetal breech presentation. Ultrasound scan diagnoses an appropriately grown fetus in frank breech presentation, with a normal amount of amniotic fluid and persistent 10-cm fibroid in the lower uterine segment. The patient would like to maximize the possibility of a vaginal delivery. Which of the following management steps is NOT appropriate?
    a. Inform the patient that the presence of a fibroid is not a contraindication for external cephalic version.
    b. Explain that a successful cephalic version may not ensure vaginal delivery because the fibroid may interfere with engagement of the fetal head into the maternal pelvis.
    c. Explain that epidural anesthesia may allow optimization of an external cephalic version and may be used for subsequent cesarean delivery in case of failed version.
    d. Plan for myomectomy at the time of the cesarean delivery.
    e. Alert the blood bank about the increased risk of postpartum hemorrhage in this patient.

29

First-Trimester Imaging

BRYANN BROMLEY | THOMAS D. SHIPP

(see *Creasy and Resnik's Maternal-Fetal Medicine, 9e: ch 29*)

Summary

The latter part of the first trimester is an ideal time to assess fetal anatomic structure and search for markers that increase the risk of genetic abnormalities. This is best accomplished with a systematic approach to evaluating the fetus. All ultrasound practitioners must be familiar and compliant with the ALARA principle (As Low as Reasonably Achievable) to obtain diagnostic-quality images at the lowest exposure possible, respecting safety parameters. The output display standard (ODS) is an on-screen display of acoustic output. A thermal index for bone should be maintained at a ratio of 0.7 or less for extended scanning. Color or spectral Doppler may be used in the anatomic evaluation of the fetus when evaluating for abnormalities. Attention must be paid to "dwell" time and particularly sensitive areas such as the fetal eyes.

Sonographic screening for common aneuploidies in the late first trimester involves measurement of the fetal nuchal translucency (NT) and evaluating the appearance of the nasal bone (NB). These sonographic markers in combination with serum analytes can be used to provide a fetal-specific risk of aneuploidy. Recently, cell-free DNA screening has improved our detection of common autosomal trisomies, and diagnostic testing with microarray analysis and in some cases gene panel assessment has expanded our understanding of the genetic basis of many conditions.

The NT is a subcutaneous fluid collection between the fetal soft tissue of the cervical spine and the skin and is measured in a standard manner, typically in a fetus with a crown-rump length (CRL) of between 45 and 84 mm. The width of the NT normally increases with increasing CRL, and normative values are available. An enlarged NT has been variably defined as ≥3.0 mm, ≥3.5 mm, ≥95%, or ≥99% for CRL. An enlarged NT has been associated with an increased risk of major autosomal trisomies, genetic conditions, and structural malformations, especially cardiac anomalies. The risk of adverse outcome increases with the degree of enlargement. Importantly, an enlarged NT may resolve with good outcome. Lack of calcification of the fetal NB is a marker for aneuploidy. The prevalence of an absent NB varies by ethnicity and gestational age and can be seen in euploid fetuses. Combining NB assessment with NT and serum biochemistry can optimize detection of common trisomies but is less frequently used given the widespread availability of cell-free DNA screening whose performance metrics are more robust.

A comprehensive sonographic evaluation of the fetus between 11 and 14 weeks' gestation results in the detection of many major structural malformations. A standardized imaging protocol, with the use of transvaginal sonography, maximizes the detection of anomalies. In singleton pregnancies, 40%–50% of major structural anomalies can be identified in this gestational age window. In those without chromosomal anomalies, 28% of malformations are detected in this age window for both singletons and dichorionic twins. Detection of abnormalities in monochorionic twins is higher, likely related to conditions correlated with this type of placentation such as conjoined twins. Some abnormalities such as acrania-anencephaly, alobar holoprosencephaly, large abdominal wall defects, and major abnormalities in fetal contour will almost always be identifiable. Others such as cardiac anomalies, facial clefts, and limb malformations may be seen, and some abnormalities such as microcephaly are not identifiable until later in gestation due to their etiology and natural history.

A detailed fetal imaging protocol should include an evaluation of the fetal skull and brain, spine, face including profile, thorax including heart and lungs, abdominal wall, gastrointestinal tract, kidney, bladder, and extremities (including movement). The falx cerebri and choroid plexus should be seen by 10 weeks' gestation, the cranial bones should be ossified by 11 weeks' gestation, and the fetal bladder should be seen by 12 weeks' gestation. The four-chamber view of the fetal heart and outflow tracts including the three-vessel trachea view should be identifiable during the latter first trimester scan and typically require directional color Doppler to optimally assess them. Physiologic midgut herniation should resolve by 12 completed weeks of gestation, although later resolution has been reported. When a structural defect or marker is identified, a careful search for other abnormalities is essential. A thorough understanding of first-trimester anatomy and the natural history of sonographic findings is critical in accurately interpreting the significance of findings on the ultrasound, and providers performing this examination should be experienced in detailed fetal anatomic imaging including communicating the results to the patient and a referring provider. Genetic counseling is important in assessing the overall risks to the pregnancy, including residual risk after a normal ultrasound evaluation. The late first-trimester sonographic evaluation of the fetus does not replace second-trimester anatomic imaging as additional anomalies may develop and become apparent in the second and even third trimesters of pregnancy.

QUESTIONS

1. A patient with class III obesity and poorly controlled diabetes is scanned at 14 weeks' gestation. On the basis of this ultrasound image of the lower extremities, which of the following is the most likely diagnosis?

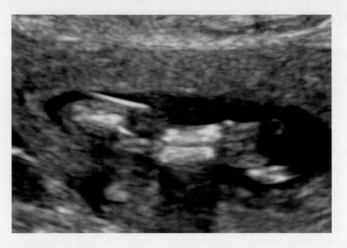

a. Lower extremities normal
b. Fused lower extremities (sirenomelia)
c. Lower extremities not well seen due to challenging imaging conditions, recommend anatomic survey at 20–22 weeks
d. Imaging the extremities is not part of an 11- to 14-week scan

2. In a patient with a normal nuchal translucency and crown-rump length appropriate for 11 weeks, which of the following is the most likely diagnosis shown here?

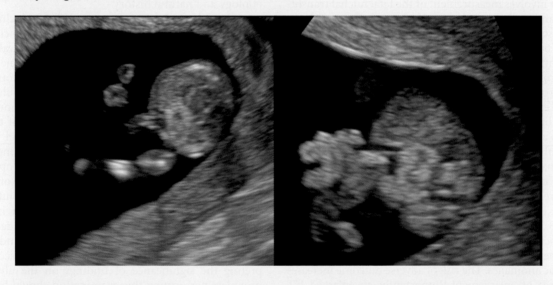

a. Prominent anterior abdominal wall bulge, omphalocele not excluded
b. Bowel containing omphalocele
c. Physiologic umbilical herniation
d. Gastroschisis

3. Which of the following settings is most appropriate while obtaining diagnostic-quality images including cardiac assessment in the first trimester?
a. Thermal Index (soft tissue), ratio 0.7 or less
b. Thermal Index (obstetrics), ratio 0.5 or less
c. Thermal index (cardiac), ratio 0.5 or less
d. Thermal index (bone), ratio 0.7 or less

4. What percentage of major cardiac defects are typically identified in the first trimester based on detailed first-trimester anatomic imaging?
a. 10%
b. 25%
c. 50%
d. 75%

5. Which of the following statements is most accurate regarding the utility of detailed first-trimester imaging in twin gestations?
   a. Congenital anomalies in twins are usually concordant between fetuses.
   b. Detection of congenital anomalies is higher in monochorionic twins than dichorionic twins.
   c. Early anatomic imaging and cell-free DNA screening is not useful in twin gestations as anomalies can't be reliably detected.
   d. Any diagnostic imaging should wait until the second-trimester anatomy scan.

6. Which of the following is the best course of action for a patient with class III obesity and poor visualization of fetal anatomy by transabdominal ultrasound examination at 13−14 weeks' gestation?
   a. Recommend transvaginal imaging as it has been shown to increase the identification rate of anatomic structures, as well as detection of structural anomalies.
   b. Discuss the limitations of your study and recommend follow-up in the second trimester.
   c. Consider the ultrasound study adequate, as long as you have identified a living fetus. Follow up as per your institutional protocol for cell-free DNA screening and subsequent imaging.
   d. Inform the patient that she is not at increased risk for congenital anomalies and should have her anatomic scan at 20−22 weeks' gestation.

7. Which of the following statements is **NOT** correct regarding first trimester detailed sonographic fetal anatomic evaluations?
   a. The detection rate of anomalies is higher in women at "increased risk" than for an unselected population.
   b. Transvaginal imaging alone is the best method of evaluating patients in the 11- to 14-week gestational age window.
   c. Using a standardized protocol results in a higher rate of anomaly detection.
   d. Identifying anomalous fetuses is higher in those with multiple anomalies than a single anomaly.

8. A patient is referred to you for an NT measurement as part of first trimester combined screening. The NT is 2.0 mm and the nasal bone is present. You obtain the following view of the fetal thorax. How do you counsel the patient?

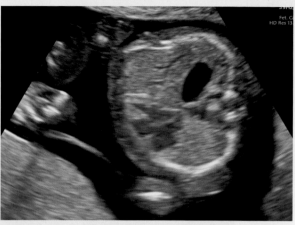

   a. Normal nuchal translucency: Wait for the results of the combined screen before making any recommendations.
   b. Congenital diaphragmatic hernia: Recommend diagnostic genetic testing including chromosomal microarray.
   c. Recommend cell-free DNA screening and follow-up second trimester anatomic evaluation.
   d. The image of the thorax is "off axis." Continue with the planned screening protocol.

9. A 31-year-old G1P0 with low-risk cell-free DNA for the major autosomal trisomies is referred to you for an early anatomic evaluation at 13 weeks' gestation. You obtain the following image. No other anatomic abnormalities are identified. What would be reasonable genetic counseling points to cover with the patient?

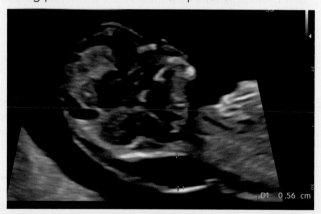

   a. Cell-free DNA screening is highly targeted for the common autosomal trisomies, but there is still a residual risk, as it is a screening test.
   b. Diagnostic genetic testing is recommended because some chromosomal abnormalities are not identified by cell-free DNA screening, and there is an additional yield of approximately 4%−7% for copy number variants.
   c. Even in the setting of a normal chromosomal microarray, there is a risk of RASopathy including Noonan syndrome.
   d. All the above

10. A patient with an isolated NT of 4.0 mm has a normal CMA and no evidence of RASopathy on diagnostic testing. The nuchal fold is normal at 16 weeks' gestation, and there are no structural malformations. Which of the following is the most appropriate recommendation?
    a. Standard second trimester anatomic examination in 2−4 weeks as genetic testing is normal.
    b. Fetal magnetic resonance imaging and fetal echocardiography should be done in 2−4 weeks.
    c. A detailed second-trimester anatomic examination should occur in 2−4 weeks, as well as fetal echocardiography.
    d. None. This ultrasound examination is adequate.

11. A patient with a low-risk cell-free DNA screen for common aneuploidies and sex chromosome aneuploidies has the following finding at 13 weeks' gestation. Which of the following is the best recommendation to the patient?

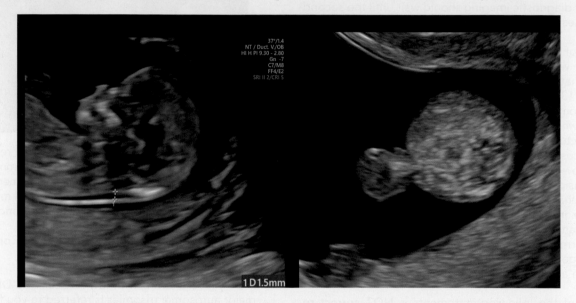

a. Bowel containing omphalocele. Recommend diagnostic testing including evaluation for Beckwith-Wiedemann syndrome.
b. Physiologic umbilical herniation. It will resolve soon.
c. Cell-free DNA screening is adequate. This may be a bowel containing omphalocele but it is not likely of clinical significance given its small size.
d. The NT and umbilical cord insertion site appear normal.

12. A patient referred to you for a 12-week scan has a normal nuchal translucency measurement; however, you notice that the fetal bladder is distended, measuring 11 mm in the sagittal plane. Which of the following statements is NOT correct?
    a. An enlarged bladder is associated with an increased risk of fetal aneuploidy.
    b. An enlarged bladder is associated with an increased risk of lower urinary tract obstruction.
    c. In the setting of a normal karyotype, a bladder length <12 mm may resolve with good perinatal outcome.
    d. There is a lower urinary tract obstruction, and the patient requires diagnostic testing and a bladder shunt.

13. A nurse midwife who works with you is not inclined to refer a patient with a low-risk, cell-free DNA screen who is at increased risk of a structural anomaly based on past obstetric history for an early anatomic scan. You discuss the clinical relevance of early anatomic imaging including all the following except:
    a. A detailed early anatomic scan can identify approximately 50% of major anomalies, 28% in chromosomally normal fetuses.
    b. A detailed early anatomic scan provides the opportunity for early diagnostic genetic testing, multidisciplinary specialty consultation, and enhanced reproductive options if an anomaly is identified.
    c. Cell-free DNA screening is highly targeted for the major autosomal trisomies and does not reliably detect other genetic or structural conditions.
    d. A detailed second-trimester ultrasound is no longer recommended after a normal first trimester anatomy scan.

14. A patient is referred to you for an early anatomic scan in the setting of medication exposure associated with an increased risk of cleft lip and cleft palate. In addition to your usual anatomic assessment, which of the following features are of additional concern?
    a. Maxilla, presence of maxillary gap
    b. Mandible, presence of mandibular gap
    c. Retronasal triangle with two nasal bones
    d. 3VT view with antegrade flow

15. During your 12-week anatomy scan on a fetus with a low-risk cell-free DNA result, you identify a normal nuchal translucency but note that the CRL lags significantly behind gestational age. What condition do you suspect based on the image below?

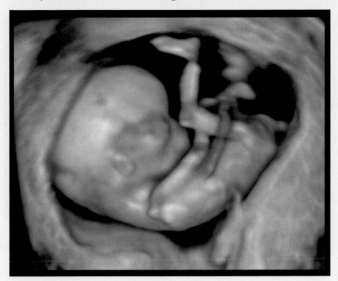

a. Normal fetus, nice three-dimensional view for parents but not necessary
b. Early fetal growth restriction, aneuploidy not likely given low-risk cell-free DNA
c. Discrepancy in size between head and body, suspicious for trisomy 18
d. Discrepancy in size between head and body suspicious for digynic triploidy

16. A patient with a low-risk cell-free DNA screen is referred for an early anatomy scan, and the following image is obtained. Which is the most likely diagnosis?

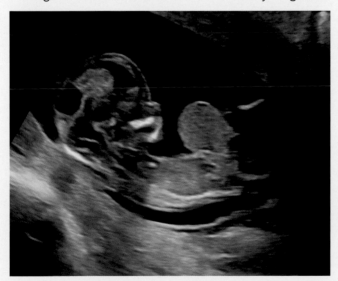

a. Arachnoid cyst
b. Anterior abdominal wall defect, either gastroschisis or omphalocele
c. Liver containing omphalocele
d. Trisomy 21

17. Your sonographer documents a CRL 72 mm and NT of 1.6 mm, in a fetus with a low-risk cell-free DNA. Which of the following is the best interpretation of the image shown?

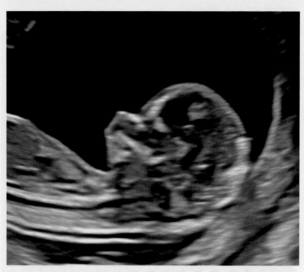

a. Profile normal
b. Nasal bone absent
c. Profile suspicious for micrognathia
d. Maxillary gap, suspicious for facial cleft

18. In scanning a 13-week fetus with a low-risk cell-free DNA screen, you suspect micrognathia based on your evaluation of the profile. What additional structures should you evaluate during this scan to increase your confidence in this diagnosis?
a. None. Recommend an anatomic survey in 18–22 weeks.
b. Obtain a modified coronal view to evaluate the mandible, noting the absence of a mandibular gap.
c. Refer her for a fetal MRI.
d. Obtain a modified coronal view to evaluate the mandible, noting the presence of a mandibular gap.

19. You are asked to evaluate a fetus at 11 weeks with a positive cell-free DNA suspicious for trisomy 13. You note the following findings on your axial scan of the fetal head. Which of the following is the best interpretation of the image?

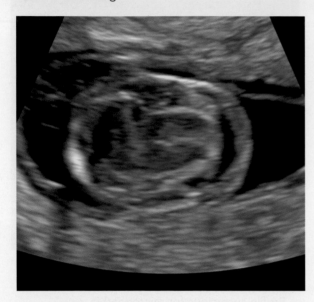

a. No calvarium is seen. The fetus has acrania.
b. The fetal head is normal.
c. The fetal head is suspicious for alobar holoprosencephaly, but this diagnosis cannot be made at 11 weeks' gestation.
d. The fetal head is abnormal due to a monoventricle and fused thalami.

20. A scan at 12 weeks' gestation shows no cardiac activity and a CRL consistent with a fetal demise at 10-week size in a patient with low-risk cell-free fetal DNA screening. Which of the following should be in your interpretation of the image below?

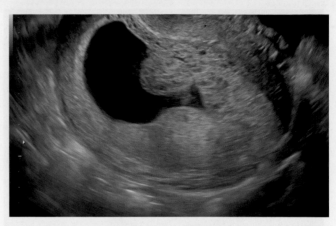

a. Fetus demise at 10 weeks. Too early to assess fetal anatomy and other features.
b. Fetus demise at 10 weeks' gestation, placenta with lacunae, suspicious for placenta accreta spectrum.
c. Fetus demise at 10 weeks' gestation, cystic appearance to placenta. Suspicious for molar pregnancy.
d. Fetus demise at 10 weeks' gestation, cystic appearance to placenta. Suspicious for partial molar pregnancy and triploidy (likely diandric).

Fetal Disorders: Diagnosis and Therapy

30

Prenatal Diagnosis of Congenital Disorders

LORRAINE DUGOFF | RONALD J. WAPNER | CAITLIN BAPTISTE | DAVID CROSBY | ANN MCHUGH

(see *Creasy and Resnik's Maternal-Fetal Medicine, 9e: Ch 30*)

Summary

The field of prenatal diagnosis has changed significantly over the past decade with improved screening technologies reducing the use of diagnostic procedures. Much of this expansion has been associated with the development of molecular technologies fostered by knowledge of the human genome. In this chapter, the approaches to screening pregnancies for genetic disease and the modalities available for in utero fetal diagnosis of congenital disorders, pretest, and posttest counseling are reviewed.

The American College of Obstetricians and Gynecologists recommends that both screening and diagnostic testing should be available to all women who present for prenatal care before 20 weeks of gestation regardless of maternal age. Screening for common fetal aneuploidies such as trisomy 13, 18, and 21 can be performed by evaluation of cell-free fetal DNA or a combination of biochemical and ultrasound nuchal translucency (NT) screening.

Cell-free fetal DNA screening, which can be performed as early as 9 weeks of gestation, has the highest sensitivity and specificity for the detection of trisomy 21, 18, and 13 and may also be used to screen for sex chromosome aneuploidies. The aneuploidy detection rates based on samples for which a result is returned are approximately 99.7% for trisomy 21, 97.9% for trisomy 18, and 99.0% for trisomy 13 with a combined false-positive rate of 0.13%. All screen-positive cases should be confirmed by invasive testing. False-positive cell-free DNA tests may result from confined placental mosaicism, an underlying maternal chromosomal abnormality, a maternal tumor or malignancy, and a vanishing twin. Approximately 0.3% to 5.3% of samples may initially result in "no-call" results for a number of reasons including a low percentage of fetal DNA, which is referred to as the fetal fraction, and assay failure. Increased rates of "no-call" results due to low fetal fraction have been associated with maternal obesity, early gestational age, increased maternal age, in vitro fertilization conception, low-molecular-weight heparin use, and fetal aneuploidy.

Carrier screening is used to screen for autosomal recessive and X-linked single-gene disorders. The goal of carrier screening is to provide individuals with information that will permit them to make informed reproductive decisions. At a minimum, the American College of Obstetricians and Gynecologists recommends carrier screening based on patient ethnicity or race for all pregnant women, as well as panethnic screening for cystic fibrosis and spinal muscular atrophy. Expanded panethnic carrier screening evaluating over 100 parental carrier states is now being introduced to replace ethnic-based screening. This approach will identify more pregnancies at risk for severe or profound conditions.

Diagnostic testing after chorionic villus sampling or amniocentesis is associated with low procedure-related loss rates when performed by experienced operators. All women considering prenatal diagnostic testing should be offered the option of fetal karyotype or chromosomal microarray. Chromosomal microarray should be recommended to all women carrying a fetus with a structural anomaly. While chromosomal abnormalities may be detected in 25% to 35% of cases with ultrasound-identified fetal anomalies, chromosomal microarray will identify an additional 5%−6% of pathogenic copy variants. Additional testing such as a sequencing panel for genes associated with the identified anomalies or exome sequencing may be warranted to detect single-gene disorders in cases with a normal microarray. Exome sequencing may result in the detection of an additional 10%−15% of genetic disorders, although the yield depends on the number of anomalies and systems involved. Cases with multiple fetal structural abnormalities are associated with detection rates as high as 25%. Cases with nonimmune hydrops and skeletal and central nervous system abnormalities have increased detection rates with exome sequencing. Due to the potential complexity associated with exome sequencing, it is strongly recommended that exome sequencing interpretation be limited to centers with extensive prenatal diagnostic experience.

QUESTIONS

1. First-trimester screening for aneuploidy (with NT and serum markers):
   Which of the following combinations of serum markers and ultrasound findings has the highest sensitivity for the detection of Down syndrome in the first trimester?
   a. NT measurement alone
   b. NT measurement, PAPP-A and β-hCG levels
   c. Absence of nasal bone, PAPP-A and β-hCG levels
   d. PAPP-A and free β-hCG levels

2. First-trimester ultrasound markers for fetal aneuploidy:
   The positive predictive value of an absent nasal bone as a screening test for trisomy 21 has been reported as:
   a. 13%
   b. 33%
   c. 54%
   d. 82%

3. Adverse obstetric outcomes and maternal serum analytes:
   The FASTER trial showed that preeclampsia, early and late fetal loss, birth weight less than the fifth percentile, and preterm birth were associated with:
   a. Increased PAPP-A levels
   b. Elevated maternal serum alpha fetoprotein levels
   c. Thickened NT in a euploid fetus
   d. Decreased PAPP-A levels
   e. Elevated β-hCG levels

4. Appropriate genetic testing for increased NT (differential diagnosis):
   Patients with a fetus with NT >3.5 mm and a normal karyotype and microarray should be:
   a. Reassured that the fetus is genetically normal
   b. Offered a fetal echocardiogram and reassured that the fetus is genetically normal
   c. Offered a fetal echocardiogram and molecular genetic testing via a panel to screen for RASopathies
   d. Offered a fetal echocardiogram and whole exome sequencing

5. Second-trimester ultrasound markers for fetal aneuploidy:
   The following second-trimester ultrasound finding has the highest positive likelihood ratio for identifying a fetus with Down syndrome:
   a. Increased nuchal fold
   b. Echogenic intracardiac focus
   c. Pylectasis
   d. Hyperechoic bowel

6. Cell-free fetal DNA screening for fetal aneuploidy factors associated with nonreportable results and low fetal fraction:
   Your patient receives a "no-call" result on cell-free fetal DNA screening. The optimal next step:
   a. Offer repeat cell-free DNA screening as there is a >90% chance that the patient will receive a test result on a repeat screen
   b. Offer repeat cell free DNA screening only if the patient has a BMI<40

   c. Offer first-trimester screening with nuchal translucency and maternal serum analytes
   d. Offer comprehensive ultrasound and diagnostic testing

7. Cell-free DNA screening—etiologies associated with false positives:
   A 29-year-old G1 presents at 11 weeks' gestation following a positive cell-free fetal DNA result for trisomy 21, and the NT scan is within normal limits (1.1 mm). Considering the possibility of a false-positive result, this may be due to all of the following except:
   a. Confined placental mosaicism
   b. Ongoing twin pregnancy
   c. Laboratory error
   d. Underlying maternal chromosomal abnormality
   e. Maternal malignancy

8. Expanded carrier screening—benefits:
   A 32-year-old G2P1 female at 10 weeks of gestation wants to discuss performing a universal panethnic expanded carrier screening test to assess for all genetic causes of a congenital anomaly. You advise her that panethnic expanded carrier screening is used to detect couples at increased risk for having a pregnancy with:
   a. Mendelian disorders
   b. Chromosomal aneuploidy
   c. Copy number variants
   d. Structural chromosomal rearrangements
   e. Adult-onset disorders

9. Expanded carrier screening—limitations:
   A 28-year-old female had a normal early pregnancy ultrasound and negative expanded carrier screening at 10 weeks of gestation. Subsequently at 29 weeks she had preterm labor and delivered a male infant who died within the first few hours of life. Whole exome sequencing was performed, revealing two heterozygous pathogenic variants in DYNC2H1, which are associated with short rib polydactyly. In counseling, she inquires how this result is possible given that they had a normal expanded carrier result. You explain the limitations of expanded carrier screening, which may include all of the following except:
   a. Residual risk
   b. Gene not present on the panel performed
   c. Low fetal fraction
   d. Laboratory error
   e. Sample mix up

10. SMA carrier screening:
    A hypotonic newborn infant is intubated shortly after birth and subsequently diagnosed with SMA type I. His 25-year-old mother had an uncomplicated pregnancy and vaginal birth at 40 weeks' gestation after negative midtrimester expanded carrier screening also negative for SMA with two copies of SMN1 noted. Which of the following is the likely explanation?
    a. Point mutation
    b. Non-paternity
    c. Laboratory error
    d. Incorrect diagnosis
    e. Parental carrier status of two copies of SMN1 in *cis*

11. Fragile X carrier screening:
    A 26-year-old woman presents to your office for pre-pregnancy counseling. She has not had menses in the last year but believes this is due to the stress of caring for her 7-year-old son who has a significant intellectual disability. Her father, at 60 years old, has tremors, progressive gait instability, and poor balance. Using expanded carrier screening, which of the following genes is most likely to reveal a causative mutation in her son and father?
    a. *CFTR*
    b. *FMR1*
    c. Dystrophin
    d. Huntington
    E. *SMN1*

12. Single-gene disorders (autosomal recessive and X-linked) that may have symptomatic carrier states:
    A 22-year-old is in her first pregnancy at 12 weeks of gestation. Expanded carrier screening reveals 70 CGG repeats in *FMR1*. She has a low-risk noninvasive prenatal test (NIPT) 46,XX result. Which of the following is she at risk of in the future?
    a. Early-onset Alzheimer disease
    b. Non-Hodgkin lymphoma
    c. Type II diabetes
    d. Premature ovarian insufficiency
    e. She is not at increased risk of any condition compared with the general population

13. Residual risk definition:
    A couple in their first pregnancy had a 100-gene expanded carrier screening panel, which returned negative for both partners. After their baby delivered vaginally at 39 weeks, newborn screening was positive for cystic fibrosis with confirmation via molecular testing. When the couple's negative expanded carrier screening report was reviewed, including the negative *CFTR* gene, the couple inquire how this was "missed." Which of the following is the likely explanation?
    a. Residual risk
    b. Pleiotropy
    c. Heterogeneity
    d. Variable expressivity
    e. Reduced penetrance

14. Risk of rhesus isoimmunization:
    A 43-year-old G1 at 14 weeks and 4 days of gestation presents for amniocentesis for "advanced maternal age." She is advised to delay the procedure until after 15 weeks' gestation due to the increased risks associated with early amniocentesis. The increased risks of early amniocentesis when compared with second trimester amniocentesis include all of the following except:
    a. Higher fetal loss rate
    b. Increased frequency of culture failure
    c. Increased risk of fetal talipes eqinovarus
    d. Increased risk of rhesus isoimmunization
    e. Increase frequency of ruptured membranes

15. CVS risk in singleton pregnancies:
    A 33-year-old woman at 11 weeks of gestation is considering chorionic villus sampling (CVS) given her prior child with Down syndrome. She has had a low-risk NIPT in this pregnancy. She is taking aspirin for a history of preeclampsia in her last pregnancy. On review of her history, the procedure is deemed to be contraindicated in her case. Which of the following would be a relative contraindication for CVS?
    a. A low-risk screening test result (NIPT) in this pregnancy
    b. Increased maternal serum alpha fetoprotein
    c. Gestational age of 11 weeks
    d. Currently taking aspirin
    e. Existing rhesus sensitization

16. Chromosomal microarray limitations:
    A 27-year-old female and her 28-year-old male partner have a history of recurrent pregnancy loss and a 4-year-old child with Down syndrome. You suspect that one of them may be a carrier of a balanced translocation. Which of the following do you recommend?
    a. Chromosomal microarray
    b. Karyotype
    c. Whole exome sequencing
    d. Noninvasive prenatal testing
    e. Expanded carrier screening

17. Chromosomal microarray yield in anomalous fetuses:
    A couple seeks genetic counseling after an anatomy ultrasound scan at 20 weeks of gestation notable for multiple fetal structural abnormalities including a ventricular septal defect, cerebellar hypoplasia, and a cleft palate. The genetic counselor discusses the option of an amniocentesis and the various genetic tests for which the sample can be sent. The couple inquire as to the benefit of sending the sample for chromosomal microarray if the karyotype is normal. A clinically relevant copy number variant can be identified in what percentage of structurally abnormal fetuses with a normal karyotype?
    a. 1%−2%
    b. 5%−6%
    c. 9%−10%
    d. 10%−15%
    e. >20%

18. Exome sequencing—yield with fetal anomalies and normal microarray:

A 36-year-old G1 has a fetal anatomy ultrasound at 20 weeks of gestation. It demonstrates fetal hydrops with a pericardial and pleural effusion, skin edema, abdominal ascites, and polyhydramnios. A nonimmune cause of fetal hydrops is suspected. The diagnostic utility of whole exome sequencing in this case is in the range of:

a. 1%–2%
b. 5%–10%
c. 10%–15%
d. 15%–20%
e. >30%

19. Exome sequencing—limitations/challenges:

Limitations for the use of whole exome sequencing for the evaluation of fetal structural anomalies include the following:

a. Lack of a registry of fetal genotype phenotype relationships
b. Phenotype expansion

c. Incomplete phenotypes in which a neurocognitive component cannot be determined
d. All of the above
e. None of the above

20. Twins—aneuploidy screening:

A 29-year-old G1 is diagnosed with a dichorionic diamniotic twin pregnancy at 12 weeks' gestation. Which screening test has the highest detection for trisomy 21?

a. NT measurement
b. First-trimester combined screen
c. Cell-free DNA screen
d. Integrated screen
e. Nasal bone measurement alone

31

Teratogenesis and Environmental Exposure

CHRISTINA CHAMBERS | JAN M. FRIEDMAN

(see *Creasy and Resnik's Maternal-Fetal Medicine, 9e: Ch 31*)

Summary

A teratogenic exposure is one that can interfere with normal structural or functional development of an embryo or fetus, producing congenital anomalies and/or lifelong behavioral or cognitive deficits in the child. Minor structural anomalies and growth impairment are frequently also seen in affected infants, and spontaneous abortion, stillbirth, and other adverse pregnancy outcomes may be more frequent than expected in the pregnancies of women with teratogenic exposures. A wide range of agents, including some prescription and over-the-counter medications, recreational drugs, and alcohol, can produce a teratogenic effect but only in certain circumstances—at a particular dose, taken by a particular route, at a particular time during pregnancy.

For most medications, information on pregnancy effects is only available from animal studies that were done as part of the regulatory approval process. Animal studies may lead to precautions or reassurance in the product labeling, but the only way we can be certain that an exposure is teratogenic in humans is to recognize that it causes structural or functional abnormalities in the children of women who were treated during pregnancy. Human studies range from case reports of adverse outcomes, clinical series, pregnancy registries, and exposure cohort (teratogen information service) studies to large population-based electronic health records or registry data linkage studies and case control studies. Each of these methods has important strengths and weaknesses. No single approach is sufficient to establish the safety of an exposure or to define the risk for the embryo or fetus fully. This means that conclusions drawn from any single study must be interpreted with caution until they are confirmed or refuted by other studies. Few human pregnancy exposures have been studied comprehensively. A major problem for pregnant women and the physicians who care for them during pregnancy is our lack of knowledge about the existence or magnitude of teratogenic risk associated with many of the exposures that may occur.

A few exposures have unequivocally been shown to be strongly teratogenic in humans (e.g., anticonvulsant therapy throughout pregnancy with valproic acid, especially in combination with other anticonvulsants, oral isotretinoin treatment early in pregnancy, or daily heavy alcohol consumption during pregnancy). Many other exposures do not appear to confer a high risk of damage overall but may increase the risk for certain kinds of birth defects. Treatment during pregnancy with some antidepressants, antipsychotics, or opioids may fall into this category, but study results are inconsistent and clinicians must share this uncertainty with patients who are concerned about such exposures. No studies have been done in pregnant women to assess the teratogenic potential of treatment with most prescription medicines, and clinically interpretable studies of many other exposures in human pregnancy are limited. A number of continually updated resources that clinicians can consult when counseling patients about potentially teratogenic exposures are available.

QUESTIONS

1. Effective approaches to reducing the risk of birth defects include ALL of the following EXCEPT:
   a. Promoting public education that encourages young women who are or may be pregnant to avoid excessive alcohol drinking
   b. Avoiding prescription of prenatal vitamins to pregnant women before the end of the first trimester.
   c. Promoting immunization of all children with measles-mumps-rubella vaccine.
   d. Discussing potential teratogenic risks of an anticonvulsant drug prior to prescribing it for a woman of reproductive age.
   e. None of the above (all of the preceding responses are correct).

2. The Principles of Teratology include all of the following EXCEPT:
   a. There is likely genetic susceptibility of the conceptus to the effects of the environmental agent
   b. Susceptibility to the teratogenic effect depends on the developmental stage when the exposure takes place
   c. Teratogenic agents increase the risk of all major birth defects
   d. Teratogenic effects are expected to increase in degree with an increase in dose

3. The best way to identify new human teratogens is:
   a. Animal studies
   b. Case reports
   c. Case-control studies
   d. Pregnancy registries
   e. Multiple methods in combination

4. Studies consistently show a statistically-significant 1.5-fold increased risk for a specific heart defect following early pregnancy exposure to a certain medication. This heart defect normally occurs in 1:5,000 pregnancies. The clinical interpretation for a patient who has already been exposed early in pregnancy should include which of the following points:
   a. She should never have taken this medication if she knew that she might become pregnant.
   b. Her risk for having a baby with a heart defect is high, and she should consider pregnancy termination.
   c. Her chance for having a baby with this kind of heart defect is increased from 1/5,000 to 1/3333.
   d. There is nothing to worry about, and she should forget about this and enjoy her pregnancy.
   e. All of the above.

5. Evidence indicates that the highest teratogenic risk for major birth defects and neurodevelopmental deficits in the child is associated with use of which of the following anticonvulsants during pregnancy?
   a. Phenobarbital
   b. Lamotrigine
   c. Valproic acid
   d. Carbamezapine

6. For treatment of seizure disorders in women, the optimum approach is:
   a. To treat with monotherapy if it is effective during pregnancy
   b. To treat with the lowest dose of an anticonvulsant medication that prevents the seizures
   c. To consider switching to valproic acid therapy prior to conception to determine its efficacy in the patient
   d. a, b
   e. None of the above

7. Treatment with methotrexate in early pregnancy
   a. Is associated with a pattern of malformations in the children
   b. Is of greater concern when used in acute high doses for treatment of ectopic pregnancy than when used in chronic lower doses for treatment of arthritis
   c. Increases the risk of spontaneous abortion
   d. All of the above
   e. None of the above

8. Prevention of pregnancy exposures to isotretinoin is managed by:
   a. Prohibition of prescribing this medication to women of reproductive age
   b. Controlled distribution of the drug through registered pharmacies and the requirement for a negative pregnancy test prior to each dispensing
   c. Requiring women to read the package insert warning and consent in writing to taking the medication
   d. Assumption of full liability for adverse pregnancy outcomes by the prescribing physician

9. Each of the following statements is true EXCEPT:
   a. Teratogenic risks may occur when a pregnant woman takes certain prescription medications during pregnancy in usual therapeutic doses.
   b. Genetic differences may exist among patients in susceptibility to an exposure's teratogenic effects.
   c. Medications that are generally considered to be safe during pregnancy may pose a teratogenic risk if taken in toxic doses.
   d. The fetus is no longer susceptible to teratogenic damage after the first trimester of pregnancy.

10. Radiation exposures of concern in pregnancy include
   a. Dental x-rays
   b. Chest x-rays in the first 4 weeks of pregnancy
   c. An ionizing radiation dose of >50 rads at 12 weeks' gestation
   d. All of the above
   e. None of the above

11. Angiotensin converting enzyme inhibitors (ACE inhibitors) or angiotensin receptor blockers (ARBs) are associated with teratogenic risk
   a. Primarily in the second half of pregnancy
   b. Primarily in weeks 6–12 of pregnancy
   c. Primarily in the first 6 weeks of pregnancy
   d. None of the above (These antihypertensive agents are safe to use throughout pregnancy.)

12. Pregnant women should be educated about fish consumption in pregnancy as follows:
   a. Avoid species of fish that are more likely to have higher levels of mercury
   b. Limit consumption of safer species of fish
   c. Recognize that nutrients in safer fish are helpful and important for fetal brain development
   d. a, b, c
   e. None of the above

13. Fetal alcohol spectrum disorders are
   a. Frequently diagnosed in the newborn nursery
   b. Only occur in women who consume 8 or more alcoholic drinks per day throughout pregnancy
   c. Common in developed countries
   d. Routinely screened for in the newborn heel-stick test

14. Most children affected by the embryonic or fetal effects of maternal alcohol use have
    a. Characteristic alcohol-related facial features
    b. Prenatal and/or postnatal growth deficiency
    c. Microcephaly
    d. Deficits in behavior, cognition or adaptive functioning that may not be recognizable until years after birth

15. Once a woman knows she is pregnant,
    a. It is safe for her to drink on special occasions, but no more than once per trimester
    b. It safe for her to drink white wine as long as she has no more than 2 glasses per day
    c. It safe for her to drink moderately after the first trimester
    d. She should avoid alcohol entirely throughout pregnancy

16. Tobacco use in pregnancy is associated with increased risks for:
    a. Miscarriage
    b. Placental abruption
    c. Certain specific birth defects
    d. Fetal growth deficiency
    e. All of the above

17. Marijuana is
    a. Rarely used in pregnancy by women who do not abuse other drugs
    b. Inherently safe because it is a natural substance
    c. Safe to use in pregnancy if it is obtained from a legal, licensed source
    d. All of the above
    e. None of the above

18. Treatment of a pregnant woman with a drug that has known teratogenic potential may be appropriate if
    a. Available safer alternatives are substantially more expensive.
    b. The woman had a normal baby in a previous pregnancy in which she received the same treatment.
    c. The benefits of treatment to the woman and her embryo/fetus outweigh the potential harm of NOT treating her during pregnancy.
    d. The woman agrees to monitor the pregnancy by serial ultrasound examination and amniocentesis.
    e. None of the above. Such treatment is never appropriate.

19. Data on short- and long-term effects of prenatal marijuana exposure are:
    a. Conclusive
    b. Often confounded by exposures to tobacco or alcohol
    c. Frequently not applicable to contemporary marijuana use
    d. b, c
    e. All of the above

20. Opioid use in pregnancy is clearly associated with:
    a. Neonatal withdrawal with exposure late in pregnancy
    b. A specific pattern of malformation with first trimester exposure
    c. Neural tube defects in about 5% of infants exposed early in pregnancy
    d. No increased risk of birth defects if taken as directed as a prescription medication

21. Children born after strongly teratogenic exposures early in pregnancy often exhibit
    a. Neurodevelopmental abnormalities
    b. Gender dysphoria
    c. Twinning
    d. Excessive growth
    e. Diabetes mellitus

22. Which of the following statements is true?
    a. Birth defects are more frequent among the children of women who are exposed through the semen of men who take a teratogenic drug than among the children of women who take the drug themselves.
    b. Drug exposures that cause miscarriage are unlikely to cause birth defects in liveborn infants.
    c. The teratogenic potential of a medication can usually be predicted on the basis of its pharmacological profile in children.
    d. The teratogenic potential of a medication can usually be predicted on the basis of its effect on human induced pluripotent stem cells.
    e. None of the above.

23. Which of the following women is at highest risk to have baby with birth defects?
    a. A woman who has been on methadone maintenance therapy for her opioid addiction for the past year
    b. A woman who smokes 2 joints of marijuana a day
    c. A woman who smokes 20 tobacco cigarettes a day
    d. A woman who drinks a bottle of wine with dinner every evening
    e. A woman who has eaten a strict vegan diet for the past 10 years

32

Assessment of Fetal Health

ANJALI KAIMAL

(see Creasy and Resnik's Maternal-Fetal Medicine, 9e: Ch 32)

Summary

Assessment of fetal health is an important part of the management of any pregnancy, but it becomes more critical when maternal and fetal complications arise. Given the wide variability in normal findings, even in the setting of abnormal test results the likelihood of an adverse outcome may be relatively low in a low-risk population. Because the primary intervention available to the obstetrician wanting to facilitate treatment of the fetus is delivery, indications of potential fetal compromise must be carefully balanced against the complications of prematurity if the decision is made to proceed with delivery.

Fetal assessment assumes that a change in fetal behavior implies a change in fetal status. Maternal evaluation of fetal activity, nonstress testing (NST), and the use of ultrasound to assess the fetal biophysical profile (BPP) rely on this principle. In the setting of placental etiologies of fetal compromise, Doppler umbilical arterial flow velocimetry and ultrasound assessment of fetal growth provide information about the short- and long-term well-being of the fetus that is useful in placing the findings of other testing modalities in context.

METHODS OF MONITORING FETAL HEALTH

Fetal Heart Rate Monitoring

Fetal heart rate (FHR) monitoring is a valuable component of virtually all multivariable fetal assessment schemes. It relies on the unique coupling of fetal neurologic status to cardiovascular reflex responses. Because many studies have shown it to be the most sensitive short-term predictor of worsening hypoxemia or acidosis, it has become part of fetal monitoring of labor and delivery. The range of FHR tracings that can be obtained for different fetuses and even for a single fetus over time is significant, which makes combination testing with ultrasound useful in many situations. The combination of fetal movements and FHR acceleration provides the basis of the NST. The classic criteria for a reactive NST result are at least two FHR accelerations lasting at least 15 seconds and rising at least 15 beats/min above the established baseline heart rate. Most term fetuses have many of these accelerations in each 20- to 30-minute period of active sleep, and the term fetus seldom goes more than 60 minutes without meeting these criteria. Modification of these criteria based on gestational age (e.g., including accelerations of 10 beats/min lasting 10 seconds in a background of normal FHR variability for fetuses <32 weeks' gestation) accepts the principle that younger fetuses have smaller accelerations but that they should always demonstrate some degree of FHR acceleration with documented/palpated fetal movements. Falsely reassuring NST results (i.e., false-negative screening test result), as defined by fetal death within 1 week, occurred at a rate of 1.9:1000 fetuses in the largest study.

Biophysical Profile

The BPP relies on the premise that multiple parameters of well-being are better predictors of outcome than any single parameter. The traditional BPP study includes five variables (amniotic fluid volume, fetal tone, fetal movement, fetal breathing, and nonstress test), with two points awarded for each variable for a total possible score of 10. A score of 6/8 does not constitute a full BPP. When the four ultrasound variables are measured first, but at least one of them is absent, the NST must be performed before the BPP is complete and the score is then reported as 6/10 or 8/10. The only score that is allowed to stand alone after only the ultrasound variables have been evaluated is 8/8. In that case, an NST is not required because the outcomes for a BPP of 8/10 and 10/10 are considered equivalent. For high-risk fetuses or fetuses at risk for conditions that may lead to specific changes in the fetal heart tracing (e.g., sinusoidal pattern of fetal anemia in an isoimmunized fetus, periodic decelerations in monoamniotic twins at risk for cord entanglement), the fetal heart tracing may provide useful information even in the setting of a BPP of 8/8. Statistically, the most likely correlate of an equivocal score is coincidental absence of expected behavior in a normal fetus. Extending the testing period, retesting after a brief interval, or adding ancillary tests can be done before moving to delivery because of equivocal scores. When a score of 0/10 to 4/10 without a correctable cause is found for a fetus whose screening results in the first and second trimesters were normal, and especially when biophysical parameters and anatomic review findings were normal in the recent past, expeditious delivery is usually warranted.

Contraction Stress Test and Oxytocin Challenge Test

The contraction stress test and oxytocin challenge test (OCT) are provocative tests using FHR responses to uterine activity to evaluate fetal health. They were first introduced in the 1970s based on the observation that recurrent late decelerations were associated with fetal hypoxemia; they have been used less frequently since the NST, BPP, and other testing modalities were introduced. Interpretation includes standard NST criteria (i.e., FHR accelerations, FHR baseline, and variability) and the FHR response after a contraction pattern has been established. Positive predictive values for perinatal mortality and morbidity, including low 5-minute Apgar scores, fetal distress, and cesarean delivery for an abnormal FHR in labor, show correlations but rarely justify proceeding with delivery. When BPP is the backup test for a positive contraction stress test or OCT result, at least 50% of pregnancies may be safely allowed to continue 1 week or more. The primary residual role for OCT may be in guiding the method of cervical ripening in patients with growth restriction who need delivery.

Doppler Ultrasound

Umbilical artery Doppler velocimetry reflects placental vascular resistance, providing insight into the fetal aspects of placentation. Umbilical artery Doppler findings strongly correlate with fetal growth restriction and critical fetal and neonatal outcomes, with outcomes progressively worsening in association with reduction, loss, and reversal of diastolic flow. The finding of absent end-diastolic velocity in the umbilical artery (AEDV) or reversed end-diastolic velocity (REDV) at any gestational age is an indication to prepare for delivery, including appropriate referral to a tertiary care center if needed, administration of antenatal steroids, and detailed maternal evaluation.

PRACTICAL ASPECTS OF FETAL TESTING

Who, When, and How to Test

There is a paucity of evidence to guide recommendations for indications, timing, and frequency for antenatal fetal surveillance. Maternal risk factors, such as hypertension, diabetes, substance abuse, obesity, and other sources of placental impairment can be indications for surveillance for fetuses. Clinical correlation and shared decision making between the pregnant person and the clinician is essential to determine the optimal testing strategy. When to initiate monitoring has not been established by randomized trial, nor is it likely to be. General guidelines, such as those recommended by the American College of Obstetricians and Gynecologists, suggest starting monitoring at 32 weeks' gestation or later for most indications. Timing for initiation of testing is determined by the risk of stillbirth, the likelihood of survival if intervention is undertaken, as well as the pregnant individual's preferences and goals. Testing frequency is also determined by the level of concern for change in fetal status and varies from 2 to 6 weeks for general assessment of fetal growth to continuous monitoring for severe fetal growth restriction with abnormal Doppler findings. It is important to acknowledge that fetal compromise and stillbirth may be mediated through mechanisms other than hypoxia and placental senescence, which is what the available antenatal surveillance strategies are best able to detect. Fetal compromise due to other mechanisms, as well as due to acute events (i.e., abruption, cord accident), may be less amenable to intervention and prevention.

SUMMARY

The first prenatal visit initiates a process of monitoring, and a customized plan for fetal assessment begins to emerge on the basis of identification of risk factors. Specific fetal information, including data from genetic testing and anatomic and growth evaluation, further refines the plan. As dictated by identified risk factors, management based on multivariable fetal assessment, with BPP scoring as a central element and the addition of Doppler assessment of the umbilical artery as indicated, can help prevent iatrogenic prematurity and provide reassurance regarding fetal well being. In this process, the risks of neonatal injury resulting from prematurity must be balanced against the risks of stillbirth and permanent injury from ongoing pregnancy in the setting of fetal compromise. The details of fetal testing will continue to evolve as further data become available, but the principles of multivariable testing; individualized, patient-centered management based on maternal and fetal conditions; and ongoing investigation to provide validation by reliable outcome measures will continue to apply.

QUESTIONS

1. You are designing an antenatal testing unit and planning to use the biophysical profile as your initial test. What percentage of patients should you anticipate will need NSTs?
   a. 15%
   b. 50%
   c. 10%
   d. 75%

2. A 39-year-old G3P1101 at 36 weeks' gestation with a history of chronic hypertension on labetalol presents with a 2-day history of decreased fetal movement. Which of the following aspects of her history is most concerning for an adverse outcome?
   a. Maternal age >35
   b. Chronic hypertension on medications
   c. Prior preterm birth
   d. Decreased fetal movement for 2 days

3. A 33-year-old G1P0 at 32 weeks' gestation presents for antenatal testing due to chronic hypertension. Which parameter of the biophysical profile is most likely to be abnormal?
   a. Fetal movement
   b. Fetal tone
   c. Fetal breathing
   d. Amniotic fluid
   e. NST

4. A 35-year-old G4P2 at 29 weeks' gestation has a biophysical profile of 8/8. Under what circumstances would an NST be most useful?
   a. Isoimmunization
   b. Fetal growth restriction
   c. Cholestasis
   d. Lupus

5. A 33-year-old G1P0 at 33 weeks' gestation is presenting for antenatal testing. Which of the following medications can alter the biophysical profile results?
   a. Nifedipine
   b. Sertaline
   c. Betamethasone
   d. Levothyroxine
   e. Metformin

6. A 27-year-old G3P1 at 38 weeks' gestation presents for NST. The use of vibroacoustic stim (VAS) is likely to
   a. Stimulate fetal breathing
   b. Precipitate a fetal heart rate deceleration
   c. Stimulate fetal tone
   d. Lead to a decrease in fetal heart rate variability
   e. Shorten the monitoring time

7. A 33-year-old G2P1 at 36 weeks' gestation has a BPP of 6/10 with points deducted for lack of fetal movement and nonreactive NST. The amniotic fluid volume is normal. The best next step in management is
   a. Repeat BPP
   b. Extended FHR monitoring
   c. Cesarean delivery
   d. Induction of labor
   e. Contraction stress test

8. A 32-year-old G1P0 at 27 weeks' gestation with type 1 diabetes has been diagnosed with fetal growth restriction at the second percentile. The most useful tool for monitoring her pregnancy is
   a. MCA Doppler
   b. Ductus venosus Doppler
   c. Umbilical venous Doppler
   d. BPP
   e. Umbilical arterial Doppler

9. Which adverse outcome is not predicted by an abnormal umbilical artery waveform?
   a. Cesarean delivery for fetal indications
   b. Low Apgar score
   c. Ventilator requirement
   d. Anemia
   e. Hypoglycemia

10. A 42-year-old G2P1 at 30 weeks' gestation is being followed for fetal growth restriction at the fifth percentile and absent end diastolic flow in the umbilical artery. BPP/NST are reassuring. The most useful finding on the ductus venosus waveform would be
    a. A diminished a-wave
    b. An absent a-wave
    c. A normal a-wave
    d. A reversed a-wave

33

Intrapartum Fetal Surveillance

VIVIANA DE ASSIS

(see Creasy and Resnik's Maternal-Fetal Medicine, 9e: Ch 33)

Summary

Uncompromised fetuses with adequate oxygenation can have a fetal heart rate (FHR) average of 110–160 beats/min. Over the course of the pregnancy the FHR tends to slow down, reflecting a maturation of vagal tone. Like the adult heart, the fetal heart has intrinsic pacemaker activity via the sinoatrial node, atrioventricular node, and His-Purkinje system. A partial or complete blockage of the electrical system of the heart can produce variations in the heart to include bradycardia.

The fetal heart rate's variability and rate are modulated by signals from the autonomic nervous system, via the vagus nerve. When the vagus nerve is stimulated, it causes decreased firing of the sinoatrial node, resulting in a decrease of the FHR. Conversely, an oscillatory blockage of the vagus nerve in a healthy fetus leads to an increase in FHR and variability. Sympathetic stimulation on the cardiomyocytes via norepinephrine release also causes an increase in heart rate and the strength of the cardiac contractions, increasing cardiac output. Sympathetic tone increases twofold during stressful situations such as fetal hypoxia.

Chemoreceptors and baroreceptors also influence the fetal heart. The interactions of central and peripheral chemoreceptors in the fetus are poorly understood. Baroreceptors are sensitive to blood pressure changes. Baroreceptors decrease the heart rate via the vagus nerve in response to the rapid rise in blood pressure.

Within the central nervous system, the medulla oblongata contains integrative vasomotor centers that process all the central and peripheral inputs and generate irregular oscillatory vagal impulses, which produce FHR variability.

The adrenal medulla, like in the adult, produces epinephrine and norepinephrine in response to stress, both of which have a chronotropic effect on the heart.

The maternal mean arterial pressure is almost twice that of the fetus. Through delicate balancing mechanisms, the placenta prevents rapid fluid shifts between the mother and fetus.

The fetal heart, unlike the adult heart, has lower intrinsic capacity to alter its contraction efficiency. Modest variations of the FHR within normal range produce small effects on cardiac output. In the extremes, however, both cardiac output and umbilical flow can be substantially compromised. Severe hypoxia can affect umbilical blood flow.

With hypoxemia or acidemia of a previously healthy fetus, there is a redistribution of blood flow in favor of vital organs (brain, heart, adrenal glands). This response allows a fetus to survive up to 30 minutes with a limited oxygen supply without compromise or decompensation. Severe acidemia or sustained hypoxemia leads to decreased cardiac output, blood pressure, and blood flow to the brain and heart, which can eventually lead to fetal death.

A low pH is a prognostic factor for adverse neonatal outcome. It is even more prognostic than a base deficit in depressed neonates at birth. Low arterial cord pH correlated to neonatal mortality and composite morbidity, as well as long-term outcomes such as cerebral palsy.

In acidemic near-term (>36 weeks' gestation) neonates, therapeutic hypothermia is generally initiated for management of neonatal encephalopathy if they are within 6 hours of delivery and meet one of the following criteria: umbilical cord pH of <7.0, base excess >16 mMol/L, or having moderate to severe encephalopathy on clinical examination.

The American College of Obstetricians and Gynecologists (ACOG), Royal College of Obstetricians and Gynecologists, and Royal College of Midwives recommend routine cord blood measurements for all cesarean deliveries and instrumented deliveries for "fetal distress." In addition, the ACOG recommends cord blood measurements for a low 5-minute Apgar score, severe fetal growth restriction, an abnormal fetal heart tracing, maternal thyroid disease, multifetal gestation, and intrapartum fever.

Fetal heart rate tracing can have baseline features which are recorded between uterine contractions. Additional features include period or episodic changes. Periodic changes occur in association with uterine contractions, whereas episodic changes do not.

Periodic FHR patterns are the alteration in fetal heart rate associated with uterine contractions or changes in blood flow within the umbilical cord vessels. The patterns included in this category would include late decelerations, early decelerations, variable decelerations, and accelerations.

Fetal tachycardia differs from an acceleration by being a sustained FHR baseline of greater than 160 beats per minutes for at least 10 minutes. Fetal tachycardia differs from fetal tachyarrhythmia in that the latter presents with an FHR greater than 240 beats per minute, it may be intermittent or persistent, and it may need to be treated with medical therapy or delivery because it can be associated with a deterioration of the fetal status.

A late deceleration is presumed to be late because the circulation time of the deoxygenated blood from the fetal placental site to the chemoreceptors and the progressively decreasing PO_2 must reach a certain threshold before vagal activity decreases the heart rate. If the late deceleration is accompanied by moderate or normal FHR variability, then reassurance of normal central nervous system integrity is present. If the late deceleration is not accompanied by moderate variability, then fetal decompensation is present (inadequate cerebral and myocardial oxygenation). The latter is typically seen in states of decreased placental reserve or after prolonged hypoxic stress.

QUESTIONS

1. A 25-year-old G2P1 at 28 weeks' gestation with a pregnancy complicated by positive anti-RO antibodies presents to triage for suprapubic pain. The fetal heart tracing has a baseline of 70 beats/min and moderate variability, and accelerations are present. The maternal heart rate is 95 bpm. What is your most likely diagnosis?
   a. Maternal medication use
   b. Complete heart block
   c. Fetal premature atrial contractions
   d. Low baseline

2. Persistent blockage of the fetal vagus nerve would cause which of the following changes in the fetal heart tracing pattern?
   a. Increase of the fetal heart rate of 20bpm
   b. Late decelerations
   c. Absent variability
   d. Early decelerations

3. The mean arterial pressure of the fetus is approximately 55 mm Hg, and the maternal mean arterial pressure is 100 mm Hg. The mean arterial pressure in the intervillous space is
   a. higher than the maternal mean arterial pressure
   b. higher than the fetus mean arterial pressure
   c. lower than the spiral arteries mean arterial pressure
   d. none of the above

4. The fetal scalp electrode measures the true beat-to-beat variability of the fetal heart tracing by
   a. measuring the R wave on the fetal ECG
   b. measuring the P wave on the fetal ECG
   c. measuring the T wave on the fetal ECG
   d. modulating the signal generated by movement of a cardiovascular structure

5. In a previously healthy fetus, hypoxemia causes redistribution of blood flow to which organs?
   a. Brain
   b. Spleen
   c. Kidneys
   d. Gut

6. A 33-year-old G2P1 at 39 weeks with an uncomplicated antepartum course presents to obstetric triage area for evaluation of rupture of membranes that occurred 25 minutes before arrival. On examination, you note a pulsatile segment of umbilical cord at the cervical os and the fetal heart tracing has recurrent variable decelerations. At the time of delivery, which of the following is the most likely finding on the umbilical cord gases?
   a. Respiratory acidosis
   b. Respiratory alkalosis
   c. Metabolic acidosis
   d. Mixed acidosis

7. Which of the following values in acid base analysis of cord blood is most predictive for adverse neonatal outcomes in the fetus?
   a. Low arterial pH
   b. Base deficit
   c. CO_2 level
   d. PO_2 level

8. Which of the following is not a criterion to initiate therapeutic hypothermia for prevention neonatal encephalopathy in a fetus with acidemia?
   a. Umbilical cord blood pH <7.0
   b. Base excess >16 mMol/L
   c. Delivery occurred within 6 hours
   d. Moderate to severe encephalopathy on clinical examination
   e. 5-minute Apgar <6

9. All the following are situations where umbilical cord blood sampling should occur at the time of delivery except
   a. maternal thyroid disease
   b. severe fetal growth restriction
   c. multifetal gestation
   d. intrapartum fever
   e. repeat cesarean delivery

10. Which of the following is not associated with causes of decreased or absent fetal heart rate variability?
    a. Absence of the cerebral cortex
    b. Morphine administration
    c. Fetal normoxia
    d. Atropine administration
    e. Complete heart block

Invasive Fetal Therapy

SARAH OBICAN | ANTHONY ODIBO | CLAUDIO SCHENONE

(see *Creasy and Resnik's Maternal-Fetal Medicine, 9e: Ch 34*)

Summary

Optimization of ultrasound and endoscopic equipment have made the fetus more easily accessible for fetal intervention by increasing the number of treatment modalities available for prenatally diagnosed conditions.

During open fetal surgery, the uterus is exposed by a large laparotomy incision and the fetus is partially exposed or exteriorized. Enabling complex surgical procedures, such as the ex utero intrapartum treatment, a multistage cesarean delivery in which the fetus is partially delivered to preserve uteroplacental circulation until a functional fetal airway is established. Most other fetal conditions can be treated by way of minimally invasive fetoscopic procedures that reduce maternal morbidity and the need for cesarean delivery.

As technology has advanced, so has the number of conditions amenable for fetal intervention. Monochorionic twin pregnancies have characteristic vascular anastomoses crossing between the placental districts that may create unique complications, including twin-to-twin transfusion syndrome (TTTS), a significant cause of mortality affecting 10% to 15% of monochorionic twins. Untreated, TTTS is associated with mortality of 80% to 90%. However, with the advent of laser photocoagulation of anastomotic vessels, the survival rate has improved significantly while also reducing the frequency of short-term disability. Other management alternatives for this complication include serial amnioreduction, septostomy, and selective feticide via umbilical cord coagulation.

Fetal therapy is also useful in cases of amniotic band syndrome, in which fetoscopic release of amniotic bands that may otherwise lead to fetal digit or limb amputation. After in utero intervention for amniotic bands, functional salvage of the involved limb is achieved in two-thirds of cases.

Percutaneous fetoscopic endoluminal tracheal occlusion has demonstrated the potential for increasing survival and reducing morbidity in cases of congenital diaphragmatic hernia, especially among fetuses with severe pulmonary hypoplasia. Other congenital thoracic malformations such as congenital airway pulmonary malformation and bronchopulmonary sequestration, also put fetuses at risk for pulmonary compression and hydrops. Antenatal interventions for these conditions include aspiration or shunting of macrocysts, thermocoagulation, and lobectomy via hysterotomy. Similarly, serial thoracocenteses, thoracoamniotic shunting, and sclerosing agents are available in selected cases of fetal pleural effusion.

Lower urinary tract obstruction is a descriptive term for several heterogeneous conditions that affect 1:5000 males. The goals of fetal intervention are to avoid further renal damage and prevent pulmonary hypoplasia and its consequences. Specifically, ultrasound-guided vesicoamniotic shunting allows diversion of urine from the obstructed fetal bladder into the amniotic cavity, promoting lung development and reducing physical deformations.

Half of long-term survivors in cases of hypoplastic left heart (HLHS) have suboptimal neurodevelopmental outcomes. This may be partially due to preferential return of oxygenated blood toward the right ventricle and lower body that may lead to suboptimal brain oxygenation in utero. In this regard, fetal cardiac intervention has arisen as an alternative to improve postnatal repair outcomes for conditions like restrictive atrial septum in HLHS, aortic stenosis with evolving HLHS, and pulmonary atresia in hypoplastic right heart syndrome.

Myelomeningocele is associated with irreversible damage to the nervous system despite immediate postnatal surgical repair. Among long-term survivors, major disabilities include lower extremity paralysis and bowel, bladder, and future sexual dysfunction. Prenatal closure of these defects was proposed to protect the fetus from the uterine environment and improve postnatal outcomes. This hypothesis was proven during the Management of Myelomeningocele Study (MOMS) trial, and longer-term follow-up studies also suggested prolonged clinical benefit.

Sacrococcygeal teratoma represents the most common neoplasm in newborns, and although most cases are uneventful, preterm labor with sacrococcygeal teratoma dystocia can occur, particularly in the context of polyhydramnios, as well as fetal anemia, and high-output cardiac failure leading to fetal demise. Prenatal interventions for these cases include in utero resection, drainage of polyhydramnios, correction of fetal anemia, and shunting of secondary urinary obstruction. Similarly, interruption of the vascular supply by either ultrasound-guided or endoscopic techniques and use of injectable sclerosing agents has been documented for other tumors like large chorioangiomas.

Fetal surgery is not exempt from inherent fetal and maternal risks, namely preterm contractions, maternal morbidity from tocolysis, rupture of membranes, uterine dehiscence, and fetal distress. After open procedures, cesarean delivery is mandatory to avoid uterine rupture.

In summary, as both diagnostic and surgical techniques continue to evolve, so does the ability of fetal therapy to manage antenatal conditions, providing prenatal resolution, alleviating severe pediatric developmental or functional deficiencies, or optimizing the fetal transition to extrauterine life.

QUESTIONS

1. A 24-year-old primigravid woman with a twin gestation at 20 weeks is referred to the fetal care center to confirm chorionicity and amnionicity and further evaluate abnormal amniotic fluid volume found on prior sonographic evaluation by outside provider. Ultrasound shows a monochorionic-diamniotic pregnancy complicated by polyhydramnios on twin A, and in twin B intermittently absent end-diastolic velocity in the umbilical artery, oligohydramnios, and inability to visualize the bladder. Which of the following is the most likely underlying cause of this patient's condition?
   a. Twin anemia-polycythemia syndrome
   b. Twin reverse arterial perfusion sequence
   c. TTTS
   d. Selective fetal growth restriction

2. A 28-year-old multigravida woman with a singleton pregnancy at 36 weeks' gestation complicated by fetal myelomeningocele with open repair earlier in pregnancy presents to the emergency department with complaints of recurrent abdominal cramping pain despite being compliant with her oral nifedipine. She reports being examined 2 days earlier during prenatal visit after complaining of abdominal discomfort and being told by the provider that her cervix was closed. On physical examination today, her cervix is 2 cm dilated. Which of the following is the most appropriate next step in management?
   a. Admit her for observation.
   b. Perform a cesarean delivery.
   c. Allow the patient to deliver vaginally since she is laboring spontaneously.
   d. Discharge home if unchanged on subsequent cervical examinations.

3. A 32-year-old primigravid woman with a singleton pregnancy at 22 weeks' gestation undergoes a comprehensive anatomy scan at a fetal care center after referral for abnormal cardiac findings during routine evaluation. During her referral sonographic examination, small bowel is seen adjacent to the fetal heart in the fetal thorax. The condition is classified as severe after further ultrasonographic evaluation. Which of the following is the most appropriate next step?
   a. Follow-up ultrasonographic evaluation in 2 weeks
   b. Referral for fetoscopic endotracheal occlusion
   c. Exclude additional abnormalities
   d. Offer termination of pregnancy

4. A 21-year-old multigravid woman with twin pregnancy at 18 weeks' gestation presents for a fetal anatomy survey. Prior ultrasonographic evaluation in the first trimester demonstrated a multifetal gestation. This examination reveals a monochorionic pregnancy with viable twin A with a moderate amount of pericardial fluid in one sac and in the other sac a large, amorphous mass with no cardiac structures identifiable. In the twin B sac there is reversed direction of flow in the umbilical artery. The patient should be advised to do which of the following?
   a. Fetoscopic photocoagulation of placental anastomoses
   b. Conservative management with close follow-up
   c. Umbilical cord coagulation of a cardiac mass
   d. No further workup is needed

5. A 27-year-old primigravida presents for her anatomic survey at 20 weeks' gestation. Ultrasonographic evaluation reveals what appears like amniotic bands constricting the right upper forearm, as well as club foot on the left lower extremity. Mild lymphedema is noted with otherwise normal vascular Doppler studies. The remaining anatomic survey appears normal, and prior invasive genetic testing was negative for genetic abnormalities. The patient should be advised to do which of the following?
   a. No further workup needed
   b. Fetoscopic release of amniotic bands now
   c. Pregnancy termination due to low probability of survival
   d. Close follow-up and offer fetoscopic release of amniotic bands if progressive deterioration is noted

6. A 35-year-old multigravida is referred to the fetal care center due to findings of an enlarged fetal bladder during anatomy survey at 18 weeks. Detailed sonographic evaluation at 21 weeks confirms a significantly enlarged bladder plus enlarged ureters bilaterally, echogenic multicystic kidneys, and oligohydramnios. If untreated, which of the following complications is most likely to limit survival at birth?
   a. Lung hypoplasia
   b. Kidney failure
   c. Skeletal deformities
   d. Bladder dysfunction

7. A 22-year-old primigravida at 22 weeks' gestation has been referred to the fetal care center for evaluation after findings of a fetal pelvic mass during routine anatomic survey at an outside provider. Detailed sonographic evaluation at the fetal care center confirms a fetus with sacrococcygeal teratoma. Which of the following is the underlying mechanism of this condition that would put the fetus at highest risk of demise?
   a. Arteriovenous shunting and/or bleeding leading to high-output cardiac failure
   b. Direct anatomic effects of tumoral mass
   c. Polyhydramnios-related preterm labor
   d. Labor dystocia

8. A 27-year-old multigravida with monochorionic twins at 24 weeks' gestation presents for ultrasonographic evaluation following findings of polyhydramnios in one of the twins by outside provider. On evaluation, her pregnancy is diagnosed with stage 3 TTTS. While counseling the patient, she asks about the management alternatives and expectations. Which of the following statements is most accurate?
   a. Overall, postoperative single intrauterine fetal demise occurs in about 33% of pregnancies following laser photocoagulation.
   b. Persistent TTTS complicates approximately 30% of cases 1 week after laser treatment.
   c. There is enough evidence to support amniotic septostomy as a primary therapeutic technique.
   d. Survival rates following fetoscopic laser treatment do not seem to be influenced by the stage of TTTS before the procedure.

9. A 29-year-old multigravida presents for detailed evaluation of a monochorionic-diamniotic pregnancy at 25 weeks' gestation. Ultrasound survey of twin A is unremarkable. Twin B's evaluation reveals estimated fetal weight <1st percentile, intermittent absent end-diastolic velocity in the umbilical artery, and oligohydramnios. A bladder is present in both fetuses. Which of the following is the most likely diagnosis?
   a. Twin anemia-polycythemia syndrome
   b. Stage III twin-to-twin transfusion syndrome
   c. Selective fetal growth restriction of fetus B
   d. Twin reverse arterial perfusion sequence

10. A 32-year-old primigravida with history of abnormally elevated maternal serum alfa-fetal protein levels presents for her routine anatomy survey at 18 weeks' gestation. Ultrasound shows a cystic mass protruding from the dorsal lumbar vertebral bodies, ventriculomegaly, microcephaly, and concave shape of the frontal calvaria. As you explain the diagnosis and management alternatives, the patient inquires about the fetal risks associated with exposure to halogenated agents. Which of the following is the most accurate statement?
   a. Studies did show a small risk for teratogenicity; however, since these procedures are performed well ahead of organogenesis, benefits still outweigh the risks.
   b. There is enough evidence to rule out neurodevelopmental impairment in fetuses exposed to anesthetic agents.
   c. Neither animal nor human studies on halogenated agents show teratogenic effects in the usual clinical doses.
   d. Only animal studies that show no risks of teratogenicity in fetuses exposed to halogenated agents are available.

35

Hemolytic Disease of the Fetus and Newborn

ERIN E. MOISE

(see Creasy and Resnik's Maternal-Fetal Medicine, 9e: Ch 35)

Summary

- An antibody screen should be undertaken at the first prenatal visit in all pregnancies.
- In the RhD-negative patient without alloimmunization, a repeat antibody screen should be performed at 28 weeks' gestation, followed by the administration of 300 μg of rhesus immune globulin (RhIG). RhIG should be given after delivery, with the dosage based on the results of routine testing for fetomaternal hemorrhage.
- In the first alloimmunized pregnancy, maternal titers can be used to guide the need for fetal surveillance. A critical titer of 16 for anti-D and other antibodies and a critical titer of 4 for anti-Kell antibodies should be used as a threshold to begin surveillance with serial middle cerebral artery peak systolic velocity (MCA PSV) Doppler ultrasound.

- Fetal RhD genotype testing through cell-free fetal DNA in the case of heterozygous paternal genotype can eliminate 50% of patients who are unaffected. Amniocentesis to obtain fetal DNA can be used to determine the fetal genotype in cases of alloimmunization to other red cell antibodies associated with hemolytic disease of the fetus and newborn (HDFN).
- In alloimmunized pregnancies, a value of greater than 1.5 multiples of the median for the MCA PSV Doppler scan indicates the need for cordocentesis and possible intrauterine transfusion.
- In previously affected pregnancies, maternal titers should not be used to guide fetal surveillance—MCA PSVs should be empirically initiated as early as 15 weeks' gestation.

QUESTIONS

1. Which of the following is the best monitoring study for fetal anemia for a patient at 30 weeks' gestation with newly diagnosed RhD alloimmunization at a critical titer?
   a. Amniotic fluid bilirubin measurement
   b. Chorionic villus sampling
   c. MCA Doppler
   d. Cell-free DNA test

2. You are teaching a medical student class about hematologic complications of pregnancy. After the lecture, a student asks you what antibodies other than anti-D can be associated with severe fetal anemia. Which of the following antibodies has been associated with a severe HDFN?
   a. Anti-c *(little c)*
   b. Anti-C *(big C)*
   c. Anti-e *(little e)*
   d. Anti-E *(big E)*

3. A G3P2 with known Rh alloimmunization is being followed with weekly MCA-PSV Dopplers after her titer increased to 64. Your sonographer says she is looking for signs of hydrops at each ultrasound when she performs the MCA Doppler. Where would you expect to see the first sonographic signs of fetal hydrops?
   a. Scalp edema
   b. Pericardial effusion
   c. Ascites
   d. Pleural effusion

4. Which of the following is the best gestational age to recommend induction for a patient whose last infant required phototherapy and whose MCA PSVs have all been <1.5 multiples of the median (MoM)?
   a. 36 weeks
   b. 38 weeks
   c. 39 weeks
   d. 40 weeks

5. A G5P4 has undergone six intrauterine transfusions in the current pregnancy and is now 36 weeks' gestation. Which of the following maternal medications could be considered in the 7 to 10 days before delivery to decrease the chance that the neonate will need exchange transfusions for hyperbilirubinemia?
   a. Phenobarbital
   b. Phenytoin
   c. Betamethasone
   d. Carbamazepine

6. A G4P3 with anti-Kell alloimmunization has been followed with weekly MCA-PSV Dopplers. Today the MCA-PSV has risen to 1.7 MoM. You plan the first intrauterine transfusion tomorrow. Which of the following fetal medications should be used to decrease the risk of procedure-related complications during the transfusion?
   a. Succinylcholine
   b. Curare
   c. Vecuronium
   d. Pancuronium

7. A G4P3 has Kell alloimmunization and the last pregnancy was complicated by the need for intrauterine transfusions at 24 weeks' gestation. The partner is homozygous for Kell. At 14 weeks' gestation in the current pregnancy, the anti-Kell titer is 128. When should serial MCA-PSV Dopplers be initiated?
   a. 15 weeks
   b. 16 weeks
   c. 18 weeks
   d. 20 weeks

8. A G4P3 is seen at 10 weeks' gestation with an anti-Kell titer of 512. In the last pregnancy, the anti-Kell titer was 64 and intrauterine transfusions started at 22 weeks' gestation. You are discussing the use of intravenous immune globulin. Which of the following common side effects should you educate your patient on?
   a. Nausea/Vomiting
   b. Diarrhea
   c. Headache
   d. Phlebitis

9. You are a referral center for intrauterine transfusions (IUTs). A community maternal-fetal medicine specialist has been performing serial MCA-PSV Dopplers in a patient with Rh alloimmunization who is now 28 weeks' gestation. The value for the MCA-PSV was 1.65 MoM. When you see the patient the following day, the MCA-PSV that you obtain is 1.4 MoM. There are no signs of hydrops. Which of the following is the best course of action?
   a. Ignore today's MCA value and proceed with IUT.
   b. Repeat MCA in 48 hours.
   c. Proceed only with diagnostic cordocentesis.
   d. Repeat the MCA in 1 week.

10. A 22-year-old G2P1 is seen for her first prenatal visit at 10 weeks. Her previous pregnancy was complicated by postpartum hemorrhage requiring the transfusion of two units of packed red cells. This pregnancy was conceived with her same partner. Her antibody screen returns positive for anti-K1 (Kell) with a titer of 16. Which of the following is the next step in her evaluation?
    a. Repeat her titer.
    b. Check the paternal Kell type.
    c. Start MCA PSV Dopplers at 18 weeks.
    d. Obtain free fetal DNA for Kell typing now.

11. A G2P1 at 10 weeks' gestation is RhD neg with a titer of 128. Her partner is heterozygous for RHD on previous testing. A cell-free fetal DNA test is drawn and reveals an RHD-negative fetus. Which of the following is the next best step in the management of this patient?
    a. Ultrasound with MCA Doppler measurement.
    b. Draw labs for antibody titer.
    c. Refer to maternal-fetal medicine alloimmunization specialist for prenatal care.
    d. Refer back to primary obstetrician for prenatal care.

12. A G1 has initial blood work drawn at 8 weeks' gestation. The blood type returns RhD negative. At the next prenatal visit, you discuss these results and the patient produces a blood donor that says the patient is RhD positive. Which of the following is the most likely explanation for this discrepancy?
    a. The blood drive typing was in error.
    b. The prenatal typing is in error.
    c. Other red cell antibodies are present and interfering with the correct typing.
    d. The patient is a weak D phenotype.

13. A G4P3 is referred at 22 weeks' gestation with an anti-D titer of 512, MCA PSV 1.8 MoM and no evidence of hydrops on ultrasound. An intravascular transfusion is unsuccessful. Using the Bowman formula for calculating intraperitoneal transfusion volume, how much volume should this fetus receive for an intraperitoneal transfusion?
    a. 5 mL
    b. 15 mL
    c. 20 mL
    d. 30 mL

14. A G4P3 at 12 weeks' gestation is RhD negative and reports previous pregnancies affected by HDFN. She also admits that she is uncertain of paternity in the current gestation. Which of the following is the best test to determine fetal RhD status?
    a. Chorionic villus sampling
    b. Amniocentesis
    c. Cell-free fetal DNA
    d. Cordocentesis

15. At an intravascular transfusion at 20 weeks' gestation, the initial fetal hematocrit is 6%? Which of the following is the optimal final target hematocrit?
    a. 10%
    b. 20%
    c. 30%
    d. 40%

16. In the previous case, which of the following is the best timing for the next intravascular transfusion to be scheduled?
    a. 2 days
    b. 5 days
    c. 7 days
    d. 14 days

17. For providers trained in the treatment and management of HDFN, what is the optimal number of IUTs that should be performed annually to maintain competence?
    a. 5
    b. 10
    c. 15
    d. 20

36

Nonimmune Hydrops

ROSEMARY J. FROEHLICH | ISABELLE WILKINS

(see *Creasy and Resnik's Maternal-Fetal Medicine, 9e: ch 36*)

Summary

Hydrops fetalis is a clinical syndrome of the fetus or newborn characterized by generalized edema and fluid collections within two or more serous spaces (pleural, pericardial, or abdominal compartments). Associated findings may include polyhydramnios or placentomegaly. Nonimmune hydrops (NIH), with many possible causes and associations, is now far more common than immune hydrops, caused by maternal red cell alloimmunization. NIH can be easily diagnosed antenatally by sonographic evaluation. Cases may be found on routine imaging or due to referral for another indication, such as uterine size greater than dates. Once the diagnosis is made, efforts should be focused on determining the cause, as treatment, prognosis, and recurrence risk in future pregnancies will be determined by the underlying fetal condition.

A broad range of conditions may lead to NIH including structural/anatomic malformations, arrhythmias, chromosomal abnormalities, infections, and metabolic disorders. Nonimmune causes of fetal anemia, chondrodysplasias, and some single-gene disorders, such as Noonan syndrome, are also associated with NIH. Others may be unique to twin pregnancies, such as hydrops associated with twin-twin transfusion syndrome. Many of these conditions are theorized to result in fetal cardiovascular compromise; however, the precise pathophysiologic mechanism of hydrops is not well understood in most cases. It should also be noted that overlap between these conditions is common (e.g., fetal structural malformations and chromosomal abnormalities).

Evaluation of a patient with hydrops should include a detailed maternal history (including obstetric, family, and genetic histories), review of antenatal medications, infections or other exposures, and a detailed fetal anatomy ultrasound including middle cerebral artery (MCA) Dopplers. Those with congenital heart disease or another major anomaly and those with a suspected arrhythmia should be referred for fetal echocardiography. Abnormal MCA Dopplers should prompt an evaluation for common causes of fetal anemia. Most patients should be referred for genetic counseling and offered invasive prenatal testing, which may include genetic analysis, infectious testing, or lysosomal enzyme testing. Approximately 30% of cases of unexplained NIH may have diagnostic genetic variants, which can be identified through exome sequencing. Thus, patients with unexplained NIH should be referred to a genetics specialist.

Management approaches are difficult to generalize. Some causes, such as fetal SVT, may be amenable to fetal therapy with reversal of hydrops and improved prognosis. However, in most cases, the cause of NIH may not be determined antenatally. If the diagnosis of NIH is made before viability, the prognosis is often grim regardless of the etiology, with high rates of fetal loss. Thus, parents should be counseled appropriately, as some may consider pregnancy termination. For those with continuing pregnancies or those diagnosed later in gestation, close monitoring is warranted. Patients are at increased risk of developing polyhydramnios, which may result in preterm labor and delivery. Preeclampsia and/or mirror syndrome can also occur, warranting preterm delivery in some cases. Maternal monitoring should include blood pressure monitoring and frequent laboratory assessments of liver enzymes and platelet count. Monitoring of fetal well-being may include sonography and/or nonstress testing.

The recommended timing of delivery may vary by cause. In idiopathic cases, expectant management may be considered until ~34 weeks, at which point delivery is often indicated. Later gestational age at delivery is associated with improved survival, thus continued expectant management until 37 weeks may be considered in some cases. Delivery should be attended by an experienced pediatric team. Cesarean delivery is not clearly indicated. In some cases, predelivery thoracentesis or paracentesis has been advocated to facilitate vaginal delivery or enable immediate postnatal resuscitation.

After delivery, if not yet determined, investigation to elucidate the cause of NIH should continue. If the fetus is stillborn or dies during the early neonatal period, postmortem examination should be encouraged. Without a determined cause, counseling the patient and her family about the recurrence risk in future pregnancies is difficult. Though rare, recurrent pregnancies with hydropic fetuses have been described in numerous case reports. Thus, it is inappropriate to counsel families that idiopathic hydrops is unlikely to recur and future pregnancies should be monitored carefully.

QUESTIONS

1. A 24-year-old G1P0 has uncomplicated prenatal care, although she declined genetic serum screening. At 20 weeks, a routine anatomic survey shows hydrops fetalis. No anatomic anomalies are identified on that examination. Fetal movement is normal, and the fetal heart rate appears normal. She is of Thai descent, as is her husband. At your request, the sonographer performs an MCA Doppler evaluation. The peak systolic velocity is 45 cm/sec (mean at this GA is 25). The *first* step in her further evaluation is:
   a. Review of her CBC
   b. Draw a multiple marker screen
   c. Biophysical profile (BPP) and umbilical artery Doppler
   d. Redraw her indirect Coombs
   e. Schedule for follow-up ultrasound in 2 weeks

2. A 28-year-old G3P2002 at 30 weeks is sent to your clinic for an urgent ultrasound for a larger than expected fundal height and decreased fetal movement. Previous prenatal care has been uncomplicated, and a 20-week anatomic survey performed by your center was normal. On today's examination, hydrops fetalis is diagnosed with significant ascites and pleural effusions, and skin edema is noted. There is polyhydramnios. Fetal size is larger than expected. You inform the referring physician that you intend to perform/refer/suggest all of the following except
   a. Fetal echocardiogram
   b. Repeat glucose screen
   c. BPP
   d. Amniocentesis
   e. MCA Doppler velocities

3. A 34-year-old G2P1001 at 31 weeks presents for a follow-up examination due to a large fundal height. Previous laboratory results and a sonographic evaluation were normal. The ultrasound examination shows ascites and skin edema. Over the next few weeks, multiple tests fail to disclose an etiology. You administer corticosteroids and perform weekly BPPs. At 34 weeks, she complains of stress and now has headaches. Her blood pressure is 150/100. Your next action is
   a. Outpatient management of possible mild preeclampsia
   b. Antihypertensive medications
   c. Headache relief with analgesics and repeat blood pressure assessment in 1 week
   d. Immediate admission for delivery

4. A 28-year-old G2P1001 is at 24 weeks and has a BPP for decreased fetal movement. The BPP is scored as 8/8. No NST is performed, but the sonographer mentions a pleural effusion. A targeted examination is ordered and reveals an isolated right fetal pleural effusion. Further evaluation includes close follow-up with weekly scans, which reveal worsening, and 3 weeks later bilateral effusions and ascites are noted. Next steps in management include
   a. Cell-free fetal DNA screening
   b. Umbilical artery Doppler
   c. MCA Doppler velocities
   d. Fetal thoracentesis

5. A 20-year-old G1P0 at 24 weeks complains of decreased fetal movement, and further evaluation reveals a hydropic fetus. MCA Dopplers are performed and reveal velocity of 48 cm/sec (mean at this gestational age is 27.9 cm/sec). A Kleihauer-Betke test is drawn and is positive. The next step in management is
   a. Ask the laboratory to quantitate the fetal bleed
   b. Prepare for possible fetal transfusion
   c. Attempt to elicit a history of inciting event before planning treatment
   d. Expectant management as it is likely self-limited

6. A 26-year-old G1P0 schoolteacher at 18 weeks reports exposure to Fifth disease from a child in her classroom. Public health authorities suspect a localized outbreak. Immediate blood work drawn by you shows no antibodies to Fifth disease in your patient, and a week later she reports symptoms. An ultrasound performed at that time is reassuring; however, follow-up 3 weeks later shows fetal hydrops. Her symptoms have resolved. Next steps include
   a. Reassurance as this is a self-limited disease
   b. Reassurance as this is not a known fetal teratogen
   c. Appropriate antiviral medication
   d. Fetal transfusion
   e. Serial scans with delivery for worsening hydrops

7. A 35-year-old G3P2002 has low-risk cell-free fetal DNA testing, and at 20 weeks a routine ultrasound is performed. This examination reveals a congenital pulmonary airway malformation (CPAM) in the fetal right lung. The CPAM consists mainly of one large cyst with some possible echogenic areas with smaller cysts adjacent. The mediastinum appears shifted. Over the next few weeks, weekly examinations reveal worsening of the mediastinal shift and development of a small rim of ascites and now on the subsequent follow-up. Frank hydrops is noted. You advise her that
   a. Other causes of pulmonary cysts should be considered because CPAM is rarely associated with hydrops.
   b. Placement of a thoracoamniotic shunt may resolve the hydrops.
   c. Open fetal surgery to resect the CPAM is indicated.
   d. CPAM tends to resolve spontaneously in utero, and therefore expectant management is indicated.

8. A 38-year-old in vitro fertilization patient has a first-trimester ultrasound showing a probable monochorionic twin gestation. Follow-up examination at 16 weeks is reassuring, but at 18 weeks Twin A is found to have poly-hydramnios, ascites, pleural effusions, and skin edema. Twin B has oligohydramnios, and the fetal bladder is not visualized. You tell the patient that next steps include
   a. Evaluation of causes of hydrops in Twin A
   b. Targeted examination to exclude Potters syndrome in Twin B
   c. As the pregnancy is by in vitro fertilization, it is likely dichorionic and twin-twin transfusion syndrome is an unlikely explanation for these findings
   d. Referral for laser ablation of communicating placental vessels
   e. Genetic screening with cell-free fetal DNA testing or multiple marker screen

9. A 26-year-old G1P0 at 31 weeks presents to triage with lower extremity edema and a headache. She has had limited prenatal care, aside from an early first-trimester ultrasound to establish dating. On examination, she is noted to be severely hypertensive with 3+ pitting edema bilaterally to the midthighs and mildly hypoxic with an SaO_2 of 92%. Urine dip shows proteinuria. A fundal height is greater than expected at 36 cm. Fetal tachycardia with a heart rate baseline of 185 bpm is noted on monitoring. A bedside ultrasound reveals severe polyhydramnios, fetal scalp edema, pericardial effusion, and ascites. Of the following, which is the strongest indication for delivery at this gestational age?
   a. Fetal hydrops
   b. Fetal tachycardia
   c. Polyhydramnios
   d. Mirror syndrome

10. A 30-year-old G4P2012 presents for follow-up ultrasound at 16 weeks. She underwent chorionic villus sampling at 12 weeks due to a fetal cystic hygroma. On the follow-up study, a large cystic hygroma is again noted, as well as fetal anasarca and bilateral pleural effusions. Which of the following is the most likely karyotypic abnormality?
    a. 69,XXX
    b. 45,X
    c. 47,XX+21
    d. 47,XY+13

11. A 35-year-old G1P0 at 26 weeks presents for a routine prenatal care visit. Her physical examination is unremarkable, and she has no complaints; however, the fetal heart rate on Doppler is in the 220s. She is sent to triage, where persistent fetal tachycardia in this range is noted. An urgent ultrasound and fetal echocardiogram are performed. Fetal hydrops is noted with a pericardial effusion and ascites. Fetal echocardiography reveals normal anatomy and supraventricular tachycardia. Which of the following statements is TRUE?
    a. Prognosis is better for fetuses with hydrops and bradyarrhythmias compared with tachyarrhythmias.
    b. Compared with nonhydropic fetuses with tachyarrhythmias, those with hydrops are more likely to respond to a single antiarrhythmic agent.
    c. Fetal tachyarrhythmias are associated with a better prognosis than most other causes of nonimmune hydrops.
    d. In utero therapy is contraindicated for a fetus with structural heart disease and tachyarrhythmia.

12. A 20-year-old G2P1001 presents for routine anatomic survey at 20 weeks. Evaluation of the fetal heart is notable for a large, echogenic mass noted in the left ventricle. The examination is otherwise unremarkable. A rhabdomyoma is suspected. Pediatric cardiology recommends frequent monitoring for development of fetal hydrops. Which of the following would be the most likely cause of hydrops in this case?
    a. Myocarditis
    b. Arrhythmia
    c. Endocardial fibroelastosis
    d. Outflow tract obstruction

13. A 32-year-old G2P1001 presents for routine anatomic survey at 22 weeks. No anomalies are identified, but fetal hydrops is diagnosed with polyhydramnios, diffuse skin edema, and pericardial effusion. MCA Dopplers are performed, consistent with severe fetal anemia. On history, the patient reports an uncomplicated first pregnancy and no medical history. Her daughter is healthy but was recently sent home from daycare with a low-grade fever and rash. Which of the following is the most likely diagnosis?
    a. Rubella
    b. Varicella
    c. Syphilis
    d. Parvovirus B-19 infection
    e. Herpes simplex virus

14. A 24-year-old G2P0100 presents for preconception counseling. Her most recent pregnancy was complicated by nonimmune hydrops, preterm labor, and neonatal demise. Other fetal findings included growth restriction, small chest size, and severely shortened long bones. She deferred amniocentesis during the pregnancy, but genetic testing on the autopsy specimen is pending. You suspect a form of lethal skeletal dysplasia as the cause. Which of the following is the most likely inheritance pattern for lethal skeletal dysplasia?
    a. X-linked recessive
    b. Autosomal dominant
    c. Mitochondrial
    d. Autosomal recessive
    e. None of the above (most cases are sporadic)

15. A 40-year-old G4P1021 at 29 weeks presents to triage with progressive abdominal distention over the past week and shortness of breath. Bedside ultrasound shows massive polyhydramnios and fetal hydrops. Her antenatal course is notable for a suspected fetal sacrococcygeal teratoma and otherwise uncomplicated. Which of the following is the most likely cause of hydrops in this case?
    a. Rapid tumor growth with vascular compression
    b. Fetal anemia
    c. High-output cardiac failure (arteriovenous shunting)
    d. Uteroplacental insufficiency

16. A 30-year-old G1P0 presents for routine anatomic survey at 21 weeks. Trace pleural effusions are visualized bilaterally. The scan is otherwise unremarkable. Over the next 2 weeks, follow-up scans show progression to hydrops with large pleural effusions, pericardial effusion, and ascites. MCA Doppler velocity is normal. Maternal titers for cytomegalovirus and toxoplasmosis antibodies are negative. She elects for pregnancy termination and accepts genetic testing on autopsy. If the cause is related to a single-gene disorder, which of the following tests is most likely to lead to a diagnosis?
    a. Fluorescence in situ hybridization/karyotype
    b. Cell-free fetal DNA testing
    c. Gene sequencing panel
    d. Whole genome sequencing

37

Multiple Gestation: Clinical Characteristics and Management

MARY E. D'ALTON | FERGAL D. MALONE

(see Creasy and Resnik's Maternal-Fetal Medicine, 9e: Ch 37)

Summary

Multiple gestations are considered high-risk pregnancies due to the increased risk of both maternal and fetal morbidity and mortality. While the incidence of multiple gestations has declined since a peak incidence in 2014, the implications of multiple gestations, their potential complications, and management strategies is essential knowledge for all obstetric providers. In the case of higher-order multiple gestations, selective fetal reduction should be considered to reduce the risk of adverse perinatal outcomes. Referral to a specialist center is recommended as consideration for reduction includes the need to assess for genetic anomalies and confirmation of chorionicity. Hypertensive disease of pregnancy is one such complication frequently seen in multiple gestations. Preeclampsia tends to occur more frequently and at an earlier gestational age compared with singletons. Aspirin prophylaxis is therefore recommended by the Amercian College of Obstetricians and Gynecologists (ACOG) for all multiple gestations to be initiated between 12 and 28 weeks of gestation to continue until delivery. Gestational diabetes, urinary tract infections, and nutrient deficiencies are also more likely to occur in multiple gestations, making vigilance with screening an essential component of prenatal care.

Ultrasound plays a pivotal role in the management of these pregnancies throughout gestation. The importance of accurate diagnosis of chorionicity cannot be understated due to the unique complications that may arise in a monochorionic gestation. Chorionicity is best established in the first or early second trimester. Genetic testing and consultation with subspecialists such as fetal interventionists, neonatologists, and maternal-fetal medicine specialists is often required, and referral to a tertiary care center may be necessary. A comprehensive anatomy ultrasound is advised for all multiples due to an increased risk of structural abnormalities. First-trimester anatomy ultrasound may be available in some centers and may aid in the early identification of anomalies. In monochorionic gestations, serial ultrasound surveillance for the development of unique complications such as twin reversed arterial perfusion, twin-to-twin transfusion syndrome, twin anemia and polycythemia sequence, and unequal placental sharing is necessary from 16 weeks onward. Fetal echocardiogram is recommended for monochorionic multiples due to an increased risk of fetal cardiac anomalies. Early referral to a fetal therapy center is recommended when concern for the aforementioned complications exists as interventions such as fetoscopic laser surgery or radiofrequency ablation may prevent adverse outcomes such as single or dual fetal demise. Serial sonographic surveillance for growth should continue throughout pregnancy with fetal surveillance (e.g., twice-weekly nonstress test, once- or twice-weekly biophysical profile, Doppler studies) should a significant growth discordance be diagnosed. Other special considerations such as monoamniotic twin gestations and conjoined twins are considered in this chapter.

Multiple gestations are at increased risk of preterm delivery. However, there is no single test or intervention that accurately predicts or prevents preterm birth, although there is some evidence to support cerclage for those with asymptomatic cervical dilation in the second trimester. For those at risk of preterm birth, either spontaneous or iatrogenic, where birth is predicted to occur within 7 days at a gestational age of 24–34 weeks, corticosteroids are recommended. Similarly, magnesium sulphate is recommended for fetal neuroprotection for those at risk of preterm delivery at <32 weeks' gestational age. Long-term tocolytic use is not recommended. Delivery timing of multiple gestations requires individualization. However, all twins should be delivered by 39 weeks' gestation, and recommendations for timing based on chorionicity are available from professional bodies and are outlined in this chapter. Induction of labor and trial of labor after cesarean are available for suitable candidates with methods of induction following that of singletons. Analgesia is recommended during labor and delivery due to the possibility of breech extraction or a combined delivery. A planned cesarean delivery is recommended for most higher-order multiple gestations or nonvertex presenting twin deliveries.

In conclusion, complicated multiple gestations are best cared for in consultation with maternal-fetal medicine specialists, prenatal genetic specialists, and pediatric teams. Close assessment of maternal and fetal health is required to optimize outcomes and prevent the increased perinatal morbidity and mortality associated with these pregnancies.

QUESTIONS

1. A 30-year-old Para 1 presents to the ultrasound unit reporting a new diagnosis of pregnancy. She is currently 13 weeks' gestation and recently discovered she was expecting twins. She was sent for confirmation of chorionicity. On ultrasonographic assessment, one gestational sac is seen containing two fetuses, both appearing active. However, no intertwin membrane is identified, and on color Doppler there is obvious cord entanglement. When counseling this patient, at what gestational age would you recommend delivery for monoamniotic twins if the fetal course is otherwise uncomplicated?
   a. 28–30 weeks
   b. 32–34 weeks
   c. 34–36 weeks
   d. 38 weeks
   e. 40 weeks

2. A 28-year-old para 0 presents to the emergency department with vaginal spotting. She has a positive pregnancy test but an uncertain LMP. A junior resident calls you for consultation after detecting a single gestation sac containing two fetal poles with active cardiac activity. However, the resident reports being unable to fully assess the fetuses, as they appear "stuck together." When discussing conjoined twins with your resident, what will you state is the most common type of conjoined twins?
   a. Thoracopagus
   b. Omphalopagus
   c. Craniopagus
   d. Ischiopagus
   e. Parapagus

3. A 41-year-old Para 0 presents to a fetal therapy center after being referred from an outside institution. This is an in vitro fertilization (IVF) pregnancy. In the first trimester, a single placenta was noted with a T sign at the site of the intertwin membrane insertion. She is currently 18 weeks' gestation. Her most recent ultrasound revealed a fluid discordance between the twins with Twin A demonstrating oligohydramnios and Twin B, polyhydramnios. Twin A's bladder is unable to be visualized, and on Doppler assessment a persistent absent end diastolic flow is noted. Twin B is noted to have a decreased A wave in the ductus venosus. You make the diagnosis of stage 3 twin-to-twin transfusion syndrome and discuss management options. You also review the risks of neurologic morbidity in survivors post laser. Which of the following options most closely approximates the risk of neurologic disability, based on current evidence, in survivors post fetoscopic laser ablation for twin-to-twin transfusion syndrome?
   a. 80%
   b. 5%
   c. 60%
   d. 15%
   e. 25%

4. A 39-year-old Para 2 at 22 weeks' gestation presents to the ultrasound unit for a second opinion. This is an IVF pregnancy after many years of secondary infertility. She has been diagnosed with monochorionic twins and has been undergoing serial sonographic surveillance. Her physician informed her of a growth discrepancy between her twins and recently recommended she consider termination of pregnancy. On your assessment, you note that Twin A is normally grown while Twin B is growth restricted with an estimated fetal weight <1st centile. On color Doppler assessment, there is persistent reversal of flow in the umbilical artery. On assessment of the umbilical vein, intermittent pulsations were noted. You discuss the options for management and, in doing so, review the risk to the normal-grown twin should the growth-restricted fetus demise. What is the risk of co-twin death when a demise occurs in a monochorionic gestation?
   a. Approximately 15%
   b. Approximately 30%
   c. Approximately 50%
   d. Approximately 65%
   e. Approximately 25%

5. A 22-year-old Para 0 presents to the fetal therapy center at 12 weeks' gestation. This pregnancy was conceived via an unmonitored ovulation stimulation cycle with timed intercourse. The patient was shocked to learn she is expecting quadruplets. She has a brother who was born preterm at 27 weeks and has residual neurologic deficits that impact his quality of life. The patient understands that multiple pregnancies are considered "high risk," and she is considering a multifetal pregnancy reduction. She wishes to know what the rate of preterm delivery is for singletons, twins, and triplets. What do you inform her about this risk based on the most recent birth data in the United States about rates of preterm birth in singletons, twins, and triplets?
   a. Singleton 8.4%, Twins 61%, Triplets 99%
   b. Singleton 8.4%, Twins 85%, Triplets 85%
   c. Singleton 10%, Twins 99%, Triplets 85%
   d. Singleton 15%, Twins 69%, Triplets 99%
   e. Singleton 10%, Twins 40%, Triplets 60%

6. A 36-year-old para 2 presents to your office at 12 weeks' gestation. She underwent fertility treatment and had an unspecified number of embryos implanted. A bedside ultrasound revealed a higher-order multiple gestation. On today's assessment, you note four gestational sacs with three placentas. One fetus appears to have a cardiac defect and abnormally positioned lower limbs. You discuss multifetal pregnancy reduction (MFPR). The patient is reluctant and asks if only the fetus with suspected cardiac defect can be reduced. When counseling her, how do you explain the difference between MFPR and selective termination?
   a. MFPR aims to reduce a complicated monochorionic pair to a singleton, and selective reduction is the choosing of which twin to reduce as part of MFPR.
   b. MFPR aims to reduce higher-order multiple to a singleton and selective reduction is targeting a specific fetus on the basis of gender diagnosed on noninvasive testing.
   c. MFPR and selective termination are synonyms for the same procedure with the same indications.
   d. MFPR targets a specific fetus of a multiple gestation due to a known or suspected fetal anomaly, and selective reduction aims to reduce higher-order multiples to twins or a singleton.
   c. MFPR aims to reduce a higher-order multiple to twins or a singleton in order to improve live birth rates and perinatal outcomes. A selective termination targets a specific fetus of a multiple gestation due to a known or suspected fetal anomaly.

7. A 43-year-old para 0 presents to your office at 14 weeks' gestation with dichorionic twins. The patient has previously been counseled regarding the risk of spontaneous preterm delivery in twin gestations, and she is concerned about experiencing preterm birth. This pregnancy was achieved after three cycles of IVF, and she is anxious to experience an uncomplicated pregnancy. The patient informs you that her friend experienced a 19-week loss but in her next pregnancy was given a cervical cerclage and subsequently delivered at term. The patient asks you about a cerclage or some other means to prevent preterm birth in twins. What do you inform her about cervical cerclage and preterm birth prevention in twins?
   a. There is no evidence that prophylactic cervical cerclage is helpful to prevent spontaneous preterm birth in twin gestations.
   b. Cervical cerclage placement is recommended at 13 weeks in twin gestations to prevent spontaneous preterm birth.
   c. Cervical cerclage placement is recommended after 24 weeks in the setting of short cervix in twins.
   d. Abdominal cerclage is recommended to prevent preterm birth in twins.
   e. Cerclage placement has been shown to reduce preterm birth in twins only with adjuvant use of progesterone supplementation.

8. A 27-year-old para 0 at 16 weeks' gestation presents to your ultrasound unit with a new diagnosis of pregnancy for her first ultrasound. On assessment, you notice two gestational sacs and two fetal poles. The dividing membrane is thin, and a "T sign" is seen with fetal cord insertions both noted close to the dividing membrane. Twin A is normal appearing, but twin B is anomalous with an abnormal cranium, absent upper limbs, and generalized anasarca. No fetal heart rate is detected, and no obvious cardiac structure is visualized. When color flow Doppler is applied to Twin B, there appears to be pulsatile retrograde flow in the umbilical arteries. What is the diagnosis in this case?
   a. Twin anemia polycythemia sequence
   b. Twin-to-twin transfer syndrome
   c. Twin reversed arterial perfusion sequence
   d. Twin-to-twin transfusion syndrome
   e. Anomalous acardiac twin sequence

9. A 35-year-old para 3 at 36 weeks with a dichorionic twin gestation presents to labor and delivery with complaints of uterine contractions. On examination, her cervix is 5 cm dilated, membranes are intact, and the presenting part is at zero station but palpates as a breech presentation. A bedside ultrasound confirms a breech presentation of Twin A and a vertex presentation of Twin B. The fetal heart rate tracings are category 1. The patient strongly desires a vaginal delivery and has had two prior successful vaginal deliveries of >3500 g babies. What do you advise the patient is likely the safest mode of delivery in terms of perinatal outcomes in this case?
   a. Breech extraction of Twin A in the operating room with Twin B allowed to delivery vaginally if remains cephalic
   b. Breech extraction of Twin A followed by an internal podalic version of Twin B and breech extraction of Twin B
   c. Internal podalic version of Twin A to allow for a vaginal delivery
   d. Caesarean delivery
   e. Breech extraction of Twin A with forceps to control delivery of the aftercoming head. Twin B allowed to descent without augmentation with plan for a vaginal delivery

10. A 29-year-old para 0 at 28 weeks with a dichorionic twin gestation presents for follow-up prenatal care. She reports feeling a little short of breath. She first noticed it when speaking on the phone, and then she realized she sounded out of breath after climbing the stairs to her fourth-floor walk-up apartment. She denies chest pain, orthopnea, paroxysmal nocturnal dyspnea, palpitations, or ankle swelling. She is able to walk up to a mile without stopping but admits she moves slower than before pregnancy. On examination, her lung sounds are clear, heart sounds S1 and S2 are normal, and a flow murmur is heard over the aortic valve, but it does not radiate. An electrocardiogram shows sinus tachycardia with a heart rate of 101. Her labs show a mild anemia with a hemoglobin of 9.9 g/dL. What is the average increase in maternal cardiac output when pregnant with twin gestations compared with a singleton gestation?
   a. 80%
   b. 50%
   c. 40%
   d. 30%
   e. 20%

11. A 37-year-old Para 0 at 12 weeks of gestation with a dichorionic pregnancy presents to your office for her first visit in this pregnancy. She has a body mass index of 35, her examination is normal, and you note two viable fetuses on bedside ultrasound assessment. You discuss the risks associated with twin gestation and methods used to mitigate those risks. At the end of the visit, you prescribe her a prenatal vitamin and a "baby" aspirin. What is the purpose of prescribing aspirin in this patient?
    a. Prophylaxis against fetal growth restriction
    b. Prevention of spontaneous preterm delivery
    c. Prophylaxis against preeclampsia
    d. Prophylaxis against both preeclampsia and fetal growth restriction
    e. Prophylaxis against venous thromboembolism

12. A 41-year-old Para 3 presents to your office with a new diagnosis of pregnancy. Her third child was affected by neurofibromatosis with a de novo mutation diagnosed on postnatal assessment following presentation with refractory seizures. She is currently 11 weeks' gestation and is pregnant with dichorionic twins. This is a spontaneously conceived pregnancy. She is anxious to determine if this pregnancy is affected by a major genetic disorder. Regarding genetic testing in multiple gestations, which of the following is the most accurate statement?
    a. Chorionic villus sampling (CVS) is not recommended for multiple pregnancies due to the risk of pregnancy loss.
    b. CVS is safe in multiples, but care must be taken to be sure of separate sampling of the placentas in a dichorionic pregnancy or in higher-order multiple gestations.
    c. Both placental samples should be taken from the same approach (e.g., transcervical or transabdominal) to reduce confusion between the placentas sampled in a dichorionic gestation.
    d. Amniocentesis is recommended to confirm CVS findings in dichorionic multiple gestations due to the risk of sampling error at the time of CVS.
    e. Genetic testing is not required for multiple gestations as noninvasive prenatal testing has eliminated the need for invasive genetic testing in multiple gestations.

13. A 39-year-old Para 1 at 22 weeks of gestation is referred to your office to discuss the findings on her most recent anatomy ultrasound. This is a spontaneous pregnancy of a dichorionic gestation. The pregnancy was uncomplicated until a routine anatomy scan was notable for severe, early-onset fetal growth restriction of twin B measuring <1st centile. Doppler assessment was notable for persistent absent end diastolic flow in the umbilical arteries. The genitalia appear ambiguous, the corpus callosum was unable to be visualized, the lateral ventricles were enlarged, and there is evidence of a ventricular septal defect. In addition, the MVP for Twin B reached the upper limits of normal. You counsel the patient that these findings are suspicious for CHARGE syndrome, likely due to a de novo mutation, and you recommend genetic analysis. Twin A has normal anatomy and growth. When counseling the patient, what do you discuss regarding the risks of expectant management with a single anomalous fetus in a twin gestation?
    a. There is a 20% increase in risk for preterm delivery, as well as an increased risk for caesarean delivery and low birth weight.
    b. There is no increased risk for preterm delivery, but there is an increased risk of dual fetal demise.
    c. An asynchronous delivery is necessary if preterm birth occurs over 26 weeks in order to protect the nonanomalous fetus.
    d. There is a 40% increase in risk for preterm delivery.
    e. There is a 30% increased risk of placental abruption but no increase in the rates of caesarean delivery.

14. A 36-year-old Para 4 at 21 weeks' gestation is referred to the fetal therapy unit. She is pregnant with a monochorionic gestation affected by stage III twin-to-twin transfusion syndrome and unequal placental sharing. She has been counseled about the options of fetoscopic laser ablation, expectant management, or selective termination. She opts to undergo selective fetal reduction of the growth-restricted donor and asks about how this will be performed. She has read that intracardiac potassium chloride (KCl) injection is a safe option for selective termination and expresses a desire to have this performed on the donor twin. How do you counsel this patient?
    a. KCl is safe in all pregnancies providing it is performed under ultrasound guidance in order to avoid maternal circulation.
    b. KCl is the primary method for termination of pregnancy in the setting of monochorionic gestations.
    c. KCl is not to be used in monochorionic gestations due to a shared placental circulation.
    d. KCl is more effective than radiofrequency ablation in selective termination in a monochorionic gestation.
    e. KCl is used in conjunction with radiofrequency ablation in the selective termination of a monochorionic gestation.

15. A 29-year-old Para 2 presents for her first visit this pregnancy. Her last menstrual period was 9 weeks ago. She reports daily nausea and vomiting. On bedside ultrasound you diagnose a twin pregnancy. There are two gestational sacs with a lambda sign. The patient asks if the twins are genetically "identical." When do you tell her is the best time to diagnose chorionicity?
    a. Chorionicity is best assessed at birth with visual inspection of the placenta.
    b. Chorionicity is best assessed in the third trimester at the time of the anatomy ultrasound.
    c. Chorionicity is best assessed in the first trimester.
    d. Chorionicity is best assessed by both first trimester ultrasound and noninvasive prenatal testing.
    e. Chorionicity is best assessed in the third trimester.

Disorders at the Maternal-Fetal Interface

38

Prevention and Management of Preterm Parturition

RUPSA C. BOELIG | VINCENZO BERGHELLA | HYAGRIV N. SIMHAN

(see *Creasy and Resnik's Maternal-Fetal Medicine, 9e: Ch 38*)

Summary

Preterm birth is the leading cause of perinatal and infant mortality for infants born to women of all races and ethnic backgrounds, particularly for non-Hispanic black women. Like other multifactorial disorders, spontaneous preterm birth is preceded by the interaction of multiple endogenous and exogenous factors. The complexity of spontaneous preterm birth is such that there are no single prediction, prevention, and treatment options. In this chapter, we describe the use of historical and clinical factors, as well as biochemical and imaging clinical tools to delineate preterm birth risk and guide use of therapies to reduce the risk of preterm birth or ameliorate its consequences.

PRIMARY PREVENTION OF PRETERM BIRTH

Primary prevention of preterm birth includes strategies that can be employed universally either before or early in pregnancy to prevent development of disease processes that lead to preterm birth. Screening for specific risk factors that warrant intervention include the following:

- Prior spontaneous preterm birth: This identifies patients who may benefit from progesterone therapy, cervical length screening, and/or cerclage. Singleton pregnancies with a history of spontaneous preterm birth would benefit from progesterone therapy (vaginal progesterone daily or 17-hydroxyprogesterone caproate weekly) from 16–36 weeks. Additionally, those with a history of cervical insufficiency or prior cerclage may benefit from cerclage placement or serial cervical length screening in the current pregnancy. Certain patients may be candidates for abdominal cerclage placement before the next pregnancy.
- Preeclampsia risk: Multiple risk factors for preeclampsia, a leading cause of indicated preterm birth, can identify patients who would benefit from low-dose aspirin prophylaxis to reduce the risk of preeclampsia and preterm birth.
- Medical comorbidities: Optimizing medical comorbidities before pregnancy, such as chronic hypertension or diabetes, reduces the risk of perinatal complications including preterm birth.
- Smoking: Smoking is a leading risk factor for preterm birth. Smoking cessation before pregnancy is an important modifiable risk factor to reduce the risk of preterm birth.
- Multiple gestation: For patients seeking assisted reproductive technologies to achieve pregnancy, strategies to minimize the risk for multiple gestations can help reduce the risk of preterm birth.

SECONDARY PREVENTION OF PRETERM BIRTH

Secondary prevention of preterm birth involves the use of screening strategies in pregnancy to identify early, asymptomatic disease pathology that could lead to preterm birth.

- Cervical length screening: Short cervical length in the mid-second trimester identifies individuals at increased risk of preterm birth. For singletons with a prior preterm birth, serial cervical length screening from 16–24 weeks is recommended, and a cervical length <25 mm is an indication for cerclage. For singletons without prior preterm birth, one-time cervical assessment is suggested at 18–22 weeks at the time of anatomic survey, and cervical length ≤25 mm is an indication for vaginal progesterone therapy. A short cervical length in a twin gestation is also a possible indication for vaginal progesterone therapy; the benefit of cerclage in this setting is unclear.
- Cervical dilation: Regardless of pregnancy history, asymptomatic midtrimester cervical dilation in a singleton or twin gestation is an indication to consider exam-indicated cerclage, which has been demonstrated to increase latency to delivery.

TERTIARY PREVENTION OF PRETERM BIRTH

Tertiary prevention strategies for preterm birth prevention are limited. Once the diagnosis of preterm labor is made, there are no therapies that reduce the risk of preterm birth, but some interventions may increase latency and/or reduce neonatal morbidity.

- Diagnosis of preterm labor: A combination of cervical examination, cervico-vaginal fetal fibronectin (fFN), uterine tocodynamometry, and cervical length ultrasound can be used as adjunctive tools to delineate the risk of preterm delivery.
- Strategies to reduce neonatal morbidity:
  - Antenatal corticosteroids: A 48-hour course of betamethasone or dexamethasone has been demonstrated to reduce neonatal morbidity and mortality in the event of preterm delivery <34 weeks.
  - Magnesium sulfate: An intravenous bolus (4 gm or 6 gm) and then continuous infusion (1–2 gm/hour) for patients at risk for imminent preterm birth <32 weeks' gestation reduces the risk of cerebral palsy.
  - Tocolytics: Tocolytic therapy (nifedipine or indomethacin most commonly) is effective in delaying delivery up to 48 hours to achieve a complete course of antenatal corticosteroids but does not prevent preterm delivery. Beta-mimetics are effective tocolytics and increase latency to delivery; however, they are associated with more significant adverse events and are not preferred agents.

QUESTIONS

1. A 35-year-old G2P0010 has a transvaginal ultrasound cervical length (TVU CL) of 20 mm at her 20-week anatomy scan. She is asymptomatic and does not have a prior spontaneous preterm birth (SPTB). The next best step in management is:
   a. cerclage
   b. vaginal progesterone
   c. pessary
   d. activity restriction

2. A 28-year-old G2P0100 has a TVU CL of 20 mm at her 20-week anatomy scan. She is asymptomatic and does have a prior SPTB, for which she is on 17-alpha hydroxy-progesterone caproate. The next best step in management is:
   a. cerclage
   b. vaginal progesterone
   c. pessary
   d. activity restriction

3. A 21-year-old G3P0020 at 29 weeks has confirmed prelabor preterm rupture of membranes (PPROM). She is not contracting, is 2 cm dilated on speculum examination, vertex, and has received betamethasone and latency antibiotics. When she progresses to active labor, the next best step in management is:
   a. amnioinfusion
   b. magnesium sulfate
   c. extra antibiotics for presumed chorioamnionitis
   d. plan for shortened second stage

4. A 40-year-old G3P0201 presents at 28 weeks with contractions. She denies leakage of fluid, and speculum examination is negative for rupture of membranes. On the monitor, she is contracting every 5–10 minutes, is not dilated on exam, and the fetal heart tracing is category 1. To best manage her threatened preterm labor, the next best step in management is:
   a. tocolysis
   b. steroids for fetal maturity
   c. transvaginal ultrasound cervical length
   d. magnesium for neuroprotection
   e. antibiotics to increase latency

5. A 39-year-old G3P0202 presents at 36 weeks with preterm labor. Her membranes are intact, and her cervix is 4 cm dilated. Fetal presentation is vertex. Her GBS is positive as of earlier in the week. Her next best step in management is:
   a. magnesium
   b. tocolysis
   c. GBS prophylaxis
   d. caesarean section

6. A 39-year-old G10P0727 presents for a preconception consult. She had seven prior spontaneous preterm births. Her last pregnancy involved history indicated cerclage at 12 weeks and subsequent 25-week vaginal delivery after PPROM. What should be recommended before her next pregnancy to minimize the chances of a recurrent early SPTB?
   a. Antibiotics
   b. Prophylactic tocolysis
   c. Transabdominal cerclage
   d. Pessary insertion

7. A 27-year-old G1P0 at her anatomy scan inquires what guidance the American College of Obstetricians and Gynecologists and the Society for Maternal-Fetal Medicine have regarding universal transvaginal ultrasound cervical length screening. You reply that they:
   a. recommend it
   b. are against it
   c. do not have a stance on it
   d. suggest it as reasonable

8. A 38-year-old G1P0 with a dichorionic twin pregnancy has a TVU CL of 20 mm at her 20-week anatomy scan. She is asymptomatic, and on examination, the cervix is 2 cm dilated. The next best step in management is:
   a. cerclage
   b. vaginal progesterone
   c. pessary
   d. activity restriction

9. A 28-year-old G1P0 with a singleton pregnancy presents at 26 weeks with regular contractions, intact membranes, and cervical dilation of 3 cm. Which intervention has the greatest benefit to the neonate?
   a. Antenatal steroids
   b. Tocolytics
   c. Cesarean delivery
   d. Magnesium sulfate

10. A 26-year-old G3P1011 at 30 weeks has confirmed prelabor preterm rupture of membranes. The most effective therapy to maximize latency from rupture of membranes to delivery is:
    a. antibiotics
    b. tocolytics
    c. hospitalization
    d. cerclage

39

Premature (Prelabor) Rupture of the Membranes

BRIAN M. MERCER I KELLY S. GIBSON

(see Creasy and Resnik's Maternal-Fetal Medicine, 9e: Ch 39)

Summary

Rupture of the fetal membranes is an integral part of parturition at term and is expected in the process of both term and spontaneous preterm birth. Whereas membrane rupture at term usually results from progressive physiologic membrane weakening, the pathologic weakening associated with preterm premature (prelabor) rupture of the membranes before the onset of contractions ("PROM") can result from several causes. Although delivery soon after preterm PROM is often inevitable, the physician will frequently need to decide whether to actively pursue delivery or conservatively manage the pregnancy.

Active and conservative management of PROM impose both common and unique risks to the fetus and newborn, including complications resulting from immaturity, as well as from intrauterine infection, abruptio placentae, and umbilical cord accidents, which are more frequent in this setting. No single management scheme is applicable to all circumstances.

The fetal membranes consist of the amnion, which lines the amniotic cavity, and the chorion, which adheres to maternal decidua. Together, the amnion and chorion form a stronger unit than either layer individually. With advancing gestational age, physiologic membrane remodeling leads to structural weakening, which is more evident in the membranes near the internal cervical os.

Preterm PROM can arise through a number of pathways that ultimately result in accelerated membrane weakening. Urogenital tract infection and colonization have been associated with preterm PROM. Physical effects related to preterm contractions and prolapsing membranes with premature cervical dilation can predispose the fetal membranes to rupture. Clinical associations include low socioeconomic status, lean maternal body mass (<19.8 kg/m^2), nutritional deficiencies (e.g., copper, ascorbic acid), and prior cervical conization. During pregnancy, maternal cigarette smoking, the presence of a cervical cerclage, second- and third-trimester bleeding, ascending genital tract infection, acute pulmonary disease, prior episodes of preterm labor or contractions, and uterine overdistension from polyhydramnios or multiple gestations have also been linked to preterm PROM.

Considerable attention has been focused on the prediction and prevention of preterm PROM. Those who have had an early preterm birth have the highest risk for a recurrence. Identification of a short cervical length on transvaginal ultrasound also confers an increased risk. Broad-based preventive strategies such as progesterone supplementation are of uncertain efficacy. Vitamin C supplementation to prevent preterm birth resulting from PROM is not recommended.

PROM affects 8% of pregnancies at term. Preterm PROM is responsible for about one-quarter of preterm births overall. Preterm PROM is associated with brief latency from membrane rupture to delivery and, on average, latency increases with decreasing gestational age at membrane rupture.

Conservative management of PROM provides the opportunity for subclinical deciduitis to progress to overt infection and for ascending infection to occur. Placental abruption is diagnosed in 4% to 12% of pregnancies complicated by PROM and can occur before or after the onset of membrane rupture. The risks to the fetus after PROM are primarily those related to intrauterine infection, umbilical cord compression, and placental abruption. Gestational age at membrane rupture and at delivery is the primary determinant of the frequency and severity of neonatal complications after PROM. Fetal lung development and growth can be especially adversely affected when PROM occurs in the periviable period.

In more than 90% of cases, the diagnosis of PROM can be confirmed by clinical assessment, including the combination of history, clinical examination, and laboratory evaluation. If the diagnosis remains unclear after initial evaluation, documentation of oligohydramnios by ultrasound, in the absence of fetal urinary tract malformations or significant growth restriction, is suggestive of membrane rupture.

Management of PROM is based primarily on the estimated maternal, fetal, and neonatal risks with immediate delivery weighed against the potential risks and benefits of conservative management to extend the pregnancy to allow time for fetal growth and maturation. Available data indicate that women with PROM at term who are not in labor on arrival at the hospital should have labor induced, usually with an oxytocin infusion.

When a patient presents with late preterm PROM at 34 to 36 weeks, consideration should be given to assessment of fetal pulmonary maturity and active delivery if maturity is demonstrated. Many institutions do not have testing to assess fetal lung maturity. The American College of Obstetricians and Gynecologists' Practice Bulletin (2020) acknowledges that either expectant management or immediate delivery in patients with preterm PROM between 34 0/7 weeks of gestation and 36 6/7 weeks of gestation is a reasonable option if no maternal or fetal contraindications for expectant management exist. If conservative management is pursued, administration of antenatal corticosteroids to accelerate fetal maturation should be considered, as should antibiotic administration to reduce intrauterine infection. After time for fetal maturation has been achieved, delivery before the onset of overt infection may be appropriate.

With PROM and documented fetal pulmonary maturity at 32 to 33 weeks' gestation, delivery should be considered. If fetal pulmonary testing reveals an immature result, amniotic fluid cannot be obtained for assessment, or fetal lung maturity testing is unavailable, conservative management with antenatal corticosteroid administration for fetal maturation and antibiotics to reduce the risk of intrauterine infection during conservative management is an appropriate choice. Delivery should be considered after antenatal corticosteroid benefit has been achieved.

Patients with PROM between 23 and 31 weeks' gestation should usually be managed expectantly to prolong pregnancy unless there is evidence of intrauterine infection, suspected placental abruption, advanced labor, or nonreassuring fetal testing.

Conservative management of preterm PROM includes initial continuous fetal heart rate and maternal contraction monitoring to assess fetal well-being and identify occult contractions and evidence of umbilical cord compression.

A single course of antenatal corticosteroids should be considered if conservative management is pursued. Betamethasone (2 doses of 12 mg IM, given 24 h apart) or dexamethasone (4 doses of 6 mg IM, given 12 h apart) is considered appropriate. Antibiotic therapy is given during conservative management of preterm PROM to treat or prevent ascending decidual infection in order to prolong pregnancy and to reduce gestational age–dependent morbidity while limiting the risk for neonatal infection. Broad-spectrum antibiotic (ampicillin/amoxicillin plus erythromycin) therapy prolongs pregnancy before 32 weeks sufficiently to reduce neonatal gestational age–dependent morbidities and reduce the frequencies of maternal and neonatal infections. Administration of magnesium sulfate to improve long-term infant outcomes is recommended when preterm PROM occurs before 32 weeks' gestation, regardless of attempts at conservative management.

Pending further study, tocolysis and progesterone therapy for pregnancy prolongation are not advised during conservative management of preterm PROM. Cerclage retention after preterm PROM has not been shown to improve perinatal outcomes, and there are potential risks related to leaving the cerclage in situ. Removal is recommended when PROM occurs.

QUESTIONS

1. Management of PROM is based primarily on the estimated risks for fetal and neonatal complications. Providers must weigh immediate delivery against conservative management to extend the pregnancy after membrane rupture. This management should:
   a. Be uniform for all pregnancies, regardless of gestational age
   b. Take into consideration local and regional factors, as well as the gestational age
   c. Be based only on the gestational age at presentation
   d. Attempt conservative management for women at high risk for intrauterine infection and at advanced gestational age

2. A 27-year-old G2P0010 presents at 40.2 weeks' gestation complaining of leaking fluid. The examination is consistent with PROM. The patient's cervix is closed, and no contractions are palpated or seen on the tocometer. The fetal tracing is reactive and reassuring. The group B strep culture was negative 4 weeks ago. You recommend:
   a. Expectant management. You discharge the patient home to await labor and lower the risk of needing a cesarean delivery.
   b. Induction of labor. You recommend a Foley bulb, as multiple studies have shown this significantly shortens the time to delivery.
   c. Induction of labor. You recommend prostaglandins but you do inform the patient of the increased risk of chorioamnionitis and neonatal intensive care unit admission with prostaglandin use.
   d. Induction of labor. You recommend oxytocin, as it is associated with lower risks of chorioamnionitis and neonatal antibiotic therapy.

3. The most common acute neonatal morbidity after conservatively managed previable preterm premature rupture of membranes is:
   a. Respiratory distress syndrome
   b. Intraventricular hemorrhage
   c. Sepsis
   d. Bronchopulmonary dysplasia

4. A multiparous patient is admitted for preterm PROM and is a candidate for expectant management. You are writing orders for antibiotics and select the option of 2 gm ampicillin every 6 hours and 250 mg of erythromycin every 6 hours for 48 hours, followed by 250 mg of amoxicillin PO every 8 hours and 333 mg of enteric-coated erythromycin base PO every 8 hours for 5 days. You counsel the patient that this regimen has been associated with:
   a. Increased likelihood of continued pregnancy after 3 days of treatment by fivefold
   b. Latency of only the week of the treatment with no continued benefit
   c. Reduced incidence of one or more major infant morbidities (death, respiratory distress syndrome, intraventricular hemorrhage)
   d. Reduction in chorioamnionitis, neonatal sepsis, and pneumonia only in those who were Group B *Streptococcus* carriers

5. Select the statement below that is false.
   a. Administration of magnesium sulfate for neuroprotection is recommended, if feasible, for patients presenting with PROM before 32 weeks' gestation, regardless of the decision for conservative management.
   b. The use of tocolysis therapy for pregnancy prolongation is recommended during conservative management of preterm PROM to allow for antenatal corticosteroid administration.
   c. Antenatal corticosteroids are effective for induction of fetal pulmonary maturity without increasing the risk for infection; therefore, a single course of antenatal corticosteroids should be considered when preterm PROM occurs before 34 weeks' gestation if conservative management is pursued.
   d. Because cerclage retention after PROM has not been shown to improve perinatal outcomes and there are potential risks related to leaving the cerclage in situ, removal is recommended when PROM occurs.

6. A 42-year-old G4P0030 presents at 18.6 weeks with preterm PROM. When discussing management options, the patient expresses a desire for expectant management. You inform the patient that:
   a. The abnormal maternal serum AFP result at 17 weeks has been associated with improved outcomes with expectantly managed previable PROM.
   b. You recommend admission now until delivery for bedrest and pelvic rest.
   c. You recommend serial ultrasound evaluation of the amniotic fluid, as persistent, severe oligohydramnios is the strongest predictor of subsequent lethal pulmonary hypoplasia.
   d. She should have a consult with your fetal surgery colleagues to discuss membrane resealing agents.

7. You are admitting a patient for conservative management of preterm PROM. While reviewing the orders with the resident, you review your rationale for fetal monitoring by explaining that:
   a. Nonstress testing is performed to assess fetal well-being and identify placental abruption or cord prolapse.
   b. Fetal assessment should be performed continuously for those with initially reassuring test results.
   c. Biophysical profile assessment can identify subtle changes in the fetal heart rate and well-being.
   d. A nonreactive result for a nonstress test and a biophysical profile score of 6 or less within 24 hours of delivery have been associated with perinatal infection.

8. A patient is transferred at 26.3 weeks for possible preterm PROM. Before transfer she was given a dose of betamethasone and started on magnesium sulfate. As her initial evaluation was inconclusive, you offer an amniocentesis and dye study. During the amniocentesis, before installation of the dye, a small sample of fluid is collected. Which of the following scenarios would be least concerning for an intrauterine infection?
   a. Shortly after the procedure, the patient develops fever above 38.0°C (100.4°F) with uterine tenderness and fetal tachycardia in the absence of another evident source of infection
   b. A glucose concentration of 11 mg/dL
   c. A Gram stain positive for bacteria
   d. A cell count with 44 red cells and 100 leukocytes

9. The best predictor of the frequency and severity of neonatal complications after premature rupture of membranes is
   a. Gestational age
   b. Length of the latency period
   c. Fetal sex
   d. Maternal age

40

Clinical Aspects of Normal and Abnormal Labor (Summary)

CLAIRE E. JENSEN

(see Creasy and Resnik's Maternal-Fetal Medicine, 9e: Ch. 40)

Summary

Understanding normal labor is considered foundational knowledge for all obstetricians. Defining the first and second stages of labor was conventionally described by Friedman but revised by contemporary researchers including Zhang's group to reflect slower progression of the first and second stages, likely at least in part due to increasing average maternal age and body mass index (BMI) at delivery. A partogram is a useful instrument to assess labor progression and has been shown to decrease prolonged labor, frequency of emergency abdominal delivery, and use of oxytocin augmentation.

First-stage abnormalities include prolonged, protracted, or arrest disorders. Prolonged latent phase is defined as 20 hours for primiparous patients and 14 hours for multiparous patients, and it is associated with excessive sedation, early epidural placement, unfavorable Bishop score, or myometrial dysfunction. Interventions include therapeutic narcosis, oxytocin augmentation, and active labor management. Protraction disorders are associated with cephalopelvic disproportion, conduction anesthesia, fetal malposition, and differences in cervical collagen content. Arrest is defined by no cervical change for 4 hours despite adequate uterine contractions (>200 Montevideo units in 10 minutes) or for 6 hours if inadequate contractions.

Second-stage abnormalities include abnormalities of rotation, descent, and shoulder dystocia. Half of shoulder dystocia cases occur in infants whose birth weight is less than 4000 grams (g), and brachial plexus injury of the infant is a serious complication. A Cochrane review does not support labor induction to prevent shoulder dystocia because of suspected macrosomia. When diagnosed, a coordinated team response and use of several standard maneuvers including McRoberts, suprapubic pressure, Rubin, Woods, posterior arm delivery, or Zavenelli may be effective.

Third-stage abnormalities include retained placenta, postpartum hemorrhage, and uterine inversion. Retained placenta is diagnosed if the placenta has not delivered within 30 minutes, after which manual removal is recommended. Postpartum hemorrhage is most likely due to atony if vaginal and cervical lacerations and coagulopathy are excluded. First-line treatment for prevention and treatment of hemorrhage is oxytocin, followed by uterotonics, intrauterine tamponade, selective embolization of pelvic vessels, or laparotomy. Uterine inversion requires prompt diagnosis, adequate tocolysis and analgesia, and reinversion via the Johnson method or, if unsuccessful, laparotomy.

Induction of labor has many medical, obstetric, and fetal indications, and there is mounting evidence to support elective induction beginning at 39 weeks, 0 days, most recently through the ARRIVE Trial. This study demonstrated that nulliparous patients undergoing induction in the 39th week compared with the 41st week had a lower chance of cesarean delivery regardless of initial Bishop score, maternal BMI, or receipt of midwifery care.

Fetal malpresentation can be a contraindication to labor and can also contribute to first- and second-stage abnormalities. Singleton breech presentation is generally an indication for a planned cesarean delivery if external version is unsuccessful, although among well-counseled patients meeting strict eligibility criteria, breech vaginal delivery may be attempted by an experienced obstetrician. External version may be offered in a hospital setting for breech presentation or transverse lie at or beyond 36 weeks' gestation, following administration of a tocolytic. If external version for transverse lie is unsuccessful, cesarean delivery is indicated, and use of a low vertical, classical, or high transverse uterine incision may be necessary for shoulder or back-down presentation. Brow presentation is not a contraindication to labor but is associated with an increased risk of first- and second- stage abnormalities. If persistent, mentum posterior and brow presentations are indications for cesarean delivery rather than expectant management, manual rotation, or rotational operative delivery.

The most common indications for cesarean delivery include labor dystocia, repeat cesarean delivery, breech presentation, fetal distress, and maternal request. Serious intraoperative complications such as anesthesia complications, hemorrhage, bowel or bladder injury, thromboembolic disease, and amniotic fluid or air embolism occur in 2% of cases. Surgical site infections are minimized via preoperative administration of both a cephalosporin and azithromycin. There is no long-term difference in pelvic floor dysfunction compared with spontaneous vaginal delivery. The goal prevalence for cesarean delivery by the World Health Organization (WHO) is 10% to 15%; however, this has not been achieved in part due to increasing frequency of advanced maternal age, increased maternal BMI, fetal macrosomia, gestational diabetes, multiple gestation, labor dystocia, medicolegal considerations, and changing practices surrounding trials of labor after cesarean delivery.

Forceps-assisted vaginal delivery may be performed if the leading point of the fetal skull is at +2 station (low forceps) or on the pelvic floor (outlet forceps), but midforceps is associated with lower neonatal cord pH values and a higher risk of fetal injury. Vacuum extraction has similar indications as forceps delivery but is shown to be associated with less maternal pelvic trauma, increased risk of neonatal cephalohematoma and retinal hemorrhage, and increased failure, particularly with soft extractor cups. Maternal and neonatal morbidity are increased if delivery is attempted with vacuum and forceps sequentially. Vacuum extraction can be an attractive option due to ease of provider training and need for less maternal anesthesia compared with forceps.

A labor doula reduces the need for analgesia and anesthesia and may reduce the incidence of protraction and arrest disorders. Options for analgesia include sedatives and narcotics, which reduce anxiety and result in sedation but do not relieve labor pain. Local anesthesia includes pudendal and, paracervical blocks. Spinal anesthesia is associated with sympathetic blockade, which can contribute to maternal hypotension and decreased maternal pushing effort. Epidural anesthesia, using a combination of local anesthetic and narcotic, provides analgesia with less motor blockade but can result in a longer second stage, instrument-assisted delivery, and intrapartum fever after 5 hours of infusion. Prehydration and ephedrine administration for hypotensive episodes can decrease uteroplacental insufficiency.

QUESTIONS

1. Which is true about contemporary labor curves, as described by Zhang et al.?
   a. The transition from latent to active labor is reflected by an abrupt change in slope of the curve.
   b. The average length of active labor is 5.5 hours.
   c. There is a deceleration phase in active labor.
   d. In the normal active phase, >2 hours without cervical dilation is considered active phase arrest.
   e. In the normal active phase, the fifth percentile for rate of dilation is <1.2 cm/hr.

2. A 27-year-old G1P0 at 38 weeks' gestation with painful contractions occurring every 4 minutes and lasting 30 seconds for the past 21 hours is found to be 1 cm dilated, 50% effaced, and at −2 station on vaginal examination. Her fetus is cephalic, fetal heart rate tracing is normal, and her examination is unchanged after 2 hours. There are no maternal or fetal complications in the pregnancy. What is the best next step?
   a. Observe and reassess in 2 hours.
   b. Discharge to home with return precautions.
   c. Offer augmentation of labor with a Foley bulb.
   d. Offer therapeutic narcosis.
   e. Offer an epidural for labor analgesia.

3. A 35-year-old G5P3013 at 40 weeks and 2 days was admitted in spontaneous labor at 4 cm. She progressed spontaneously to 6 cm over 3 hours and remained at 6 cm for the subsequent 3 hours. Her prenatal course has been uncomplicated, and vital signs are normal. Fetal heart rate is category I, and contractions are every 2-3 minutes. What is the best next step?
   a. Augment with oxytocin.
   b. Place an intrauterine pressure catheter.
   c. No intervention is needed.
   d. Recommend a cesarean delivery for arrest of dilation.
   e. (a) and (b).

4. Which of the following complications is associated with a second stage of labor that exceeds 3 hours?
   a. Hypoxic ischemic encephalopathy
   b. Subgaleal hemorrhage
   c. Hyperbilirubinemia
   d. Shoulder dystocia
   e. Transient tachypnea of the newborn

5. What is the appropriate initial intervention for management of a shoulder dystocia?
   a. Suprapubic pressure
   b. McRobert maneuver
   c. Delivery of the posterior arm
   d. Making an episiotomy

6. A 40-year-old G2P1001 at 34 weeks, 6 days has a spontaneous vaginal delivery complicated by the need for manual removal of the placenta. The patient's prenatal course was uncomplicated and she has had one prior uncomplicated vaginal delivery. What is the most likely primary risk factor for retained placenta for this patient?
   a. Preterm delivery
   b. Placenta accreta spectrum
   c. Maternal age
   d. Multiparity

7. Which of the following criterion is required to diagnose failed induction of labor?
   a. Absence of fetal fibronectin in cervical and vaginal secretions
   b. At least 12 hours of oxytocin stimulation after membrane rupture without cervical dilation
   c. More than 24 hours of cervical ripening
   d. Any induction of labor that results in a cesarean delivery
   e. None of the above

8. Which dating criterion would be required for a candidate for induction of labor?
   a. A self-reported ovulation date
   b. Third-trimester uterine size was consistent with estimated gestational dates
   c. Sonographic estimation of gestational age performed before 20 weeks' gestation
   d. Self-reported conception date
   e. Third-trimester femur length

9. A 29-year-old G1P0 at 36 weeks, 4 days has a singleton fetus in complete breech presentation, posterior placenta, maximum vertical pocket of 1.5 cm, estimated fetal weight of 3000 g, and fetal heart rate of 150 beats per minute. Which of the following is the best next step?
   a. External cephalic version
   b. Primary cesarean delivery at 37 weeks' gestation
   c. Primary cesarean delivery before 40 weeks' gestation
   d. Breech vaginal delivery criteria

10. A 32-year-old patient presents in labor with a fetus in breech presentation. Which of the following conditions would be a contraindication for a vaginal breech delivery?
    a. Complete breech presentation
    b. Estimated fetal weight of 2600 g
    c. Gynecoid pelvis
    d. Skilled obstetrician
    e. Extended fetal head

11. Which is not a relative contraindication to external cephalic version?
    a. Prior cesarean delivery
    b. Suspected fetal macrosomia
    c. Uterine anomalies
    d. Third-trimester bleeding

12. A 30-year-old G1P0 at 38 weeks, 5 days is admitted for spontaneous labor. Prenatal course is uncomplicated, fetal heart rate is category I, and she is contracting every 3 minutes. Compared with using intravenous fentanyl for labor analgesia, an epidural is more likely to result in which of the following?
    a. More likely to have a spontaneous vaginal delivery
    b. More likely to have a shorter duration of labor
    c. Less likely to have an instrument-assisted delivery
    d. Less likely to have an intrapartum fever
    e. Less likely to have maternal sedation

13. Which contraindication to operative vaginal delivery is unique to vacuum extraction?
    a. Station is above +2 cm
    b. Gestational age less than 34 weeks
    c. Face or brow presentation
    d. Incompletely dilated cervix
    e. Cephalopelvic disproportion

14. Compared with cesarean delivery, which outcome is associated with term, vertex low, or outlet forceps-assisted vaginal delivery?
    a. Decreased neonatal respiratory morbidity
    b. Decreased neonatal birth trauma
    c. Decreased maternal wound complications
    d. Decreased postpartum hemorrhage
    e. All of the above

15. A 31-year-old G3P2002 undergoing a trial of labor after cesarean has an arrest of dilation. Intraoperatively, a uterine wound dehiscence was incidentally noted, and the uterus was repaired with a two-layer closure. What risk factor in this patient is associated with an increased rate of uterine wound dehiscence?
    a. Intended route of delivery
    b. Presence of unknown type of scar
    c. Use of oxytocin for labor augmentation
    d. None of the above

Recurrent Pregnancy Loss

MEREDITH HUMPHREYS I D. WARE BRANCH

(see Creasy and Resnik's Maternal-Fetal Medicine, 9e: Ch 41)

Summary

Early pregnancy loss is a common reproductive complication. Recurrent pregnancy loss (RPL), defined as two or more failed clinical pregnancies, occurs in 1% to 2% of couples. Most pregnancy losses occur in the preembryonic or embryonic period.

Practitioners should refer to professional guidelines for appropriate evaluation and management of couples with RPL (Table 41.1). Prudence calls for taking a careful medical and social history. Both the American Society for Reproductive Medicine (ASRM) and European Society of Human Reproduction and Embryology (ESHRE) guidelines recommend evaluation of the uterine cavity, screening for antiphospholipid antibodies, and screening for thyroid disorders. In addition, ASRM guidelines recommend parental karyotype analysis, assessment for diabetes, and serum prolactin. ESHRE guidelines recommend testing for anti–thyroid peroxidase (TPO) antibodies but recommend against routine parental karyotype testing or routine testing for diabetes and prolactin abnormalities. Testing for hereditary thrombophilia is not recommended, nor is testing for immunologic abnormalities other than antiphospholipid antibodies. Chromosomal microarray analysis of products of conception in a recurrent miscarriage is a plausible, utilitarian approach in the evaluation of a patient having a second miscarriage that, if abnormal, may avoid further workup.

About 10% of women with RPL will be found to have a müllerian anomaly. Robust evidence that metroplasty (e.g., for uterine septum) is efficacious with regard to avoiding miscarriage is lacking, though most experts support septum takedown in women with RPL. Women with repeatedly positive antiphospholipid antibodies meeting international criteria should be treated with a heparin agent and low-dose aspirin in pregnancy. If found, endocrine disorders should be treated appropriately. Couples found to be carriers of a balanced chromosomal anomaly should seek preconception genetic counseling. In vitro fertilization with preimplantation genetic testing is an option, but in the majority of cases the prognosis for live birth from a natural conception is modestly good. Retrospective studies indicate that eventual live birth rates are similar to comparable couples with RPL not due to karyotype abnormalities. There may be a contributory, causative role in RPL for maternal use of caffeine, alcohol, tobacco, and illicit substances, as well as maternal obesity. Preconception consultation allows an opportunity to screen for these factors and recommend affected women with RPL undertake healthy lifestyle modifications.

At least 50% of couples evaluated for RPL are found to have no single, dominant etiology. The prognosis for live birth in such cases is largely favorable, with maternal age and the number of prior losses being important prognostic factors. In contrast, available evidence holds that otherwise unexplained fetal death between 10 weeks and before 20 weeks of gestation has a less favorable prognosis.

QUESTIONS

1. A 30-year-old G3P0030 woman is referred by her primary obstetrician-gynecologist to a Reproductive Endocrinology and Infertility specialist for consultation regarding RPL. She undergoes evaluation including thorough history and physical, saline sonohysterogram, laboratory workup, and karyotype for both partners, and no apparent etiology is found. The couple is dismayed that no specific etiology is found. You explain that this is the case in at least what percentage of evaluated patients?
   a. 10%
   b. 35%
   c. 50%
   d. 80%

2. A 36-year-old G3P0020 presents to her obstetrician for her first visit after finding out she is pregnant. She has regular 28-day cycles and has a sure last menstrual period dating her 8w1d, which is confirmed with bedside ultrasound. Her medical history is positive for well-controlled asthma, and her gyn surgical history includes a dilation and curettage (D&C) for her last miscarriage. She has no drug allergies, takes a prenatal vitamin daily, and uses an albuterol inhaler about once a month. She asks about any other medications she should be using given her history of two miscarriages. Which of the following is true regarding the use of progesterone?
   a. All women with a history of two or three prior miscarriages should receive progesterone.
   b. The efficacy of treatment with progesterone in women with RPL remains a matter of considerable debate.
   c. Professional guidelines recommend evaluation for possible luteal phase defect (LPD) and treatment with progesterone if LPD is identified.
   d. Progesterone supplementation is contraindicated in the first trimester of pregnancy.

TABLE 41.1	Recommended Evaluations in Couples With Recurrent Early Pregnancy Loss		
			Comments
Known or suspected cause	Specific tests or assessments	ASRM guidelines	ESHRE guidelines
History and selected physical examination	Maternal age; details of and number of prior losses; BMI; social habits		
Uterine anomalies or defects	Options: • 3D ultrasound of uterus • Sonohysterography • Hysterosalpingography • Magnetic resonance imaging	Recommended	Transvaginal 3D US preferred due to high sensitivity and specificity, and can distinguish between septate uterus and bicorporeal uterus with normal cervix (former AFS bicornuate uterus).
Cytogenetic	Parental karyotypes Products of conception array-CGH	Recommended Cytogenetic analysis of subsequent losses can be employed to evaluate whether the event was random and may be of psychologic value to the couple.	Parental karyotyping is not routinely recommended in couples due to low yield in couples without a history of a genetically abnormal fetus/newborn or a child with congenital anomalies. Individual risk assessment recommended. Genetic analysis of pregnancy tissue is not routinely recommended but it may be performed for explanatory purposes.
Autoimmune	Antiphospholipid antibodies • LA • aCL IgG and IgM • anti-β_2-glycoprotein I (aβ2GPI) IgG and IgM	Recommended. Other autoantibody tests (e.g., ANA are not generally recommended).	Screening for LA and aCL IgG and IgM recommended. Screening for aβ2GPI may be considered. Other autoantibody tests such as ANA and celiac disease markers not recommended.
Endocrinologic disorders	TSH Diabetes screen Prolactin	TSH recommended. Testing for anti-thyroid antibodies not recommended. Hemoglobin A1c (HgbA1c) recommended. Recommended.	TSH and TPO antibodies recommended. Abnormal TSH and TPO-antibody levels should be followed up by T4 testing. Assessment of fasting glucose (or insulin) not recommended. Prolactin testing is not recommended in women with RPL in the absence of clinical symptoms of hyperprolactinemia (oligo/amenorrhea).

3D, 3-dimensional; aCL, anticardiolipin; AFS, American Fertility Society; ASRM, American Society for Reproductive Medicine; BMI, body mass index; CGH, comparative genomic hybridization; ESHRE, European Society of Human Reproduction and Embryology; LA, lupus anticoagulant; RPL, recurrent pregnancy loss; TPO, thyroid pyroxidase; TSH, thyroid-stimulating hormone; US, ultrasonography.

3. A 37-year-old G2P0020 has a slightly elevated TSH of 5.7 mU/L and is concerned this is a cause of her RPL. The rest of her evaluation is negative. Regarding her thyroid status and RPL, which of the following is true?
   a. The American Thyroid Association recommends treatment for pregnant women with subclinical hypothyroidism as defined by thyroid-stimulating hormone (TSH) levels above trimester-specific ranges and TPO antibodies, or with TSH levels above 10.0 mU/L regardless of TPO antibody status.
   b. ESHRE guidelines recommend testing for TPO antibodies and treating with prednisone if positive.
   c. Treating with a low dose of levothyroxine is indicated because it promotes successful pregnancy.
   d. Treating with a low dose of levothyroxine is indicated because it prevents autism in the offspring.

4. A 25-year-old G2P0020 presents to the operating room for planned D&C after confirmation of missed abortion. The embryonic crown-rump length was consistent with 6w4d. This is her second pregnancy loss in the last year. You recommend she consider chromosomal microarray analysis (CMA) of the products of conception for which of the following reasons?

   a. The CMA results are unlikely to be abnormal given that the patient has RPL, but they might be.
   b. Array comparative genomic hybridization will detect triploidy if it is present.
   c. CMA might prove clinically utilitarian because many experts believe that finding a genetically abnormal conceptus abrogates the need for further evaluation after this, her second, miscarriage.
   d. CMA detects aneuploidy, though this genetic abnormality is uncommon in early miscarriages.

5. A 27-year-old G3P0030 is referred to Maternal-Fetal Medicine for evaluation after her most recent confirmed pregnancy loss, all of which occurred before 10 weeks' gestation. She has a medical history of anxiety, current body mass index of 31 kg/m^2, no past surgeries, and no known drug allergies. She takes sertraline and a prenatal vitamin daily. In her workup, which of the following regarding evaluating the uterine cavity is NOT true?
   a. Appropriate diagnostic studies include 3-D ultrasound and saline sonohysterography.
   b. She does not need evaluation of the uterine cavity because she has only preembryonic and embryonic losses.

c. Müllerian abnormalities are found in approximately 6% to 15% of women with RPL.

d. Professional guidelines suggest there is limited support for septum resection to decrease subsequent losses in women with RPL.

6. A 31-year-old G0 woman presents for a preconception counseling visit. She would like to conceive in the next year and is interested in discussing her risks associated with pregnancy. She is a healthy woman, with no significant medical or surgical history. She is currently using a copper intrauterine device for contraception. Her 73-year-old father had a stroke about 2 years ago and was found to be heterozygous for factor V Leiden. The patient was subsequently tested and was found to be heterozygous as well. Regarding this issue, which of the following is most accurate?
   a. Factor V Leiden is conclusively shown to be associated with miscarriage.
   b. The patient should also be tested for tetrahydrofolate reductase gene mutations.
   c. Professional guidelines recommend routinely testing women with RPL for inherited thrombophilia.
   d. A decision to use heparin chemoprophylaxis in her pregnancy should be based on an assessment of the patient's risk for thromboembolism.

7. A 32-year-old G2P0110 presents to labor and delivery for induction after she was diagnosed with an intrauterine fetal demise at 15–16 weeks' gestation. The fetus appeared morphologically normal at the time of the ultrasonic diagnosis of fetal demise. The patient has no significant medical history, and her thorough evaluation for causes of fetal death have proved negative. What is the most accurate statement regarding the likelihood of the patient's next pregnancy ending in midtrimester fetal demise?
   a. About 5%–10%
   b. About 20%–25%
   c. Negligible
   d. Perhaps as high as 55%–75%

8. A 32-year-old G4P1031 presents to her obstetrician-gynecologist's office for a preconception visit. She has a history of one-term vaginal delivery and three prior miscarriages before 10 weeks' gestation, one of which was managed with D&C. Her medical history is significant for class III obesity and subclinical hypothyroidism. Her thorough workup has proven negative, and the CMA from her last miscarriage found a normal 46,XY result. Which of the following is this patient's most likely risk factor for recurrent euploid miscarriage?
   a. Obesity
   b. There is no increased risk
   c. Subclinical hypothyroidism
   d. Prior D&C

9. A 38-year-old G3P1021 of Swedish descent presents to her high-risk obstetrician's office for preconception counseling in the setting of two prior first-trimester losses and one term delivery of a male. She is a healthy person, though in the past she was found to be weakly antinuclear antibody (ANA) positive. She would like at least two more children. What is her indication for human leukocyte antigen (HLA) status testing?
   a. Her RPL; professional guidelines suggest that all couples with RPL should undergo HLA testing.
   b. The fact that she is ANA positive.
   c. ESHRE conditionally recommends determination of HLA class II (HLA-DRB1*15:01 and HLA-DQB1*05:01/05:2) status in Scandinavian women with RPL after the birth of a boy.
   d. To determine if she and her spouse are HLA compatible.

10. Which of the following is not routinely recommended by both the ASRM and ESHRE guidelines in the evaluation of couples with RPL?
    a. Parental karyotyping
    b. Evaluation for uterine anomalies or defects
    c. Testing for antiphospholipid antibodies
    d. TSH testing

Stillbirth

LENA C. SWEENEY | UMA M. REDDY

(see *Creasy and Resnik's Maternal-Fetal Medicine, 9e: Ch 42*)

Summary

Stillbirth is defined as fetal death at 20 weeks of gestation or greater; 98% of them occur in low- and middle-income countries. The stillbirth rate in the United States is 6 per 1000 births equally distributed between "early" (20–27 weeks) and "late" (28 weeks or greater). The rate is higher than most other high-income countries and has remained relatively stable for decades.

Risk factors for stillbirth include race (higher rates in non-Hispanic black and Hispanic people are multifactorial and incompletely understood), extremes of maternal age (<15 and ≥35 years), extremes of parity (one prior pregnancy conveys lowest risk), multiple gestation, and assisted reproductive technology (particularly in vitro fertilization). Obesity and tobacco/drug use increase risk with dose-response relationship. Prior stillbirth is associated with a higher rate of stillbirth but is at least partially related to increased risk of pregnancy complications such as preeclampsia and abruption. Stillbirth risk is also increased with prior delivery of a preterm or growth restricted infant.

Stillbirth classification is important but difficult. Systems with more detail favor accuracy but apply less broadly.

Pathogenesis (cause of stillbirth) in a large American cohort with comprehensive stillbirth evaluation was attributed as follows: 29% obstetric conditions, 24% placental abnormalities, 14% fetal genetic/structural abnormalities, 13% infection, 10% umbilical cord abnormalities, 9% hypertensive disorders, and 8% other maternal medical conditions. Twenty-five percent remained unexplained.

Infection is more common in low-income countries and more frequently found in early stillbirths. Ascending or hematogenous infection causes maternal illness, preterm birth, and fetal or placental inflammation and dysfunction. Pathogens include bacteria (group B *Streptococcus, Escherichia coli, Listeria,* syphilis, malaria) and viruses (parvovirus, cytomegalovirus, Zika virus, SARS-CoV-2).

Maternal conditions cause and contribute to stillbirth, often related to degree of control. Hypertensive disorders of pregnancy are most risky if severe disease or underlying chronic hypertension is present. Pregestational diabetes is a greater risk when associated with poor glycemic control and resultant fetopathy, placental insufficiency, and labor complications. Well-controlled gestational diabetes overall is not associated with increased risk. Increased stillbirth risk in thyroid disease is seen only with fetal thyrotoxicosis (Graves disease) and overt hypothyroidism. Active systemic lupus erythematosus increases risk, especially with SS-A/Ro and SS-B/La or antiphospholipid antibodies. Renal impairment, particularly if severe or complicated by hypertension, increases risk, which is mitigated by successful transplant. Intrahepatic cholestasis of pregnancy increases risk with serum bile acids ≥100 μmol/L. Antiphospholipid syndrome (APS) can cause stillbirth, but no other coagulopathies or thrombophilias clearly relate to stillbirth risk.

Fetal conditions include red blood cell and platelet alloimmunization, fetomaternal hemorrhage, and heterogeneous structural abnormalities. Genetic etiologies are especially important to investigate, particularly with concurrent malformations, and include aneuploidy (most commonly trisomy 21 and monosomy X), confined placental mosaicism (particularly trisomy 16), and single-gene disorders (such as prolonged QT syndrome). Fetal growth restriction, particularly if severe or with concurrent conditions, and being large for gestational age increase risk. Placental abnormalities include abruption (considered causative if >75% of the placenta is disrupted), insufficiency, inflammation, previa, and thrombi. Umbilical cord abnormalities include vasa previa, velamentous insertion, occlusion, prolapse, torsion, and thrombosis. Isolated finding of nuchal cord or true knot is not explanatory without concurrent pathology findings. In multiple gestations, monochorionicity is particularly an increased risk, but higher rates of obstetric complications also contribute. Intrapartum stillbirth is relatively rare in high-income countries and usually occurs with severe prematurity or rare labor complications.

Diagnosis and evaluation can be difficult for providers and families. Thorough medical and obstetric history is critical. The most useful testing is placental and umbilical cord pathology and fetal autopsy with limitations per family preference. Other recommended tests include genetic evaluation (amniocytes, cord segment, or internal fetal tissue specimens preferred over skin) via microarray as a first line test, with exome sequencing as indicated; flow cytometry or Kleihauer-Betke; indirect Coombs; and APS testing (anticardiolipin antibodies IgM, IgG; β2-glycoprotein antibodies IgM, IgG; lupus anticoagulant). Infectious and thrombophilia testing are not routinely recommended.

Management relies on patient preferences. Most (80%–90%) enter spontaneous labor within 2 weeks, but expectant management carries small risk of coagulopathy, limits stillbirth evaluation, and requires close monitoring. A dilation and evacuation procedure at <24 weeks has the lowest risk of complications, is more cost-effective, and is likely similar for grief response, but autopsy and bereavement options are limited and a trained provider is necessary. For labor induction <28 weeks, misoprostol is preferred; for >28 weeks, use standard obstetric protocol. Individualize with prior uterine scar given the risk uterine rupture. Misoprostol can be used <28 weeks with prior low-transverse incision. Repeat cesarean delivery is appropriate if there is a prior classical uterine incision given the potential increased risk of labor-associated rupture. Induced or spontaneous labor has high success for vaginal delivery: 98% without prior cesarean and 91% with prior cesarean. Comprehensive bereavement options, keepsake items, and psychosocial support should be offered. Follow-up for result of stillbirth evaluation and implications should be arranged.

Stillbirth prediction is difficult, as it must be universally applicable, since most stillbirths occur in patients with no risk factors. Low pregnancy-associated plasma protein-A (PAPP-A), elevated maternal serum alpha-fetoprotein (MSAFP), elevated beta−human chorionic gonadotropin (β-hCG), and abnormal uterine artery Doppler have all been associated with increased risk of stillbirth but with low positive predictive value. Increased fetal growth restriction detection via universal third-trimester assessment by ultrasound has promise but is not currently recommended. Decreased fetal movement is nonspecific but occurs more commonly with stillbirth.

Stillbirth prevention remains elusive. Improved management of underlying conditions including diabetes and hypertension decreases risk. Anticoagulation and aspirin in APS decrease risk. Low-dose aspirin may have modest benefit in at-risk women. Antepartum testing for risk factors alone has limited evidence. Currently, antepartum testing recommendations are individualized for advanced maternal age (AMA) and obesity. Utility of kick counts is unclear in low-risk patients. Elective induction of labor at 39 weeks' gestation, particularly if risk factors are present, should be considered and does not increase cesarean delivery risk.

For management of subsequent pregnancy, data are sparse but recommendations include achievement of normal maternal weight, optimization of comorbid conditions, avoidance of toxic exposures, serial ultrasound for growth ≥28 weeks, maternal monitoring of fetal movement ≥28 weeks, and antenatal testing ≥32 weeks (or earlier with concurrent conditions). Delivery should be planned at 39 0/7 if there are no other indications, and early-term delivery is appropriate with shared decision making.

QUESTIONS

1. A 45-year-old gravida 2, para 1001 at 38 weeks' gestation comes to triage with 2 days of decreased fetal movement. She has well-controlled hypothyroidism and diet-controlled gestational diabetes. Her prior pregnancy was delivered via cesarean. Her temperature is 37.2°C (99.0°F), pulse is 84/min, respirations are 16/min, and blood pressure is 112/75 mm Hg. Her abdomen is soft and nontender. Ultrasound demonstrates a fetal demise. Which of the following factors has consistently been associated with an increased risk of stillbirth?
   a. Parity
   b. Hypothyroidism
   c. Gestational diabetes
   d. Prior cesarean
   e. Maternal age

2. A 26-year-old, primigravida at 34 weeks' gestation presents for a routine prenatal visit. She has no medical history. Her midwife is unable to auscultate the fetal heart rate. An ultrasound is performed and demonstrates a fetus measuring 30 weeks in breech presentation with no fetal cardiac activity. Her temperature is 37°C (98.6°F), pulse is 100/min, respirations are 18/min, and blood pressure is 160/94 mm Hg. Her cervix is closed and long. Which of the following is the most appropriate next step in management?
   a. Send her home to await labor
   b. High-dose misoprostol
   c. Mechanical ripening and oxytocin (Pitocin)
   d. Dilation and evacuation
   e. Cesarean delivery

3. A 30-year-old gravida 4, para 2, is diagnosed with stillbirth at 26 weeks' gestation. She has a history of hypertension on no medications. She denies any serious illness or toxic exposures during pregnancy. She works as a daycare teacher. She undergoes induction and delivers a hydropic fetus with a nuchal cord. On autopsy, the fetus has findings of severe anemia and myocarditis. The placenta is hydropic. Which of the following is most likely to definitively establish the cause of stillbirth?
   a. Travel history
   b. Maternal Coombs testing
   c. Maternal infectious serologies
   d. Histologic staining of placenta
   e. Umbilical cord pathology

4. A 19-year-old primigravida is diagnosed with a stillbirth at 37 weeks. She had an amniocentesis during the pregnancy with a prenatal diagnosis of trisomy 21. She is otherwise healthy. She is group B *Streptococcus* positive and is not treated. She undergoes induction and has an uncomplicated delivery. She develops gestational hypertension 8 days postpartum. Her placental pathology demonstrates abruption of 30% of the placental surface and mild inflammatory changes. What is the most likely etiology of the stillbirth?
   a. Fetal aneuploidy
   b. Maternal age
   c. Gestational hypertension
   d. Placenta abruption
   e. Ascending infection

5. A 38-year-old gravida 5, para 1, presents to the emergency department for vaginal spotting and contractions at 36 weeks. She has a history of asthma, type 2 diabetes, and stage 1 diabetic nephropathy. She had one uncomplicated full-term vaginal delivery and three early pregnancy losses. Her temperature is 37.5°C (99.5°F), pulse is 97/min, respirations are 16/min, and blood pressure is 128/81 mm Hg. Pelvic examination demonstrates scant blood and cervical dilation of 5 cm with bulging membranes. Tocometry shows regular contractions, but no fetal heart tones are auscultated. Ultrasound confirms a fetal demise and extensive placental calcifications. She wants to do everything she can to determine the cause of stillbirth. Which of the following is the least likely to be useful in her evaluation?
   a. Hemoglobin A1c
   b. Factor V Leiden mutation analysis
   c. Antiphospholipid antibody testing
   d. Flow cytometry
   e. Placental pathology

6. A 26-year-old gravida 3, para 1 presents to your office for her first prenatal visit at 12 weeks. She has a history of migraine headaches and eczema. Her BMI is 24. She had one uncomplicated full-term cesarean for breech presentation of a 2800 gm (6 lb 2 oz, 8% percentile for gestational age) boy who is healthy. Her temperature is 36.8°C (99.5°F), pulse is 78/min, respirations are 17/min, and blood pressure is 98/71 mm Hg. Her best friend recently experienced a stillbirth, and she is anxious about her risk. Which of the following should be incorporated into her pregnancy plan to screen for stillbirth risk?
   a. Thyroid-stimulating hormone
   b. Third-trimester growth ultrasound
   c. Uterine artery Doppler screening
   d. Fetal kick counts three times daily
   e. Repeat cesarean delivery at 38 weeks

7. A 28-year-old primigravida is diagnosed with a stillbirth at 35 weeks. Her BMI is 37. She has a history of polycystic ovarian syndrome and was hospitalized for pyelonephritis during this pregnancy. She had normal fetal anatomy on ultrasound and low-risk aneuploidy screening. Her younger brother has severe developmental delay, and her mother was recently diagnosed with diabetes. She is interested in all recommended testing to determine the cause of stillbirth including genetic evaluation. Which of the following is the least useful type of specimen to collect for genetic testing?
   a. Amniotic fluid
   b. Placental block
   c. Umbilical cord segment
   d. Fetal skin section
   e. Fetal patellar tissue

8. A 30-year-old gravida 1, para 1 presents to your office for consultation. She has a history of systemic lupus erythematosus, chronic kidney disease on hemodialysis, hypertension, and anemia. Her last lupus flare was 8 months ago. She currently uses hydroxychloroquine, azathioprine, and labetalol. Her prior pregnancy resulted in a stillbirth at 25 weeks' gestation. A severely growth-restricted fetus was delivered via an uncomplicated dilation and evacuation in the setting of preeclampsia with severe features requiring maternal intensive care unit admission. Which of the following is advisable preconception to reduce her stillbirth risk in subsequent pregnancy?
   a. Discontinue azathioprine
   b. Low-dose aspirin

   c. Prophylactic anticoagulation
   d. Iron supplementation
   e. Renal transplant

9. A 24-year-old gravida 5, para 3 presents to your office for a routine prenatal visit at 30 weeks. She has a history of Crohn disease and vitiligo. Her first two pregnancies were uncomplicated full-term vaginal deliveries. In her most recent pregnancy, she had a stillbirth at 38 weeks due to an unprovoked large-volume maternofetal hemorrhage. Prenatal care for this pregnancy has been unremarkable. Fetal growth is normal today, and she will start antenatal testing at her next visit. She sees a therapist and has initiated medications, but she has daily panic attacks and insomnia centered on her concerns about fetal well-being. She requests delivery now. When is the earliest induction of labor may be considered if this pregnancy remains uncomplicated after detailed counseling regarding neonatal risks compared with potential benefit?
   a. 35 weeks
   b. 36 weeks
   c. 37 weeks
   d. 38 weeks
   e. 39 weeks

10. A 20-year-old primigravida presents to the emergency department after a bicycle accident and is newly diagnosed with pregnancy and a stillbirth measuring 24 weeks. She has a history of depression. Her temperature is 37.1°C (98.8°F), pulse is 80/min, respirations are 15/min, and blood pressure is 110/81 mm Hg. Her abdomen is soft and nontender, and she has no vaginal bleeding. Her trauma survey is otherwise notable only for humeral fracture. Her laboratory studies demonstrate hemoglobin 13.2 (hematocrit 39.6), platelets 210, normal Kleihauer-Betke test, and normal coagulation studies. Which of the following is the most appropriate next step in management?
   a. Induction of labor
   b. Genetic counseling
   c. Consent for autopsy
   d. Toxicology testing
   e. Psychological support/services

Placenta Previa and Accreta, Vasa Previa, Subchorionic Hemorrhage, and Abruptio Placentae

ANDREW D. HULL | ROBERT RESNIK | ROBERT M. SILVER

(see *Creasy and Resnik's Maternal-Fetal Medicine, 9e: Ch 43*)

Summary

- Reporting of placental location should use the National Institute of Child Health and Human Development terminology—the terms *marginal* and *partial* placenta previa should be abandoned.
- All women with a placenta less than 2 cm from the cervix on a late third trimester scan should have cesarean deliveries.
- All women with placenta previa should be evaluated for placenta accreta.
- Vaginal examination should not be performed in any woman at greater than 20 weeks' gestation before ensuring that placenta previa has been excluded with ultrasound.
- Abruption remains a clinical diagnosis—imaging is useful only to exclude placenta previa.

QUESTIONS

1. In most cases of bleeding complicating the second half of pregnancy, the most common etiology is
   a. Placenta previa
   b. Placenta accreta
   c. Placental abruption
   d. Early labor or local lesion of the lower tract or no source identified

2. A 26-year-old G2 P1001 presents at 30 weeks' gestation with a complaint of "painless vaginal bleeding." Her prenatal course has been uncomplicated. Her vital signs are normal. The fetal heart rate is category 1, and she is having no contractions. The most reliable way to diagnose a placenta previa is
   a. Transabdominal ultrasound
   b. Transvaginal ultrasound
   c. Digital examination
   d. Sterile speculum examination

3. The sonographic features of placenta accreta include all of the following except
   a. Sonolucencies in the placenta
   b. A homogeneous appearance to the placenta
   c. Loss of normal hypoechoic boundary between the bladder wall and uterus
   d. Increased vascularity in the placenta-uterus interface

4. A 36-year-old G5 P3013 presents at 36 weeks' gestation with a complaint of "vaginal bleeding." Her prenatal course has been complicated by late entry to care. She has a history of two prior cesarean deliveries. Her vital signs are normal. The fetal heart rate is category 1. She is having no contractions. A formal ultrasound shows a complete placenta previa. The placenta has multiple lucencies, there is loss of the normal bladder and myometrial interface, and there is also marked vascularity noted in the placenta-uterus interface. After betamethasone administration, what is the next step in management?
   a. Delivery via cesarean hysterectomy, given that there is sonographic evidence of placenta accreta
   b. Observation in the hospital for 48 hours
   c. Discharge home
   d. None of the above

5. A 32-year-old G3 P1011 presents at 32 weeks' gestation with a complaint of "painless vaginal bleeding." Her prenatal course has been complicated by velamentous cord insertion. Her vital signs are normal. The fetal heart rate was initially consistent with tachycardia and decelerations, but subsequently a sinusoidal rhythm was noted. She is having no contractions. The most likely diagnosis of the abnormal fetal heart rate rhythm is
   a. Placenta accreta
   b. Placenta previa
   c. Vasa previa
   d. Low-lying placenta

6. The Society for Maternal Fetal Medicine recommends delivery of patients with vasa previa at:
   a. 37 weeks
   b. 36 weeks

c. Between 34 and 35 weeks with amniocentesis
d. Between 34 and 35 weeks

7. Subchorionic hemorrhages generally occur in the first half of pregnancy and are associated with
   a. Spontaneous abortion
   b. Preterm delivery
   c. Placental abruption
   d. All of the above

8. Known risk factors for placental abruption include
   a. Prior history of abruption
   b. Hypertension
   c. Smoking
   d. Factor V Leiden mutation
   e. Choices a through c

9. A 38-year-old G5 P4001 presents at 28 weeks' gestation with contractions and vaginal bleeding. Her prenatal course has been complicated by smoking. Her vital signs include a blood pressure of 140/95 mmHg. The fetal heart rate category 1. She is having contractions every 2 minutes. Laboratory studies are significant for normal complete blood count, creatinine, and liver function tests. There is no protein in her urine. A Kleihauer-Betke test was negative. The most likely diagnosis for the clinical picture is
   a. Placenta previa
   b. Placental abruption
   c. Preterm rupture of membranes
   d. Preeclampsia

10. Factors associated with coagulopathy with placental abruption include
    a. Massive abruption
    b. Initial presentation with contractions
    c. Fetal demise
    d. Both a and c

44

Fetal Growth Restriction

GIANCARLO MARI | ROBERT RESNIK

(see Creasy and Resnik's Maternal-Fetal Medicine, 9e: Ch 44)

Summary

Initial evaluation of suspected fetal growth abnormality (estimated fetal weight [EFW] and/or abdominal circumference <10th percentile) includes accurately determining gestational age and then distinguishing between a fetus that is constitutionally small but normal and a fetus with true fetal growth restriction (FGR), including an EFW usually <3rd percentile, and evidence of abnormal umbilical artery diastolic flow impedance. Ultrasound evaluation of the fetus is the preferred and accepted modality for diagnosis of inadequate fetal growth.

The cause of FGR is not always recognized. "Placental insufficiency" is often viewed as the primary cause of FGR. However, "placental insufficiency" is more often the manifestation of a process whose etiology and pathogenesis remain to be fully elucidated.

Two phenotypes of FGR have been described, and they have been termed *early* (≤32 weeks) and *late* (>32 weeks) FGR on the basis of gestational age at diagnosis. However, a clinical classification that allocates FGR cases into (A) previable, (B) very early (between 25 and 28 weeks), (C) early (between >28 and 32 weeks), and (D) late (>32 weeks) categories better reflects perinatal outcomes.

The risk of perinatal morbidity and mortality is higher in a growth-restricted fetus, and the risk increases with the severity of the restriction. The risks do not end at birth, because FGR is a significant risk factor for subsequent development of chronic hypertension, ischemic heart disease, type 2 diabetes, and obstructive lung disease.

Management of FGR in the United States is different than in other areas of the world, based on different definitions and guidelines. Therefore, a classification has been proposed that allows investigators from different areas of the world to communicate.

The first step in the assessment of the FGR starts with a detailed anatomic survey to detect the presence of any structural abnormalities. If there is any suggestion of risk of aneuploidy, fetal karyotype and chromosomal microarray should be determined. If there is risk of fetal infection, maternal serum should be evaluated for seroconversion, and, if indicated, amniotic fluid analysis of viral DNA should be performed. Ultrasound is used for measurement of fetal growth trajectory, Doppler interrogation of fetal vessels, and biophysical profile (BPP); surveillance frequency is determined by severity of fetal growth restriction.

Treatment with antenatal betamethasone is indicated if delivery occurs between 24 and 34 weeks' gestation. Magnesium sulfate administration decreases the risk of neurodevelopment impairment at less than 32 weeks' gestation.

Timing of delivery is determined by gestational age and fetal status, as well as the underlying etiology and coexisting maternal morbidity. Normal findings by ultrasound and antenatal testing indicate the fetus can be delivered near term. The extent of abnormal findings helps determine whether the fetus needs to be delivered preterm.

Doppler ultrasonography has a paramount role in the management of FGR. If umbilical artery diastolic flow is absent between 33 and 34 weeks or beyond, or is reversed between 30 and 32 weeks, the fetus should be delivered. In a very preterm fetus (<30 weeks) with absent or reversed diastolic flow, additional daily testing (e.g., NST, BPP) is indicated and the management is individualized. After 36 weeks, delivery is indicated if fetal growth velocity has tapered significantly (EFW <3rd percentile), decreased umbilical artery diastolic flow is observed (pulsatility index >95th percentile), or worsening of maternal status occurs. If diastolic flow is normal, delivery may occur at 39 weeks' gestation.

Mode of delivery depends on several factors. It is reasonable to allow a trial of induction and vaginal delivery with meticulous fetal monitoring in most cases. However, in premature FGR with reversed flow of the umbilical artery and an unfavorable cervix, it is reasonable to give the patient the option of a scheduled cesarean birth because many of these fetuses will not tolerate labor and it may prevent an acute insult in a fetus with chronic hypoxia.

The experience of the team that manages FGR is paramount for the best possible outcome. Therefore, multidisciplinary collaboration among obstetricians, neonatologists, anesthesiologists, other consultant specialists, and nursing staff is the key to best management of FGR.

This chapter reviews the factors that influence normal fetal growth and lead to various causes of fetal growth restriction and considers the methods of antepartum recognition and diagnosis, as well as clinical management.

QUESTIONS

1. A healthy 28-year-old primigravid woman, at 37 weeks' gestation, is referred for an ultrasound because of size less than dating. An ultrasound shows an abdominal circumference at the 4th percentile. The EFW is at the 15th percentile. Biophysical profile is 8/8. Which of the following is the most appropriate next step in evaluation?
   a. Reassure the patient and recommend routine prenatal care.
   b. Reassess fetal growth in 3 weeks.
   c. Perform Doppler of the umbilical artery.
   d. Recommend delivery.
   e. Admit to hospital for further monitoring.

2. A healthy 35-year-old primigravid woman, at 37 weeks' gestation by first-trimester ultrasound, is referred for an ultrasound because of size less than dating. An ultrasound shows an abdominal circumference at the 11th percentile. The EFW is at the 2nd percentile. Which of the following is the most appropriate recommendation?
   a. Reassurance and continuation with routine prenatal care
   b. Delivery
   c. Steroids and delivery
   d. Umbilical artery Doppler
   e. Hospital admission for further monitoring

3. A 33-year-old woman, gravida 2, para 1001, with chronic hypertension and a singleton fetus presents to your clinic for a follow-up ultrasound at 28 weeks' gestation. The EFW is at the 7th percentile. The umbilical artery pulsatility index is abnormal (there is umbilical artery forward diastolic flow). The amniotic fluid index is 8 cm. According to this chapter, how would you classify this FGR?
   a. Stage 1 FGR
   b. Stage 2 N FGR, chronic hypertension
   c. Stage 2, 8 cm, chronic hypertension
   d. Stage 1 N FGR, chronic hypertension
   e. Stage 3 FGR A, chronic hypertension

4. A 24-year-old primigravid woman is referred to your office because she has been diagnosed with FGR at 33 weeks' gestation. The patient would like to know when the weekly fetal weight increase peaks in a normal pregnancy. Which of the following is the most appropriate answer?
   a. Between 28 and 32 weeks
   b. Between 30 and 32 weeks
   c. Between 32 and 34 weeks
   d. Between 34 and 36 weeks
   e. Between 38 and 40 weeks

5. A 33-year-old woman, gravida 1, para 0101, with a history of severe FGR that was delivered at 32 weeks' gestation because of reversed flow of the umbilical artery, presents for preconceptional counseling and inquires whether there are medications that can decrease her risk of having another FGR baby. Which of the following is the most appropriate answer?
   a. Vitamins and iron supplementation
   b. Indomethacin started before the next pregnancy
   c. Low-molecular-weight heparin when the heart rate is visualized
   d. Sildenafil started at 12 weeks' gestation
   e. None of the above

6. A 33-year-old woman, gravida 2, para 1, with FGR (EFW = 1st percentile) and umbilical artery reversed diastolic flow, has been admitted to the hospital at 27 weeks' gestation. According to this chapter, which of the following is the most reasonable antenatal testing modality?
   a. BPP every day
   b. Nonstress test every other day
   c. Biophysical profile every day and nonstress test every 12 hours
   d. BPP and nonstress test twice a week
   e. Doppler of the ductus venosus and BPP every day

7. A 23-year-old Hispanic woman, gravida 4, para 3003, has been referred to your office for an ultrasound to confirm a FGR diagnosed in the office of her primary ob/gyn. The referring physician inquires whether you use the National Institute of Child Health and Human Development (NICHD) curve that incorporates racial-ethnic specific standards. Which of the following is the most appropriate answer?
   a. The NICHD curve is superior to the Hadlock curve.
   b. The NICHD curve is superior to improve the detection and outcome of FGR to the World Health Organization curve.
   c. The NICHD curve does not improve the detection and outcome of FGR when compared with the Hadlock formula.
   d. Both the NICHD and World Health Organization curves are equivalent, and they are superior for the detection and outcome of FGR when compared with the Hadlock formula.
   e. None of the above.

8. A 37-year-old woman, gravida 5, para 4004, presents at 23 weeks for an ultrasound to assess fetal growth. The patient is a heavy smoker (2 packs/day). You tell her that smoking decreases birth weight by approximately 135 to 300 gm. Which of the following interventions may reduce this adverse effect on birthweight?
   a. Starting aspirin
   b. Smoking cessation
   c. Exercise
   d. Bed rest
   e. All of the above

9. A 40-year-old woman, gravida 3, para 2002, has been diagnosed with FGR at 37 weeks' gestation. Her two previous pregnancies were uncomplicated vaginal deliveries. Which of the following parameter(s) is an indication for delivery?
   a. Absent umbilical artery end-diastolic velocity Doppler
   b. EFW at 2nd percentile
   c. Reversed diastolic flow of the umbilical artery
   d. Abnormal umbilical artery pulsatility index
   e. All of the above

10. A 35-year-old woman, gravida 2, para 1001, has been admitted to the hospital for delivery at 35 weeks' gestation secondary to FGR and preeclampsia with severe features. The primary ob/gyn inquires whether the fetus would benefit from antenatal corticosteroids. According to this chapter, which of the following is the most appropriate answer?
    a. Antenatal corticosteroids are indicated.
    b. Antenatal corticosteroids would increase the rate of neonatal hypoglycemia.
    c. Antenatal corticosteroids increase the need for respiratory support.
    d. FGR benefit from late preterm antenatal corticosteroids.

11. A healthy 20-year-old primigravid woman has been admitted to the hospital for delivery at 36 weeks' gestation because of FGR (EFW = 5th percentile). The umbilical artery Doppler is normal. The amniotic fluid index is 9 cm. The maternal uterine arteries have been abnormal at 24 weeks' gestation. The BPP is 10/10. The charge nurse calls you and questions the indication for delivery at 36 weeks in this patient. According to this chapter, which of the following is the most appropriate answer?
    a. Deliver immediately because of FGR.
    b. Delivery is indicated at 36 weeks in absence of other complications.
    c. Delivery is indicated at 37 weeks in absence of other complications.
    d. Delivery is indicated at 39 weeks in absence of other complications.

12. A 23-year-old primigravid woman has been admitted to the hospital for delivery at 39 weeks' gestation because of FGR (AC = 1st percentile; EFW = 2nd percentile). The umbilical artery pulsatility index is normal. The AFI is 11 cm. The NST is reactive. She has a Bishop score of 3. The patient would like to deliver vaginally, if possible. The primary ob/gyn, who would like to perform a cesarean delivery because of FGR and unfavorable cervix, calls you for a second opinion. Which of the following is the most appropriate management?
    a. Cesarean section should be performed because of FGR.
    b. Vaginal delivery is contraindicated.
    c. Wait for spontaneous labor.
    d. Ripen the cervix and induce labor.

13. A 23-year-old primigravid woman, at 28 weeks' gestation with FGR (AC = 5th percentile) and preterm premature rupture of membranes for 1 week, starts to contract regularly every 5 minutes. Vaginal examination is 1 cm/30%/−3/cephalic. She has completed the latency antibiotics and one course of antenatal corticosteroids. The fetal heart rate is category 1. Which of the following is the most appropriate intervention at this time?
    a. Cesarean section
    b. Magnesium sulfate for neuroprotection
    c. Tocolysis
    d. Operative vaginal delivery

14. A 31-year-old primigravid woman has been diagnosed with FGR, stage 2N, idiopathic, at 30 weeks' gestation. She is concerned about the effect of FGR on brain development.
    Which of the following is the most appropriate statement?
    a. FGR is associated with reduced total brain volume.
    b. FGR is associated with decreased number of neurons.
    c. FGR is associated with myelinization deficits.
    d. All of the above.

15. A 30-year-old primigravid woman has been diagnosed with FGR (EFW = 6th percentile) at 24 weeks' gestation. Her NIPT was negative. A detailed personal and family history is unremarkable. A detailed ultrasound examination reveals no abnormalities. According to this chapter, which of the following is the most appropriate diagnostic study at this time?
    a. Cytomegalovirus
    b. Toxoplasmosis
    c. Antiphospholipid antibody panel
    d. All of the above
    e. None of the above

16. A 19-year-old primigravid woman has been diagnosed with FGR (EFW = 8th percentile) at 27 weeks' gestation. Her NIPT was negative. A detailed personal and family history is unremarkable. A detailed ultrasound examination reveals no abnormalities. According to this chapter, which of the following is the most appropriate diagnosis based on gestational age?
    a. Very early FGR
    b. Late FGR
    c. Early FGR
    d. Periviable FGR
    e. Symmetric FGR

17. A 19-year-old woman, gravida 2, para 1001, has been diagnosed with FGR (EFW = <1st percentile) at 26 weeks' gestation. She declined aneuploidy testing. A detailed personal and family history is unremarkable. A detailed ultrasound examination reveals no abnormalities. The umbilical artery has reversed flow in diastole. There is "brain-sparing effect." According to this chapter, which of the following is the most likely etiology?
    a. Placental insufficiency
    b. Fetoplacental insufficiency is the most likely cause of FGR
    c. Idiopathic FGR
    d. Aneuploidy
    e. None of the above

18. A 25-year-old woman, gravida 3, para 2002, has been diagnosed with recurrent FGR (EFW: 5th percentile) at 28 weeks' gestation. In her two previous pregnancies she developed preeclampsia and delivered two small babies (birthweight of first baby at the 2nd percentile; birthweight of the second baby at the 5th percentile) by cesarean section at 28 and 29 weeks, respectively. She has again developed preeclampsia. She has not taken baby aspirin in this pregnancy. She inquires whether FGR diagnosed in patients with preeclampsia is like FGR diagnosed in patients who do not have any maternal/fetal pathology. According to this chapter, which of the following is the most appropriate answer?
    a. In patients with preeclampsia, FGR is usually early-onset FGR.
    b. FGR is called idiopathic when there is no maternal/fetal pathology.
    c. FGR is not a homogeneous group.
    d. Cardiovascular changes in FGR that develops in patients with preeclampsia are unpredictable.
    e. All of the above.

19. A healthy 26-year-old primigravid woman has been diagnosed with FGR (EFW = 8 percentile) at 28 weeks' gestation. Her NIPT was negative. A detailed ultrasound examination reveals no abnormalities. You inform the patient that you are going to study the umbilical artery (UA) Doppler because her pregnancy is a high-risk pregnancy. The patient asks if it is necessary. Which of the following is your best answer based on the current literature?
    a. The information of UA Doppler in high-risk pregnancies is associated with fewer perinatal deaths.
    b. The use of UA Doppler in high-risk pregnancies is associated with fewer unnecessary induction of labor.
    c. The information of UA Doppler in high-risk pregnancies is associated with fewer cesarean deliveries.
    d. All of the above.

20. A 22-year-old primigravid woman with dichorionic twins has been diagnosed with FGR at 35 weeks' gestation. Twin A EFW is at the 9th percentile, whereas twin B EFW is at 7th percentile. The umbilical artery Doppler is normal in both twins. A detailed personal and family history is unremarkable. The patient asks you, "Why are my babies FGR"?
    Which of the following is the most appropriate answer?
    a. Twins grow similarly to singletons up to 32 weeks' gestation. After that, growth rates diverge.
    b. There is fetal-placental insufficiency.
    c. There is an increased risk of aneuploidy in the twins.
    d. An infection is a likely cause of FGR in this pregnancy.
    e. Twins grow similarly to singletons up to 28 weeks' gestation. After that, growth rates diverge.

45

Pregnancy-Related Hypertension

LORIE M. HARPER | S. ANANTH KARUMANCHI | ALAN T.N. TITA

(see *Creasy and Resnik's Maternal-Fetal Medicine, 9e:* Ch 45)

Summary

Although imperfect, the American College of Obstetricians and Gynecologists (ACOG) nomenclature is straightforward and available worldwide. The classification system includes the following diagnoses:

- Hypertension in pregnancy: Any blood pressure ≥140/90 mm Hg, as measured on at least two occasions at least 4 hours apart
- Chronic hypertension: Hypertension diagnosed before 20 weeks' gestation or that is newly diagnosed during pregnancy and persists for at least 6 weeks postpartum
- Gestational hypertension: New-onset hypertension after 20 weeks' gestation in the absence of proteinuria
- Preeclampsia-eclampsia: New-onset hypertension accompanied by proteinuria or other signs in pregnancy, typically after 20 weeks
- Chronic hypertension with superimposed preeclampsia: A diagnosis of preeclampsia in women with preexisting chronic hypertension

Chronic Hypertension. Women with chronic hypertension are at increased risk of preeclampsia, preterm birth, small for gestational age, perinatal death, maternal mortality, and cardiovascular morbidity. The initial antepartum evaluation of women with chronic hypertension focuses on assessing end organ damage, particularly renal disease, with serum creatinine and urine protein assessment. ACOG recommends that during pregnancy, antihypertensive therapies should be used to achieve a goal blood pressure of less than 140/90 mm Hg. First-line agents include labetalol and nifedipine. Serial assessments of fetal growth and antenatal testing are generally recommended. The recommended timing of delivery is between 36 and 39 weeks, based on blood pressure control and comorbidities.

Gestational Hypertension. Because gestational hypertension may predate the onset of preeclampsia, women with newly elevated blood pressures after 20 weeks' gestation should be monitored closely for preeclampsia. Women with gestational hypertension are also at increased risk of small for gestational age and perinatal death. Serial assessments of fetal growth and antenatal testing is generally recommended. The recommended timing of delivery is 37 weeks.

Preeclampsia-Eclampsia. Preeclampsia occurs as a spectrum that is divided into those with or without severe features. The diagnosis of preeclampsia with severe features is made for any of the following criteria: blood pressure of 160 mm Hg systolic or higher or 110 mm Hg diastolic or higher on two occasions at least 4 hours apart, new-onset cerebral or visual disturbances, pulmonary edema, persistent epigastric or right upper quadrant pain, impaired liver function, thrombocytopenia, and progressive renal insufficiency.

Risk factors for preeclampsia include nulliparity, family history of preeclampsia, in vitro fertilization, extremes of childbearing age, obesity, chronic hypertension, renal disease, and diabetes. Multiple maternal organ systems are affected by preeclampsia including the liver, kidney, brain, eye, and heart.

Once the diagnosis of preeclampsia has been made, the initial evaluation should attempt to distinguish between preeclampsia with severe features and preeclampsia without severe features by assessing patient symptoms and laboratory values. In addition, fetal well-being should be assessed including fetal weight, amniotic fluid index, and antenatal testing. Once fetal well-being and severity have been established, decisions to deliver or expectantly manage the pregnancy can be made, taking into consideration the gestational age. Management seeks to balance risks to maternal health versus prematurity.

QUESTIONS

1. A 29-year-old, nulligravid woman at 19 weeks' gestation presents to the obstetric office for a routine prenatal visit. She has no medical history. Her blood pressure is 163/102 mm Hg. Which of the following is the most appropriate next step in diagnosis?
   a. Review prenatal records for prior blood pressures to determine if she has chronic hypertension.
   b. Order a 24-hour urine protein and serum labs to assess for preeclampsia.
   c. Obtain an ultrasound for fetal growth.
   d. Obtain a maternal renal ultrasound to assess for secondary causes of hypertension.

2. A 39-year-old multigravida presents for a routine prenatal visit at 33 weeks and is found to have a blood pressure of 172/93 mm Hg. She has no medical history, and her blood pressures before this visit have been normal. She denies headache, changes in her vision, and abdominal pain and reports good fetal movement. Which of the following is the most appropriate next step in diagnosis and management?
   a. Order a 24-hour urine protein and serum labs to be returned at her next prenatal visit.
   b. Administer betamethasone and admit to the antepartum floor for expectant management of preeclampsia with severe features.
   c. Send to obstetric emergency department and administer IV hydralazine if blood pressure is >160/110 mm Hg on arrival.
   d. Administer betamethasone and admit to labor and delivery for 24-hour urine, serum labs, and fetal monitoring with a plan for delivery if blood pressure is >140/90 mm Hg.

3. A 31-year-old nulligravid woman at 27 weeks' gestation is admitted to the antepartum unit for expectant management of preeclampsia. She was admitted and diagnosed with preeclampsia 2 days ago with blood pressures of 161/91 and 163/94 mm Hg, on two occasions 4 hours apart. A 24-hour urine protein was sent and resulted as 450 mg. Her serum labs on admission included platelets of 145, aspartate transaminase (AST) 46, and creatinine of 0.9. She received antenatal corticosteroids on admission and blood pressures are currently 140s-150s/90s. Which of the following is the most appropriate next step in management?
   a. Repeat the 24-hour urine every week to monitor for increasing proteinuria, as this would impact the timing of delivery.
   b. Order daily antenatal testing (nonstress test, contraction stress test, or biophysical profile) with a plan for delivery if nonreassuring fetal status is detected.
   c. Discharge home with twice-weekly antenatal testing, blood pressure checks, and serum labs.
   d. Deliver for preeclampsia with severe features.

4. A 32-year-old nulligravid woman at 24 weeks' gestation presents to the emergency department with abdominal pain. Her blood pressures on admission are 190/104, 195/107, and 201/102 mm Hg. She receives 20 mg IV labetalol and is transferred to labor and delivery. On arrival to labor and delivery, her repeat blood pressure is 181/106 (20 minutes after receiving labetalol) and fetal heart tones are detected in the 120s. A complete blood cell count, type and screen, liver function tests, and creatinine are ordered. An ultrasound is performed, confirming cephalic presentation, a fetal weight of 602 g, and amniotic fluid index of 7 cm. Which of the following is the most appropriate next step in diagnosis and management?
   a. Labetalol 20 mg IV push. Plan to deliver if any serum laboratory abnormalities.
   b. Hydralazine 5 mg IV push. Plan for cesarean delivery when type and screen results are available.
   c. Magnesium sulfate 6 g IVPB. Start antenatal corticosteroids. Plan for induction of labor when type and screen results are available.
   d. Labetalol 40 mg IV push. Start antenatal corticosteroids. Plan to deliver and start magnesium sulfate if evidence of DIC.

5. A 25-year-old multigravida woman at 26 weeks' gestation is admitted with preeclampsia with severe features. Which of the following is a contraindication to expectant management for 48 hours in order to administer betamethasone?
   a. A fetal diagnosis of anencephaly
   b. Platelets of 85,000
   c. An amniotic fluid index of 3 cm
   d. Blood pressure of 167/92 mm Hg

6. A 38-year-old multigravida at 19 weeks' gestation presents for a routine prenatal visit. Below is the flowsheet from her prenatal care.

Gestational Age	Fetal Heart Tones	Blood Pressure	Fundal Height	Urine Protein	Urine Glucose	Urine Ketones
8	+	138/87	–	1+	–	–
12	+	141/89	–	Trace	–	1+
16	+	137/84	–	–	–	–
19	+	142/94	–	Trace	–	–

Which of the following is the next most appropriate step in her care?
a. Obtain a detailed anatomy scan.
b. Initiate aspirin 325 mg Qday.
c. Initiate labetalol 200 mg twice daily.
d. Refer to dietitian for counseling on a low-salt diet.

7. A 31-year-old multigravida at 30 weeks presents for a routine prenatal visit. Below is the flowsheet from her prenatal care. She currently takes no medications.

Gestational Age	Fetal Heart Tones	Blood Pressure	Fundal Height	Urine Protein	Urine Glucose	Urine Ketones
8	+	125/82	–	–	–	–
12	+	137/91	–	Trace	–	–
16	+	143/88	–	–	–	–
20	+	138/81	–	Trace	–	–
24	+	140/86	24	–	Trace	–
28	+	136/90	28	Trace	Trace	–
30	+	151/92	29	–	Trace	Trace

Which of the following is the likely diagnosis and most appropriate next step in her care?
a. This is likely chronic hypertension with a return to normal prepregnancy blood pressures as she reaches the maximum volume of pregnancy. Discharge home with follow-up in 2 weeks for routine prenatal visit.
b. This is likely superimposed preeclampsia given the newly elevated blood pressures. Admit to the hospital for expectant management and potential delivery.
c. This is likely gestational hypertension given the newly elevated blood pressures. Will monitor for progression to preeclampsia with serum labs (platelets, AST, creatinine) and weekly urine protein/creatinine ratios.
d. This may be chronic hypertension with a return to normal prepregnancy blood pressures as the maximum volume of pregnancy is reached, but superimposed preeclampsia must be ruled out. Obtain 24-hour urine protein and serum labs (platelets, AST, creatinine) and base further management on those results.

8. A 28-year-old multigravida at 27 weeks presents for a routine prenatal visit. Below is the flowsheet from her prenatal care. She currently takes no medications.

Gestational Age	Fetal Heart Tones	Blood Pressure	Fundal Height	Urine Protein	Urine Glucose	Urine Ketones
8	+	125/82	–	–	–	–
12	+	137/91	–	Trace	–	–
16	+	143/88	–	–	–	–
20	+	138/81	–	Trace	–	–
24	+	140/86	24	–	Trace	–
27	+	172/101	29	+	–	–

Which of the following is the likely diagnosis and most appropriate next step in her care?
a. This is likely chronic hypertension with a return to normal prepregnancy blood pressure as she reaches the maximum volume of pregnancy. Discharge home with follow-up in 2 weeks for routine prenatal visit.
b. This is likely superimposed preeclampsia given the newly elevated blood pressures. Admit to the hospital for evaluation with quantitative urine protein, serum labs (platelets, AST, creatinine). Consider betamethasone and magnesium sulfate for neuroprophylaxis.
c. This is likely gestational hypertension given the newly elevated blood pressures. Will monitor for progression to preeclampsia with serum labs (platelets, AST, creatinine) and weekly urine protein/creatinine ratios.
d. This may be chronic hypertension with a return to normal prepregnancy blood pressures as the maximum volume of pregnancy is reached, but superimposed preeclampsia must be ruled out. Obtain 24-hour urine protein and serum labs (platelets, AST, creatinine) and base further management on those results.

9. A 27-year-old nulligravid presents at 28 weeks to the OB emergency department with complaints of decreased fetal movement and vaginal bleeding. She denies contractions, leakage of fluid, or abdominal pain. On evaluation, her blood pressures are 168/102, 159/111, and 173/105 mm Hg. She receives 20 mg IV labetalol with decrease in her blood pressures to 140s/90s. On examination, she has minimal blood in the vaginal vault. Ultrasound demonstrates a fundal placenta, amniotic fluid index 4 cm, and estimated fetal weight at the third percentile, cephalic presentation. Fetal heart tones are 130s, minimal variability, and no decelerations with contractions every 5-10 minutes. Serum labs demonstrate platelets of 105, AST of 93 (normal 40 IU/mL), and creatinine of 1.0. Which of the following is the next most appropriate step in management?
   a. Initiate magnesium sulfate for maternal and fetal neuroprophylaxis, administer betamethasone, and attempt to expectantly manage through betamethasone window with a plan for delivery for nonreassuring fetal status or continued vaginal bleeding.
   b. Initiate magnesium sulfate for maternal and fetal neuroprophylaxis, administer betamethasone, and start nifedipine immediate release for both tocolysis and blood pressure control. Plan for expectant management with a plan for delivery for nonreassuring fetal status or any laboratory abnormalities.
   c. Initiate magnesium sulfate for maternal and fetal neuroprophylaxis and proceed with urgent cesarean delivery for a National Institute of Child Health and Human Development category 3 tracing.
   d. Initiate magnesium sulfate for maternal and fetal neuroprophylaxis, administer betamethasone, and begin an induction of labor for oligohydramnios and elevated AST.

10. A 38-year-old nulligravid at 38 weeks presents to the OB emergency department for contractions and rupture of membranes. On examination, she is confirmed to be ruptured and is 5 cm dilated. Her blood pressures on arrival are 148/93, 151/89, and 147/91 mm Hg. Her urine dip was negative for protein. The next most appropriate step in management is:
   a. Start magnesium sulfate for maternal neuroprophylaxis.
   b. Obtain quantitative urine protein and serum labs (platelets, AST, creatinine); begin magnesium sulfate for maternal neuroprophylaxis if any serum abnormalities are present or if any blood pressures >160/110.
   c. Repeat blood pressures after epidural placement and, if they continue to be elevated, start magnesium sulfate for maternal neuroprophylaxis.
   d. Repeat blood pressures after epidural placement and if they continue to be elevated, obtain quantitative urine protein and serum labs (platelets, AST, creatinine). Begin magnesium sulfate for maternal neuroprophylaxis if any serum abnormalities, urine protein/creatinine ratio >0.3, or blood pressures >160/110.

11. A 19-year-old primigravida presents on postpartum day 3 to the emergency department with complaints of headache and lower extremity swelling. Her pregnancy and delivery were uncomplicated. On arrival, her blood pressures were 168/110, 172/101, 167/99 mm Hg. Her urine dip was negative for protein. What is the next most appropriate step in management?
   a. Consult anesthesia to rule out a postepidural puncture headache.
   b. Obtain quantitative urine protein and serum labs to assess for preeclampsia.
   c. Administer 10 mg of IV hydralazine.
   d. Start magnesium sulfate for maternal neuroprophylaxis.

12. A 22-year-old nulligravida at 34 weeks' gestation presents to a routine prenatal visit. She has no history of chronic hypertension. She has been followed during this pregnancy for A1 gestational diabetes (GDM) and has normal blood glucose logs. On presentation in the clinic, she has a blood pressure of 142/89 mm Hg and denies headache, changes in her vision, or right upper quadrant pain. She has good fetal movement. You order a 24-hour urine protein, serum labs (complete blood cell count, AST, creatinine), and an ultrasound. Her serum labs are all within normal limits, fetal weight is appropriate for gestational age, amniotic fluid is normal, and 24-hour urine protein is 231 mg. A repeat blood pressure when she returned her 24-hour urine protein was 143/92. The next most appropriate step in management is:
   a. Admission for betamethasone and delivery after completion of antenatal corticosteroids
   b. Outpatient expectant management with weekly visits for blood pressure checks, serum labs, and antenatal testing
   c. Inpatient expectant management with administration of antenatal corticosteroids, at least twice-weekly serum labs, and daily antenatal testing
   d. Schedule an induction of labor at 37 weeks

13. A 27-year-old multigravida and 31 weeks' pregnant presents to the emergency department and has a witnessed general tonic-clonic seizure while in the waiting room. No IV is in place. The next most appropriate step in management is:
   a. Magnesium sulfate 10 g IM
   b. Transfer to an operating room for emergency cesarean under general endotracheal anesthesia
   c. After stabilization, obtain a head CT to rule out intracranial bleeding or mass as an organic cause of seizure
   d. Labetalol 20 mg IV to control blood pressures

14. A 41-year-old nulligravid patient is admitted at 32 weeks for expectant management of preeclampsia with severe features. She received antenatal corticosteroids 5 days ago. Her blood pressures have been well controlled with nifedipine XL 30 mg. Today, her blood pressures are 178/92, 186/103, and 192/108 mm Hg. She is asymptomatic. The next most appropriate step in management is:

   a. Increase nifedipine XL to 60 mg and repeat antenatal corticosteroids.
   b. Increase nifedipine XL to 60 mg and start magnesium sulfate for neuroprophylaxis.
   c. Administer IV antihypertensives and proceed with cesarean delivery for preeclampsia with severe features.
   d. Administer IV antihypertensives, evaluate patient symptoms, evaluate fetal status, and obtain serum laboratory values (platelets, AST, creatinine).

Maternal Complications

Patient Safety and Quality Improvement in Obstetrics

CHRISTIAN PETTKER | WILLIAM GROBMAN

(see *Creasy and Resnik's Maternal-Fetal Medicine, 9e: Ch 46*)

Summary

Patient safety and quality improvement efforts aim to reduce harm and optimize care. In obstetrics, these concepts are of critical importance because threats to life and health are often unexpected and excellent outcomes are the norm. The patient safety movement has matured, and regulatory agencies are paying increasing attention to obstetric care. While many efforts have been directed to the inpatient setting, the application of principles of patient safety to outpatient settings is just beginning. However, evidence of the benefit of these approaches is only slowly emerging. Few randomized clinical trials exist because these types of interventions tend to focus not on building a corpus of evidence but rather timely quality improvement. In fact, as suggested by Berwick, the type of study design most commonly found in the literature may arguably be the most feasible for studying the "complex, unstable, [and] nonlinear social change" characterized by quality improvement initiatives.

Nevertheless, the application of the techniques described in this chapter is beginning to show improved obstetric care in a variety of areas, and some of these results have occurred with more impact, less effort, less expense, and certainly less time than traditional basic science and translational approaches to advancing care. Engaging in these processes can help an obstetric unit evolve into a high-reliability organization, where safety is a paramount end, teams are valued over the individual, effective and transparent communication is constantly reinforced, and the unexpected becomes expected.

QUESTIONS

1. All the following are obstetric quality measures proposed and used by The Joint Commission EXCEPT:
   a. low-risk, i.e., nulliparous women, at term with singleton fetus in a vertex presentation (NTSV) cesaren delivery rate
   b. episiotomy rate
   c. early elective delivery without a medical indication (before 39 weeks) rate
   d. exclusive breastmilk feeding at discharge rate

2. According to The Joint Commission Sentinel Event Alert report on patient safety and infant death, the most common root cause of sentinel events involving perinatal death is:
   a. poor communication.
   b. insufficient staffing.
   c. inadequate staff competency.
   d. lack of appropriate training.

3. On the basis of a review of cases, more than 50% of paid liability claims involve alleged misuse of:
   a. misoprostol
   b. nonstress tests
   c. oxytocin
   d. obstetric forceps and vacuum

4. Simulation work addressing shoulder dystocia education and teamwork training has demonstrated:
   a. no impact on outcomes
   b. reduced incidence of neonatal brachial plexus palsies
   c. reduced incidence of neonatal encephalopathy
   d. reduced incidence of obstetric anal sphincter injuries

5. Sets of evidence-based interventions grouped together under a care target and aimed to be implemented together or in part are called:
   a. checklists
   b. bundles
   c. care pathways
   d. guidelines

6. According to a survey by the American College of Obstetricians and Gynecologists, what percent of obstetricians in the United States experience at least one liability claim during their careers?
   a. 20%
   b. 50%
   c. 80%
   d. 90%

7. The beginning of the patient safety movement can be traced back to:
   a. the Annenberg Conference
   b. the founding of the Institute for Healthcare Improvement
   c. the founding of the National Patient Safety Foundation
   d. publication of "To Err is Human" by the National Academy of Medicine

8. Script concordance theory testing, which can test both knowledge and judgment, has been applied to certification and credentialing for the practice of:
   a. electronic fetal monitoring
   b. operative vaginal delivery
   c. cesarean delivery
   d. amniocentesis and chorionic villus sampling

9. The 'Donabedian model' of quality measures includes all of the following EXCEPT:
   a. process measures
   b. structural measures
   c. outcome measures
   d. indicator measures

10. A foundation of the patient safety movement is nonjudgmental recognition of:
    a. near miss and adverse events
    b. normalized deviance
    c. the ubiquity of human and system error
    d. liability claims and their resolutions

11. A system that identifies and addresses issues as system failures but creates accountability for unsafe and reckless behaviors is called:
    a. retributive justice
    b. restorative justice
    c. just culture
    d. culture of blame

12. The terms *second victim* and *secondary trauma* refer to instances when:
    a. a fetus is impacted during the course of a maternal adverse event
    b. a partner is affected by a maternal adverse event
    c. a physician experiences the trauma of litigation for a legal claim
    d. a person witnesses a traumatic event

13. The acceptance of events that are not supposed to happen due to a general drift in practice, in which failures are not recognized as unexpected but rather as routine, is called:
    a. normalization of deviance
    b. a near-miss event
    c. root cause analysis
    d. situational awareness

14. A compendium of obstetric care bundles, such as those for obstetric hemorrhage, severe hypertension in pregnancy, and reducing peripartum racial/ethnic disparities, has been organized by:
    a. The Joint Commission
    b. Council on Patient Safety in Women's Health Care
    c. Agency for Healthcare Research and Quality
    d. Institute for Healthcare Improvement

15. All of the following are part of the obstetric Adverse Outcome Index (AOI) proposed by Mann except:
    a. uterine rupture
    b. postpartum hemorrhage
    c. maternal intensive care unit admission
    d. maternal return to the operating room

Maternal Mortality

ROBERT M. SILVER | TORRI D. METZ

(see *Creasy and Resnik's Maternal-Fetal Medicine, 9e: Ch 47*)

Summary

Maternal mortality is a tragedy for the woman and her family, as well as for health care providers and society. Reports of trends or causes of maternal mortality invariably receive much attention in the media and on the internet. Although the maternal mortality rate is now very low in resource-rich countries (MMRCs), these deaths reflect much larger numbers of mothers with near misses or severe morbidity. In addition, it is likely that further reductions are possible in many high-resource countries including the United States.

There are various definitions of maternal mortality. Definitions from the Centers for Disease Control and Prevention (CDC) subdivide maternal deaths into pregnancy related and pregnancy associated. Pregnancy-related deaths are those resulting from obstetric complications or deaths from aggravation of an unrelated condition by the physiologic effects of pregnancy. In contrast, pregnancy-associated deaths are those occurring during pregnancy or within a year of the end of pregnancy, regardless of cause.

In 2012, the National Center for Health Statistics suspended national reporting of maternal mortality ratios for several years. After an extensive review to improve data quality and adoption of new coding procedures based on this review, the National Center for Health Statistics released a maternal mortality ratio for 2018, which was 17.4 deaths per 100,000 live births. This rate exceeds that of other developed countries. An analysis of US National Vital Statistics data from 2003−2016 revealed that approximately one-third of pregnancy-related deaths occur outside of a medical facility, emphasizing that prevention of maternal deaths will require a multipronged approach that extends into the community.

State level MMRCs have been established in the vast majority of US states and can provide detailed data on maternal deaths through case reviews of autopsy reports, medical records, police reports, birth certificates, and death certificates. Reviews have been standardized across committees through the use of the CDC Maternal Mortality Review Information Application (also known as "Maria"), which leads MMRCs through key decisions related to cause of death, pregnancy relatedness, preventability, contributing factors, and recommendations. Multidisciplinary engagement in MMRCs is critical.

Obstetric hemorrhage is the most common cause of maternal death globally. With the advent of modern blood banking, intensive care, and interventions for control of uterine atony, mortality has fallen. However, hemorrhage still accounts for more than 10% of maternal deaths in the United States. Case reviews demonstrate that institutional issues, such as failure to have a response team with a plan, delay and denial, and lack of availability of and familiarity with blood component therapy are potential targets to reduce deaths. In addition, the increasing frequency of multiple prior cesarean births has led to an epidemic of placental implantation issues, including placenta previa and placenta accreta spectrum, which can result in life-threatening postpartum hemorrhage, and should be managed at a tertiary center.

Amniotic fluid embolism (AFE) is no longer believed to be universally lethal. Population-based series note a frequency of AFE of 2−6 per 100,000 live births, with a mortality rate of 15%−40%. The majority (70%) of AFEs occur during labor, with the remainder occurring immediately after delivery. However, it is still unclear whether fetal cells in the maternal circulation is the inciting event for AFE. In case reviews, some deaths occurred after slow responses and undertreatment of coagulopathy, but others occurred despite intensive support after catastrophic cardiovascular collapse. Unfortunately, mortality may occur even in cases that are optimally managed.

Venous thromboembolism causes approximately 10% of maternal deaths, most of which occur after pulmonary emboli. Any episode of sudden onset of shortness of breath with tachypnea and tachycardia in a pregnant or postpartum woman deserves full evaluation with prompt treatment if VTE is confirmed. Over the past decade, there has been much debate about the need for VTE prophylaxis at the time of delivery, particularly after cesarean birth. Both the Royal College of Obstetricians and Gynaecologists and the American College of Chest Physicians advocate for evaluation of risk of VTE based on scoring systems. However, the efficacy of pharmacologic prophylaxis in the postpartum period remains uncertain. Until more data are available, decisions regarding pharmacologic prophylaxis will depend on the hospital patient population and resources.

Preeclampsia and eclampsia remain causes of death with potential for preventability. Most maternal deaths from preeclampsia are due to intracranial hemorrhage, liver failure, or pulmonary complications. National guidelines in the United States now recommend aggressive treatment of systolic hypertension >160 mm Hg or diastolic hypertension >110 mm Hg, if confirmed as persistent for 15 minutes or more. Prevention of maternal deaths from HELLP syndrome (*h*emolysis, *e*levated *l*iver enzymes, and *l*ow *p*latelets) depends on early recognition and prompt delivery. Given that patients with preeclampsia often present postpartum, other care providers such as emergency medicine personnel must also be aware of these conditions and prepared to promptly treat them.

Cardiovascular disease is the leading cause of pregnancy-related mortality in the United States and United Kingdom. Two-thirds of deaths from cardiovascular disease are from cardiomyopathies, with underlying structural heart disease responsible for the majority of others. It can be difficult to differentiate normal pregnancy symptoms from cardiac warning signs. The anticipated morbidity and risk of mortality with pregnancy for individuals with structural heart disease varies on the basis of the severity and location of cardiac abnormality. It is important that those with known complicated, structural heart disease undergo serial monitoring with a multidisciplinary team throughout pregnancy to reduce morbidity and mortality.

Sepsis is an increasingly common cause of maternal death in the United States and United Kingdom. Prevention of sepsis-related morbidity and mortality during pregnancy and postpartum focuses on early recognition of sepsis, followed by appropriate resuscitation and treatment. Laboratory tests such as lactate and arterial blood gases can help evaluate the degree of maternal compromise related to the infectious process and may help dictate transfer to a facility with a higher level of care. Septic shock should be managed in collaboration with infectious disease and critical care specialists.

Suicide and homicide account for more pregnancy-associated deaths than any other cause of maternal mortality. The CDC data collection tool "Maria" for use by MMRCs has a field for identification of a death as suicide, homicide, or domestic violence and whether a mental health condition contributed to the cause of death. This standardized classification will ultimately allow for more accurate assessment of the proportion of pregnancy-associated and pregnancy-related deaths

that result from suicide and homicide. Rates of suicide are likely underestimated, as they are often classified simply as drug overdose of unknown intent. Screening for intimate-partner violence, substance use disorders, and mental health disorders may help identify women at risk for death from suicide or homicide.

Racial disparities in maternal death remain significant. A report from the CDC's National Pregnancy Mortality Surveillance System from 2011–2015 demonstrated that Black and American Indian/Alaskan Native women had pregnancy-related mortality ratios that were, respectively, 3.33 and 2.5 times as high as White women. Importantly, structural racism and implicit bias likely also contribute to high rates of maternal mortality in minoritized populations. Disentangling the contributing factors related to the observed disparities is a subject of ongoing investigation. Regardless of the cause, health care providers in all disciplines should be aware of the higher risk of maternal death in these populations and thoroughly evaluate any concerning symptoms in pregnancy and the postpartum period.

Obstetrics and maternal-fetal medicine subspecialists are in an optimal position to take the lead in state or regional maternal-mortality reviews in order to help eliminate preventable maternal deaths in the United States and globally.

QUESTIONS

1. What is the accepted term to describe the number of maternal deaths per 100,000 live births?
   a. Maternal mortality rate
   b. Maternal death rate
   c. Pregnancy-related death ratio
   d. Maternal mortality ratio

2. A 31-year-old G2P1102 dies in a motor vehicle crash 4 months after delivering her baby by elective repeat cesarean delivery. Using CDC criteria, this maternal death would be best classified as
   a. pregnancy related
   b. unknown
   c. pregnancy associated
   d. Neither pregnancy associated nor pregnancy related

3. A 22-year-old G1P0 at 28 weeks' gestation dies of a hemorrhagic stroke attributed to severe-range blood pressure with a diagnosis of preeclampsia with severe features. Using CDC criteria, this maternal death would be best classified as:
   a. pregnancy related
   b. unknown
   c. pregnancy associated
   d. neither pregnancy associated nor pregnancy related

4. Best practices for review of maternal deaths by state-level maternal mortality review committees include which of the following?
   a. Identification of factors that contributed to the maternal death at the provider or system level
   b. Use of the pregnancy checkbox on the death certificate to determine pregnancy relatedness
   c. Modification of the cause of death on the death certificate for vital statistics records
   d. Calculation of a state maternal mortality rate

5. According to an analysis of US National Vital Statistics data, what proportion of maternal deaths occur outside of a medical facility?
   a. One-tenth
   b. One-quarter
   c. One-third
   d. One-half

6. A 43-year-old G1P1 who is now 2 weeks postpartum from a cesarean delivery presents with sudden onset of chest pain and shortness of breath. She has a heart rate of 130 bpm and an oxygen saturation of 91% on room air. What is the most appropriate test to order at this time?
   a. D-dimer
   b. Lower-extremity Doppler
   c. Computed tomography angiogram
   d. Ventilation-perfusion scan

7. What are the four components of the National Partnership for Maternal Safety care bundles?
   a. Assessment, Implementation, Evaluation, Modification
   b. Readiness, Recognition, Response and Reporting, Systems Learning
   c. Recognition, Evaluation, Implementation, Systems-Based Practice
   d. Readiness, Implementation, Assessment, Change

8. Risk of a cardiac complication during pregnancy for an individual with congenital heart disease can be most accurately calculated using which of the following scoring systems?
   a. APACHE II
   b. qSOFA
   c. CARPREG II
   d. CARPREG

9. A 28-year-old G3P2 dies by suicide at 18 weeks' gestation. Review of her records demonstrates a long history of bipolar disorder managed with multiple medications that were stopped when she discovered she was pregnant with subsequent relapse. Using CDC criteria, this maternal death would be best classified as
   a. pregnancy related
   b. unknown
   c. pregnancy associated
   d. neither pregnancy associated nor pregnancy related

10. What markers have been recommended by the American College of Obstetricians and Gynecologists and Society for Maternal-Fetal Medicine to identify potential cases of severe maternal morbidity?
    a. Disseminated intravascular coagulation or transfusion of fresh frozen plasma
    b. Admission to the intensive care unit or receipt of four or more units of blood products
    c. Need for subspecialist care by a cardiologist, nephrologist, or neurologist
    d. Transfer from Labor and Delivery to another unit in the hospital as an escalation of care

Bacterial and Parasitic Infections in Pregnancy

BLAIR JOHNSON WYLIE | MATTHEW A. SHEAR | TOOBA ANWER

(see *Creasy and Resnik's Maternal-Fetal Medicine, 9e: Ch 48*)

Summary

Infectious disease is frequently encountered during pregnancy. Some conditions pose a risk primarily to the pregnant patient, while others pose a risk primarily to the fetus.

Urinary tract infections are the most common medical complication of pregnancy, occurring in up to 20%. Asymptomatic bacteriuria (ASB) occurs in 2% to 11% and is associated with a 20- to 30-fold risk of pyelonephritis, preterm birth, and low birth weight. Acute pyelonephritis occurs in 1% to 2.5% of pregnancies and is characterized by high fever, chills, flank pain, dysuria, leukocytosis, pyuria, and bacteriuria and confirmed with a positive urine culture. Forty percent of pregnancies with ASB will develop pyelonephritis if untreated, with a recurrence risk of 10% to 18% within the same pregnancy. Progesterone causes a decrease in ureteral muscle tone, peristalsis, bladder tone and incomplete emptying, physiologic hydronephrosis, and static columns of urine, which predispose to ascending infection. The most common implicated organisms are *E. coli*, *Klebsiella*, *Proteus*, and *Enterobacter* sp. Patients with suspected acute pyelonephritis should be admitted and treated aggressively with intravenous (IV) fluids and antibiotics and should receive prophylaxis daily for the remainder of pregnancy.

Intraamniotic infection (chorioamnionitis) is a leading risk factor for neonatal sepsis and occurs in up to 10% of pregnancies. Diagnosis is made by a combination of maternal fever plus maternal or fetal tachycardia, uterine tenderness, foul odor or purulence of amniotic fluid, or leukocytosis. Ascending infection from the lower genital tract is the most common etiology, while hematogenous transplacental spread occurs occasionally. The most common organisms are *Bacteroides* sp., *G. vaginalis*, group B *Streptococcus* (GBS) and other streptococci, *E. coli*, gram-negative rods, or genital mycoplasmas. Treatment is with ampicillin plus gentamicin. If cesarean delivery is performed, clindamycin or metronidazole should be added for anaerobic coverage. For penicillin allergic (prior anaphylactic IgE-mediated reactions) patients substitute vancomycin for ampicillin. Treatment postpartum is limited to one dose regardless of route of delivery. If the patient has a risk for treatment failure (body mass index >30, prolonged rupture of membranes), treatment for at least 24 hours postpartum is recommended.

Puerperal endometritis is diagnosed by fever within 36 hours of delivery. It is usually a polymicrobial infection of the normal vaginal flora. Risk factors include intraamniotic infection, young age, cesarean delivery, prolonged rupture or membranes, multiple vaginal examinations, internal monitoring, bacterial vaginosis, GBS, and preexisting infection with gonorrhea. Diagnosis is often made by postpartum fever, but attention should be paid to a broader differential including perineal infection, urinary tract infection, pyelonephritis, atelectasis, and pneumonia. Multiple treatment regimens are available.

Episiotomy and perineal infections are associated with higher-order obstetric lacerations, operative delivery, smoking, and obesity. Wound infection occurs in 3%-5% of patients who undergo cesarean delivery, and risk factors include intraamniotic infection, prolonged labor, obesity, diabetes, and immunosuppression. Presence of frank pus or significant serosanguinous effusion requires the wound to be opened and drained completely. Perineal or abdominal infection that spreads along fascial planes with brawny edema, skin that is blue or brown, with bullae or frank gangrene, loss of sensation, or hyperesthesia raises concern for necrotizing fasciitis. Necrotizing fasciitis should be treated aggressively with debridement of devitalized tissue, IV fluids, and broad-spectrum antibiotics.

Pelvic abscess typically presents with persistent fever despite appropriate antibiotic therapy. The diagnosis is confirmed by ultrasound, computed tomography (CT), or magnetic resonance imaging (MRI). Treatment includes surgical drainage with image-guided drain placement, laparotomy, or laparoscopy. Antibiotics against aerobes and anaerobes are recommended until the patient is afebrile for 24-48 hours, followed by oral treatment for 10-14 days. Sepsis is covered in Chapter 71.

Septic pelvic vein thrombophlebitis is rare and occurs in 1:2000 pregnancies. It may present with new-onset abdominal pain and fever or as an enigmatic fever in patients treated for presumed puerperal endometritis. Diagnosis is made by CT or MRI showing thrombi in the major pelvic vessels. Treatment includes therapeutic anticoagulation with unfractionated heparin.

Mastitis occurs in 5% of lactating women and is typically caused by *Staphylococcus aureus* or *Streptococcus viridans*. Diagnosis is made by an erythematous tender area on the affected breast with fever or malaise. Treatment includes dicloxacillin for at least 7 days and longer depending on the response to treatment.

Group B streptococcal infection is a significant cause of fetal perinatal morbidity and mortality. Up to 30% of pregnant patients are colonized with GBS, and all pregnant patients should be screened at 36 0/7 to 37 6/7 weeks with vaginal-anorectal swab or nucleic acid amplification test. Penicillin G remains the drug of choice for intrapartum prophylaxis and should be given to all carriers at the time of labor or rupture of membranes. If the patient has a non-anaphylactic, non-IgE mediated, allergy to penicillin treat with Cefazolin. If the patient has had a prior anaphylactic, IgE-mediated allergic reaction to penicillin, perform antibiotic susceptibility testing and depending on results treat with clindamycin or erythromycin. If resistant to both, treat with vancomycin. Women with GBS bacteriuria, previous history of an infant with GBS disease, unknown GBS colonization status with ruptured of membranes >18 hours, intrapartum fever, and those at risk for imminent preterm delivery should also receive GBS antibiotic prophylaxis.

Listeriosis is 13 times more prevalent in pregnancy than in the general population and is associated with stillbirth and preterm labor. Patients may present with flulike illness, diarrhea, or other GI symptoms, especially after ingestion of contaminated food. Ascending infection from the cervix is possible, but the more common route is hematogenous dissemination to the placenta leading to placental abscesses. Treatment includes IV penicillin or ampicillin for 14 days. For patients with anaphylactic IgE-mediated allergies to penicillin substitute trimethoprim-sulfamethoxazole.

Primary syphilis is characterized by a painless chancre at the site of entry, usually on the genitals, with painless inguinal lymphadenopathy. Secondary syphilis is the stage of bacteremia dissemination where any organ and even the central nervous system can be infected. Typical manifestations are a maculopapular rash starting on the trunk and spreading to the body including palms and soles. Latent syphilis is when there is no apparent clinical disease. Transmission to the fetus may occur in any trimester or at birth and is associated with risk of perinatal death, preterm labor, and low birth weight. Early congenital syphilis presents with a maculopapular rash, desquamation, snuffles, hepatosplenomegaly, and chorioretinitis. All pregnant patients should be screened for syphilis. Treatment is benzathine penicillin G and, for those with a penicillin allergy, penicillin desensitization followed by treatment with penicillin is recommended.

Lyme disease is the most common vector-borne illness in North America and Europe and is transmitted by infected ticks. Patients present with a characteristic bull's-eye rash, arthralgia, and fever following a tick bite. Transplacental passage of the causative spirochete is rare but has been documented, and the effect during pregnancy is not completely understood. Treatment in pregnancy is recommended with cefuroxime or amoxicillin following high-risk tick bites or for identified disease.

Toxoplasmosis is a parasitic infection that may be acquired through ingestion of undercooked meat or cat feces. Forty percent of neonates born to mothers with acute toxoplasmosis have evidence of infection, and the risk of fetal injury is greatest if maternal infection occurs in the first trimester. The clinical manifestations of congenital toxoplasmosis include purpuric rash, hepatosplenomegaly, ascites, chorioretinitis, uveitis, periventricular calcifications, ventriculomegaly, and seizure. Treatment is spiramycin for the duration of pregnancy, and if fetal infection is confirmed by PCR of amniotic fluid, pyrimethamine plus sulfadiazine with folinic acid.

Pregnant women and children are the two groups most vulnerable to malaria worldwide. The disease is caused by the protozoa *Plasmodium* and transmitted by the *Anopheles* mosquito. The placenta becomes a site for sequestration of parasites and is associated with fetal growth restriction, preterm labor, and stillbirth. Diagnosis is made through peripheral blood microscopy. Treatment or preventive therapy is with sulfadoxine-pyrimethamine.

Chagas disease is caused by the parasite *Trypanosoma cruzi* spread by triatomine bugs and is more common in Mexico and Central and South America. Presenting symptoms are nonspecific, if they occur at all, including fever, malaise, myalgias, and headache. Diagnosis is made by microscopy of peripheral blood or polymerase chain reaction (PCR). Vertical transmission to the fetus is possible in 1%-2% of affected pregnancies and can have lifelong adverse consequences if not recognized. Treatment is typically delayed until after delivery.

QUESTIONS

1. A 31-year-old G4P0 presents to triage at 28 weeks' gestation with fever and abdominal pain. Initial vitals are temperature 102.1°F, heart rate (HR) 131, blood pressure (BP) 78/45, and respiratory rate (RR) 26. Review of prenatal records shows unremarkable first trimester screening. The results of a 50-g 1-hour oral glucose tolerance test were 92 mg/dL at 0 hours and 142 mg/dL at 1 hour. Examination reveals a patient with diaphoresis and rigors who is otherwise alert and oriented. There is flank tenderness but no fundal tenderness. Initial obstetrical ultrasound shows a single fetus in vertex presentation with reactive nonstress test (NST). Risk factors for pyelonephritis in pregnancy include all of the following EXCEPT:
   a. Young maternal age
   b. Previous history of pyelonephritis
   c. Asymptomatic bacteriuria
   d. Nulliparity
   e. Miscarriage

2. A 42-year-old G2P1 at 41 weeks' gestation by in vitro fertilization (IVF) dating presents for induction of labor. Medical history includes age-related infertility, hypothyroidism, and mild depression. Fetal status shows a reactive NST with the most recent estimated fetal weight in the 32nd percentile. Review of prenatal care shows anorectal-vaginal culture negative for GBS at 36 weeks' gestational age. A cervical ripening balloon and vaginal misoprostol are placed. Forty-eight hours later, despite artificial rupture of membranes for 18 hours and administration of oxytocin (Pitocin), the cervix has remained 5 cm dilated with 50% effacement over three examinations. The patient develops tachycardia with HR 125-135, and an axillary temperature is 101.2°F and 101.5°F 30 minutes later. You begin treatment with ampicillin and gentamicin. The MOST COMMON organism found in the amniotic fluid of women with chorioamnionitis (intraamniotic inflammation or infection "III") is:
   a. Aerobic streptococci
   b. *Bacteroides* sp.
   c. *Gardnerella vaginalis*
   d. *Escherichia coli*
   e. Aerobic gram-negative rods

3. A 21-year-old G1P0 undergoes scheduled cesarean delivery at 39 weeks' gestation for placenta previa. Delivery is complicated by postpartum hemorrhage of 2000 mL due to uterine atony, which resolves with administration of oxytocin (Pitocin) and methylergonovine. Postoperative day 1 she is unable to void, and an indwelling Foley catheter is placed for 900 mL of pale-yellow urine. Postoperative day 2 she develops abdominal pain and fever, and an examination reveals fundal tenderness. You initiate broad-spectrum antibiotics, but the patient remains febrile. In a patient with postcesarean endometritis and persistent fever despite therapy with clindamycin and gentamicin, the MOST LIKELY cause of treatment failure is:
   a. Occult wound infection
   b. Septic pelvic thrombophlebitis
   c. Incorrect antibiotic dosage
   d. Pelvic abscess
   e. Resistant *Enterobius* sp.

4. A 33-year-old G3P3 presents to the office 3 weeks postpartum with a chief complaint of increased vaginal discharge and pain. Her delivery was complicated by category III fetal heart tracing, operative vaginal delivery, and a third-degree laceration, which was repaired with polyglactin suture. Her medical history includes tobacco use, obesity, and pregestational insulin-dependent diabetes. On examination the margins of the perineal repair have separated and appear dusky. There is exquisite pain on examination and palpable crepitus. In a patient with a perineal wound infection and suspected necrotizing fasciitis, surgical debridement MUST be carried out to the point:
   a. The tissue appears clearly viable and tissue bleeding is encountered.
   b. The margins of the surgical field are hemostatic.
   c. The deep fascia is reached.
   d. Serosanguinous discharge appears within the tissue bed.
   e. Purulent discharge appears with the tissue bed.

5. A 22-year-old G1P1 presents for 2-week postpartum follow-up. Intrapartum, she developed severe-range hypertension treated with IV labetalol. She was diagnosed with preeclampsia with severe features, for which she received IV magnesium. At delivery, a mediolateral episiotomy was performed for a category III fetal heart tracing. She was started on oral nifedipine and discharged postpartum day 4 after antihypertensive titration. On presentation to the office, her BP is 141/61, HR 98, and temperature 99.0°F. Examination reveals normal heart sounds without murmur, and lungs are clear to auscultation. Her perineal wound has purulent exudate, tenderness to palpation, and blanching erythema. In a patient who presents with signs of marked superficial cellulitis following episiotomy, initial management should include:
   a. Wound cultures for group-A streptococci and sitz baths
   b. Exploration, debridement, and immediate repair
   c. Exploration, debridement, broad-spectrum oral antibiotics, and healing by secondary intention
   d. Exploration, debridement, and delayed repair

6. A 28-year-old G3P2 at 39 weeks' gestation presents to labor and delivery for induction of labor for oligohydramnios. Medical history includes obesity, chronic hypertension controlled on labetalol, and tobacco use. Surgical history includes LEEP for persistent cervical dysplasia and laparoscopic appendectomy. Induction proceeds with vaginal misoprostol, and the patient promptly develops painful contractions, reports leakage of fluid, and progresses to full dilation. After 2 hours of pushing, fetal station has progressed from +1 to +2 station and fetal heart tone is category II. You suspect occiput posterior presentation and counsel the patient regarding a manual rotation. After 30 additional minutes of pushing, the fetal station moves abruptly from +2 to crowning and the patient has a spontaneous vaginal delivery of a viable male neonate with Apgar scores 7 and 9. A third-degree laceration is noted and repaired. Risk factors for perineal wound infection include all of the following, EXCEPT:
   a. Obesity
   b. Operative vaginal delivery
   c. Third-degree laceration
   d. GBS colonization
   e. Smoking

7. A 29-year-old G1P0 at 40 weeks, 2 days gestational age presents in spontaneous labor. She is found to be 4 cm dilated with 60% effacement and −1 station and undergoes placement of neuraxial anesthesia. She progressed to 6-cm dilation and develops chorioamnionitis, for which she receives ampicillin and gentamicin. She makes slow progress over the next 8 hours to 9-cm dilation and receives oxytocin (Pitocin) for augmentation. An intrauterine pressure catheter is placed, demonstrating adequate uterine contractions, and a repeat examination is unchanged at 9-cm dilation. A cesarean delivery is performed for failure to progress in the active phase of labor. Clindamycin, cefazolin, and azithromycin are added for surgical prophylaxis, and the procedure is uncomplicated. Her initial postpartum course is uncomplicated, and she is discharged on postpartum day 4. She represents to triage on postpartum day 7 with subjective fever, erythema, and purulent discharge from her abdominal wound. Treatment of postcesarean wound infection should include which of the following for a patient with methicillin-resistant *S. aureus* colonization?
   a. Linezolid IV q8hr
   b. Vancomycin by mouth (PO) three times daily
   c. Azithromycin PO daily
   d. Vancomycin IV twice daily
   e. Ampicillin IV q6hr

8. A 41-year-old G2P2 with a history of lupus nephritis and chronic hypertension presents to triage on postpartum day 7 with fatigue and abdominal pain. Labor was complicated by chorioamnionitis and was treated with vancomycin, clindamycin, and gentamicin given a history of anaphylaxis to penicillin and fetal intolerance to augmentation of labor, for which she underwent cesarean delivery. Examination in triage reveals abdominal tenderness without wound erythema. A CT abdomen/pelvis reveals a 4.3 × 6.1 × 2.1 cm rim enhancing fluid collection in the posterior cul-de-sac, and the patient is admitted for interventional radiology-guided drainage and broad-spectrum antibiotics. For patients with a postcesarean pelvic abscess receiving ampicillin, gentamicin, and clindamycin who develop renal dysfunction, which of the following is the appropriate substitute?
   a. Vancomycin for ampicillin
   b. Aztreonam for gentamicin
   c. Metronidazole for ampicillin
   d. Aztreonam for clindamycin
   e. Metronidazole for clindamycin

9. A 25-year-old G2P2 at 23 weeks' gestation with spontaneous di-di twin pregnancy presents to labor and delivery with reports of several days of increased watery vaginal discharge and intermittent cramping. Her medical history is pertinent for chronic hypertension, tobacco use, obesity, and asthma. Speculum examination demonstrates a visually closed cervix, positive ferning, positive nitrazine, and pooling of flocculent fluid consistent with gross rupture. Initial examination demonstrates a patient is afebrile and in no acute distress, BP 151/95, HR 101, and RR 12. External cardiotocography shows reactive NSTs for both fetuses. After counseling, the patient opts for expectant management and is admitted to the antepartum service to begin latency antibiotics with azithromycin and ampicillin. Six hours later the patient develops an altered mental status. The patient's vitals are found to include HR 133, BP 76/33, and T 101.0°F, and a rapid response is called. For a pregnant patient with suspected sepsis, the first priority in treatment is:
   a. Broad-spectrum antibiotics
   b. Obstetrical ultrasound to evaluate fetal lie and HR
   c. IV fluid therapy
   d. Vasopressors
   e. Central line placement

10. A 44-year-old G1P0 with an IVF pregnancy undergoes scheduled cesarean delivery at 39 weeks' gestation for placenta previa. Delivery is complicated by prolonged operative time due to adhesiolysis for stage IV endometriosis. Postoperative day 2 the patient complains of dull abdominal pain and chills. An examination reveals mild fundal tenderness, and vitals show HR 104, BP 121/81, and RR 12 T 100.5°F and O_2 99% on room air. Laboratory analysis including CBC, comprehensive metabolic panel, chest radiograph, and spot urinalysis are unrevealing. Blood cultures and urine culture are sent, and broad-spectrum antibiotics with ampicillin-sulbactam are initiated for presumed endometritis. Twenty-four hours later the patient remains febrile with persistent abdominal discomfort. A CT abdomen/pelvis is performed, revealing a thickened, tortuous, ropelike structure in the proximity of the right ovarian vein. Initial empiric treatment for septic pelvic thrombophlebitis should include:
    a. Anticoagulation with anti-factor Xa inhibitors
    b. Vascular surgical consultation
    c. Placement of an inferior vena cava filter
    d. Anticoagulation with IV heparin
    e. Anticoagulation with IV heparin and administration of antibiotics

11. A 26-year-old woman, gravida 1, para 1, who had an uncomplicated vaginal delivery 3 days ago comes to OB triage after calling to report right-sided lower abdominal discomfort radiating to the ipsilateral flank, nausea, and nonbloody emesis. On arrival, her temperature is 37.8°C, her HR is 102 bpm, her oxygen saturation is 97% on room air, she is tachypneic with a RR of 21 breaths per minute, and she exhibits guarding without rebound tenderness on palpation of the right lower abdomen. Review of systems is positive for newly increased urinary frequency and urine that she reports is "a little red." Her work-up, including an electrocardiogram, labs, pelvic ultrasound, and a chest x-ray, is unremarkable, with the exception of a slight leukocytosis to 11,200 WBCs/microliter with normal differential and a urinalysis with 100 WBC/hpf, 1+ leukocyte esterase, and 2+ squamous epithelial cells. A urine culture is not available. A CT scan of the abdomen and pelvis with IV contrast shows no evidence of pelvic fluid collection, appendicitis, or nephrolithiasis. Which of the following is the most likely diagnosis:
    a. Nephrolithiasis
    b. Adnexal torsion
    c. Pelvic abscess
    d. Septic pelvic vein thrombophlebitis
    e. Chorioamnionitis

12. A 39-year-old, nulliparous woman at 25 weeks' gestation presents to the emergency department with a chief complaint of fever. She reports chills, myalgias, and back pain. Her vitals show a temperature of 102.2F, HR 120 beats per minute, BP 100/60 mm Hg, and an O_2 saturation of 97%. She has no localizing symptoms on examination. Blood cultures are collected, and an amniocentesis Gram stain exhibits gram-positive pleomorphic rods with rounded ends. This pathogen has a predilection to form placental abscesses. Which of the following is the most appropriate pharmacotherapy at this time?
    a. PO trimethoprim-sulfamethoxazole for 7 days
    b. IV ampicillin for 14 days
    c. IV ceftriaxone for 2 days
    d. IV penicillin for 3 doses
    e. PO amoxicillin for 14 days

13. A 31-year-old woman, gravida 1, para 1, who had an uncomplicated vaginal delivery 2 months prior comes to the clinic to seek advice regarding poor latching. She appears in no acute distress but is flushed and asks for the temperature to be turned down. During the conversation, she winces as her left elbow crosses her chest. Further examination reveals a cracked nipple with surrounding erythema, tenderness extending to the ipsilateral axilla, and associated mild adenopathy but without evidence of mass on deep palpation. She reports expression of slight discolored material with pumping. On intake vitals, her temperature is 39°C, her heart rate is 74 bpm, her BP is 123/76 mm Hg, and her oxygen saturation is 100% on room air. You prescribe her dicloxacillin for a tentative 7-day course. In addition, what advice should you provide the mother with?
    a. Continue nursing with careful attention to thorough breast drainage.
    b. Pump and discard milk with careful attention to thorough breast drainage.
    c. Allow the breasts to "rest" removing only enough milk to relief discomfort.
    d. Wear loose-fitting bras.
    e. Present to interventional radiology for abscess drainage.

14. A 21-year-old gravida 5, para 1, woman at 10 weeks' gestation presents for initial prenatal visit. She has no complaints. Her initial prenatal labs are notable for a positive *Treponema pallidum* particle agglutination assay. A quantitative rapid plasma reagin (RPR) is positive. Which of the following is the most likely diagnosis?
    a. Acute syphilis infection
    b. Chronic syphilis infection
    c. Insufficient information to determine acute versus chronic syphilis infection
    d. Congenital syphilis infection
    e. False-positive result

15. A 34-year-old woman, gravida 2, para 2, who immigrated to the United States from South America roughly 2 months ago, had an uncomplicated vaginal delivery 1 month ago, and carries no diagnoses appears in OB triage acutely dyspneic, with 3+ bilateral lower extremity pitting edema, bilateral pleural effusions, pulmonary vascular congestion, and cardiomegaly on a two-view chest radiograph. She is placed on 4 L of oxygen per minute via nasal cannula for hypoxia on room air, her BP is 98/52 mm Hg without associated dizziness, and she is tachycardic to 115 bpm with sinus rhythm and normal electrocardiogram. Her sodium is 127 mEq/L, her BNP is 2000 pg/mL, her total bilirubin is 2 mg/dL, her AST is 88 U/L, and her ALT is 92 U/L. A transthoracic echocardiogram is concerning for dilated cardiomyopathy. She has had two cats at home for the past 5 years. A kissing bug is a known transmitter of this disease. PCR and serum IgG tests looking to identify which organism will establish the diagnosis:
    a. *Taenia solium*
    b. *Trichinella spiralis*
    c. *Trypanosoma cruzi*
    d. *Toxoplasma gondii*
    e. *Plasmodium ovale*

16. A 35-year-old woman, gravida 0, para 0, without prior medical history who has been trying to conceive with her partner for the past 5 months comes to your clinic for a consultation regarding when to consider IVF. Her intake vitals and physical examination are unremarkable, and a full review of systems is negative. After discussion about the time interval after which unsuccessful attempts at conception should warrant concern and further investigation, she tells you that she and her partner will be living in a country in West Africa for work and are unable to defer travel. During this time, they plan to continue to try to conceive. What preventative measure is the most important to recommend to prevent local disease?
    a. Avoiding undercooked meats
    b. Use of insecticide-treated bednets and antimalarial prophylaxis
    c. Measles, mumps, rubella vaccine
    d. Daily amoxicillin-pot clavulanate (Augmentin) prophylaxis
    e. Avoiding drinking water straight from a river

17. A 35-year-old gravida 1, para 1, who is 2 weeks status post an uncomplicated spontaneous vaginal delivery takes her neonate to the pediatric emergency department for failure to thrive. The neonate is diagnosed with meningitis likely due to late-onset GBS. What is the highest risk factor for transmission?
    a. Nosocomial transmission from nursery
    b. Prolonged rupture of membranes
    c. Maternal intrapartum fever
    d. Multiple cervical examinations in labor
    e. Prematurity

18. A 21-year-old woman, gravida 0, para 0, without prior medical history comes to your clinic for a preconception visit with her fiancé. Her intake vitals are normal, and a full review of systems is negative on initial questioning. Pelvic examination reveals no lesions, cardiac and abdominal examinations are normal, but pulmonary auscultation reveals absent breath sounds at the bilateral bases. Her social history is notable for active tobacco and marijuana use, a remote history of unprotected sexual intercourse with multiple partners, and time spent in a juvenile detention center in her mid-teens. Family history is notable for rheumatoid arthritis in her mother and Sjogren disease in a maternal aunt. When asked if she has a history of similar symptoms, she reports occasional pleuritic chest pain and has been trying topical emollients for "sun sensitivity" on her face. You raise your concern for occult rheumatologic disease and ask her to stop by the laboratory for a serum antinuclear antibody (ANA) titer. She and her fiancé request sexually transmitted disease screening, which you order. Both her treponemal and nontreponemal tests return positive, and her ANA titer is 1:640. A full rheumatologic panel has been ordered. Which of the following is most likely to explain the results of her treponemal and nontreponemal testing?
   a. False negative
   b. False positive
   c. True positive
   d. True negative
   e. Insufficient information

19. A 38-year-old, gravida 2, para 1, woman at 30 weeks' gestation presents for a routine obstetric visit. She is measuring size less than dates, which prompts her provider to obtain a growth ultrasound. Her medical history is notable for poorly controlled type 1 diabetes mellitus and social history notable for working in a butcher shop. The ultrasound findings include ventriculomegaly, intracranial calcifications, hepatomegaly, liver calcifications, and severe fetal growth restriction. An amniocentesis is performed, and PCR is positive for toxoplasmosis DNA. Which of the following is the most appropriate pharmacotherapy?
   a. Spiramycin
   b. Ganciclovir
   c. Penicillin
   d. Pyrimethamine and sulfadiazine and folinic acid
   e. Mefloquine

20. A 19-year-old gravida 1 woman presents to labor and delivery with painful contractions at 39 weeks' gestation. She has had intermittent prenatal care and no GBS swab result on file. A GBS swab is collected and the results are pending. Her allergy to penicillins is anaphylaxis. When the patient is 8 cm dilated, she experiences spontaneous rupture of membranes. Which of the following is the most appropriate next step in management?
   a. Penicillin
   b. No antibiotics at this time
   c. Vancomycin
   d. Cefazolin (Ancef)
   e. Clindamycin

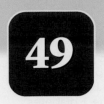

49

Maternal and Fetal Viral Infections

KARIN NIELSEN-SAINES | MARY CATHERINE CAMBOU

(see Creasy and Resnik's Maternal-Fetal Medicine, 9e: Ch 49)

Summary

Infectious diseases are the most common clinical problem encountered by obstetricians. Pregnancy is a period of immune reshaping and physiologic changes, both of which may render greater maternal susceptibility to infection. Pregnancy notoriously renders women more susceptible to acquisition of viral infections such as cytomegalovirus (CMV) or human immunodeficiency virus (HIV). Gestation can also be associated with worse maternal outcomes in the case of infections due to influenza, measles, hepatitis E, yellow fever, severe acute respiratory syndrome coronavirus 2 (SARS CoV-2), and also nonviral infections such as coccidiodomycosis (Valley fever). Viral infections, particularly, can be an important cause of adverse outcomes for the maternal-fetal pair by either leading to severe maternal morbidity or mortality or causing severe complications to the fetus and newborn infant, including significant teratogenicity or other serious complications such as prematurity, fetal growth restriction, and severe fetal anemia. This is the case with herpes simplex virus (HSV), Parvovirus B19, CMV, rubella virus, and Zika virus. Congenital CMV, congenital rubella syndrome, congenital varicella syndrome, and, more recently, congenital Zika syndrome are all important causes of severe fetal malformations leading to serious childhood disability with long-term repercussions. Serious threats to maternal-fetal health are also posed by Chikungunya virus, HIV, Ebola virus, and more recently SARS CoV-2.

When evaluating viral infections during pregnancy, it is important to distinguish between viruses that may lead to adverse fetal outcomes by severely impacting maternal health and viruses that are relatively benign to the mother but may be vertically transmitted and lead to untoward outcomes due to viral replication in the fetus. The timing in pregnancy in which women are infected is also critical to the mechanism of pathogenesis. Certain pathogens tend to cause the most damage when transmitted early in pregnancy during the time of embryogenesis; those are usually teratogenic viruses such as rubella, CMV, and Zika virus, which are generally innocuous to the mother but deleterious to fetal development. Varicella zoster virus when transmitted early in pregnancy following primary infection can also lead to congenital varicella syndrome. Other viruses are more easily transmitted later in pregnancy, as in the case of HIV and CMV (though early transmission of CMV is more likely to lead to teratogenicity). Infection later in pregnancy, especially close to delivery, can have devastating consequences to the newborn infant, as in the case of maternal varicella right before delivery, acute maternal Chikungunya infection, or primary maternal genital HSV infection. In this situation, the infant acquires the virus perinatally without passive transfer of effective maternal antibodies. This may lead to a severe sepsis-like illness in the immediate neonatal period due to disseminated HSV, varicella, or Chikungunya, for example.

The mechanism through which a virus impacts pregnancy may also differ. Some viruses can infect trophoblasts, transferring through the placenta to the fetus. The level of viremia is critical to vertical transmission in many situations such as in the case of HIV and Hepatitis B or C, for which antivirals have been shown to successfully reduce transmission. Some viruses infect the fetus through an ascending vaginal infection at the time of birth, whereas other viruses will adversely impact fetal health solely by severely impacting maternal health without necessarily ever crossing over to the fetus. Such is the case of measles, influenza, hepatitis E, and yellow fever virus. More recently, SARS CoV-2, which has a low vertical transmission rate, has been shown to have the potential to adversely affect the fetus through the induction of a hostile maternal inflammatory environment in utero. In the case of COVID-19 and possibly many other infections, altered maternal inflammatory chemokine/cytokine parameters may lead to adverse immunologic parameters in early infant life with potential repercussions to future neurodevelopment.

From an environmental perspective, global warming and population mobility have in recent years increased the geographic span of arboviral vectors such as *Aedes* species mosquitoes. This has led to an increase in arboviral infections globally, with more pregnant women becoming infected with dengue, chikungunya, and Zika viruses. There are many different species of arboviruses globally, and the threat of new outbreaks lingers, particularly since arboviral outbreaks are cyclical. There is a potential for other flaviviruses such as West Nile Virus to be teratogenic as well, so one should be cognizant of the potential risk these may confer to pregnant hosts. In addition, Zika virus, unlike most arboviral infections, can be transmitted via sexual contact, so women who are pregnant can still be infected by their partners without necessarily traveling to endemic areas.

In summary, the embryologic, fetal, and immediate neonatal periods are a window to an individual's future health, not only during childhood but also throughout adult life. Fetal health mirrors maternal health. It is critical that infections during pregnancy be surveilled; prevented when possible, through the use of vaccines; and promptly diagnosed and treated, to improve long-term maternal and fetal outcomes and prevent serious disabilities. The present chapter reviews the most common viral infections occurring during pregnancy.

QUESTIONS

1. Symptomatic disease is most frequently found in which of the following viral infections?
   a. Dengue
   b. Zika
   c. Yellow fever
   d. Chikungunya
   e. COVID-19

2. The presence of a rash suggests risk of person-to-person transmission is no longer present in which of the following diseases?
   a. Measles
   b. Varicella
   c. Herpes simplex infection
   d. Rubella
   e. Parvovirus B19 disease

3. A 40-week-old term infant born vaginally to a mother who has been HIV infected for 10 years on stable antiretroviral therapy for the past 3 years with an undetectable virus load throughout pregnancy and a CD4 cell count of 480 cells/mm^3 has a risk of acquiring HIV-infection of:
   a. 40%
   b. 25%
   c. 8%
   d. <1%
   e. No risk

4. A 36-week male is born to 20-year-old G1P0. The pregnancy was complicated by oligohydramnios, decreased fetal movement, and decreased fetal growth noted toward the end of gestation. The mother was admitted for observation, and the infant was delivered via cesarean birth. Birthweight was 1980 gm and Apgar scores were 8 $^{1 \, min}$ and 9 $^{5 \, min}$. The infant had mild respiratory distress at delivery, diffuse petechiae, and a blueberry muffin rash. Hepatomegaly and thrombocytopenia are present, as well as rapid development of jaundice. Computed tomography scan of the brain demonstrates periventricular calcifications. No seizure activity is detected. Immediate therapeutic management of this infant would most likely include:
   a. acyclovir IV
   b. pyrimethamine with sulfadiazine and folic acid
   c. crystalline penicillin G
   d. gancyclovir IV
   e. valgancyclovir

5. Third-trimester/perinatal mother-to-child transmission of this viral pathogen is unlikely with the following:
   a. Varicella
   b. Rubella
   c. HSV-2
   d. Chikungunya
   e. HIV

6. A neonatal sepsis-like picture is more likely present in an infant born to a mother with the following viral infection during pregnancy:
   a. Rubella
   b. Parvovirus B19
   c. HSV-2
   d. HIV
   e. Hepatitis C

7. An infectious cause of congenital heart disease in a newborn is most likely due to the following maternal infection in pregnancy:
   a. Measles
   b. Dengue
   c. Chikungunya
   d. Rubella
   e. West Nile

8. The most common infectious cause of sensorineural hearing loss in a young toddler is exposure to which virus in utero?
   a. CMV
   b. Rubella
   c. Measles
   d. Parvovirus B19
   e. Yellow fever

9. A 21-year-old woman who is fully immunized according to the CDC guidelines and who has never left upstate New York during pregnancy gives birth to a child with microcephaly. The following maternal infection is likely not responsible:
   a. Zika virus
   b. Chikungunya
   c. CMV
   d. West Nile
   e. All infections above could have been responsible for microcephaly in this setting.

10. In a 2-day-old newborn with several congenital defects due to a maternal infection during pregnancy, the following virus is unlikely to be identified in the infant:
    a. Zika
    b. CMV
    c. Rubella
    d. Varicella
    e. None of the above

11. The ACIP lists pregnant women as a high-priority group for the seasonal influenza vaccine. The influenza vaccine is safe in which trimester of pregnancy?
    a. First only
    b. Second only
    c. Third only
    d. During any trimester
    e. None of the above

12. A 32-year-old G3P2 presents to a clinic with cough for 3 days. Her 5-year-old son was diagnosed with COVID-19 yesterday. The preferred diagnostic test is:
    a. antigen testing
    b. IgM
    c. IgG
    d. nasopharyngeal RT-PCR
    e. none of the above

13. A 25-year-old G2P1 at 35 weeks presents to the emergency department with 7 days of fever, myalgias, and diarrhea. She returned 2 weeks ago from a 2-month trip to the Democratic Republic of the Congo, where there is currently an Ebola outbreak. Two family members have similar symptoms. You have high suspicion for Ebola. What is the estimated maternal mortality for Ebola without treatment?
    a. 2%
    b. 15%
    c. 35%
    d. 90%
    e. 100%

14. While perinatal transmission of HPV is rare, which HPV genotypes cause respiratory papillomatosis (laryngeal papilloma)?
    a. 6 and 11
    b. 16 and 18
    c. 6, 11, 16, and 18
    d. None of the above

15. Infection with mumps during the first trimester is associated with:
    a. spontaneous abortion
    b. atrial septal defects
    c. neural tube defects
    d. fetal growth restriction
    e. all of the above

Sexually Transmitted Diseases

ROBERT PHILLIPS HEINE | JOSHUA F. NITSCHE

(see *Creasy and Resnik's Maternal-Fetal Medicine, 9e:* Ch 50)

Summary

Rates of sexually transmitted diseases are increasing in women of reproductive age. Thus, pregnancies complicated by these infections have and will continue to become more prevalent. A number of these infections, such as gonorrhea, chlamydia, herpes simplex virus, and syphilis, can have a significant impact on both the women's overall health and that of her pregnancy. Others, such as trichomoniasis and bacterial vaginosis, don't pose significant long-term concerns for the mother but are linked to substantial pregnancy and neonatal complications. Thus, an understanding of the diagnosis, treatment, and prevention of these infections in pregnancy is essential for the modern obstetrician.

Vulvovaginal candidiasis (VVC) is relatively common in pregnancy, especially those also complicated by diabetes, obesity, immunosuppression, or recent use of broad-spectrum antibiotics. Such an infection is typically diagnosed on the basis of hyphae presence on a potassium hydroxide wet preparation or yeast culture if the wet preparation is normal but suspicion for a yeast infection remains high. Topical azole creams are the first-line treatment for nonrecurrent VVC, with oral fluconazole for recurrent or resistant infections. Pregnancy complications are rare with VVC.

Trichomoniasis is another cause of vaginitis that is usually characterized by pruritus, dysuria, and a malodorous, yellow-green, frothy discharge. Diagnosis is made most often on saline wet preparation showing numerous leukocytes and motile, flagellated trichomonads; however, culture and commercial testing systems for causes of vaginitis are more sensitive. Metronidazole, as either a single 2-g dose or 7-day course of 500 mg PO twice daily, is the recommended treatment. Trichomoniasis in pregnancy has been associated with an increased rate of low birth weight, preterm delivery, and preterm premature rupture of membranes (PPROM).

Bacterial vaginosis (BV), yet another cause of vaginitis, is a polymicrobial overgrowth where pathogenic species of *Gardenella*, *Mycoplasma*, *Prevotella*, *Atopobium*, *Mobiluncus*, *Sneathea*, and *Leptotrichia* outnumber the typical lactobacillus that predominate in the vagina. Like VVC and trichomoniasis, it is most often diagnosed via saline wet preparations with clue cells comprising 20% or more of the epithelial cells present. Additional diagnostic features include a positive whiff test with addition of potassium hydroxide and an elevation of the vaginal pH. A 7-day course of metronidazole 500 mg PO twice a day is the most effective treatment, as a single 2-g dose of metronidazole has significantly lower cure rates. BV has been associated with an increased rate of preterm delivery, clinical chorioamnionitis, and endometritis.

Gonorrhea is caused by the gram-negative diplococcus *Neisseria gonorrhea* and transmitted solely by sexual contact. As women with gonorrhea are typically asymptomatic, screening via nucleic acid amplification (along with chlamydia) is recommended in all pregnancies. Rescreening in the same pregnancy is recommended in areas with a high prevalence of the disease. Most maternal infections are isolated to the anus and genitalia, but pharyngeal and disseminated infections occur. In pregnancy, current Centers for Disease Control and Prevention (CDC) guidelines call for treatment with a single IM 500-mg dose of ceftriaxone, along with a single PO dose of 1 g of azithromycin as cotreatment for a chlamydial infection. While the risks of ophthalmia neonatorum in newborns exposed to *N. gonorrhea* during delivery has long been known, there is also an association with maternal gonorrhea and intraamniotic infection, PPROM, chorioamnionitis, preterm birth, fetal growth restriction, neonatal sepsis, and postpartum endometritis.

Chlamydiae are obligate intracellular bacteria that can cause cervicitis similar to that seen with *N. gonorrhea*, but they are more likely to spread beyond the cervix and progress to pelvic inflammatory disease, which in turn is associated with tubal factor infertility, ectopic pregnancy, and pelvic pain. Screening via nucleic acid amplification (along with *N. gonorrhea*) is recommended in all pregnancies. Treatment options include a single PO azithromycin dose of 1 g. Association between chlamydial infections and PPROM, low-birth-weight infants, and neonatal death has been described; however, other studies have found no association between maternal chlamydial infection and adverse pregnancy outcomes.

Human papilloma virus (HPV) has been well established as the cause of anogenital warts and cervical and vaginal cancer. While hundreds of HPV types exist, only certain types are associated with a high risk of cervical dysplasia. Low-risk HPV types are more often associated with warts. Asymptomatic anogenital warts are most often not treated in pregnancy unless the infection is extensive. The safety of podophyllin resin, podofilox, or imiquimod in pregnancy are not well known and thus are typically avoided in pregnancy. Treatment with topical trichloracetic or bicloracetic acid or excision remain possible in pregnancy. Treatment of cervical dysplasia short of microinvasive cancer is typically deferred until after pregnancy, with excision during pregnancy reserved for microinvasive disease. Other than a very low risk of neonatal pharyngeal papillomatosis, HPV infection itself poses little risk to the pregnancy. However, the use of loop electric excisional procedure or cervical conization used in the treatment of cervical dysplasia has been associated with a small risk of cervical insufficiency and preterm delivery in pregnancies that occur after these procedures.

Herpes simplex virus (HSV) most often causes a vesicular eruption in the oral or genital area. While historically HSV-1 was thought to be the predominant cause of oral infections and HSV-2 the predominant cause of genital infections, this is no longer the case, as now up to 40% of new genital herpes infections are due to HSV-1. Maternal infection is typically self-limiting and resolves spontaneously. Treatment for both primary and recurrent disease is with acyclovir or valacyclovir. The greater concern is transmission of the infection to the neonate if the mother has an active HSV outbreak at the time of delivery. Manifestations of neonatal HSV disease include skin lesions, cough, cyanosis, tachypnea, dyspnea, jaundice, seizures, and disseminated intravascular coagulation as the infection spreads from the skin and becomes more disseminated, leading to pneumonitis and encephalitis. Given the potential severity of this disease, cesarean delivery is recommended for women with an active herpes infection at the time of delivery.

Syphilis can involve nearly all organ systems and is a result of infection with the spirochete *Treponema pallidum*. This infection has a wide variety of manifestations, the first most often being the presence of a painless chancre at the site of inoculation along with lymphadenopathy. As these resolve, the spirochetes then spread throughout the body, where they can lie dormant. Ultimately, they may lead to pathology of any organ system weeks or years after the initial infection. The cardiovascular and central nervous systems are systems most commonly affected in this way, leading to aortic aneurysm, aortic insufficiency, general paresis, tabes dorsalis, optic atrophy, and meningitis. Diagnosis is typically reached through a

two-phase testing strategy, which starts with a nontreponemal specific test such as the rapid plasma reagin (RPR) or the Venereal Disease Research Laboratory (VDRL) test. If these are positive, treponemal specific tests, such as the fluorescent treponemal antibody absorption test and the *T. pallidum* particle agglutination assay, are performed, and if positive, they confirm infection. While the use of other drugs outside of pregnancy remains an option in nonpregnant women, the primary treatment of syphilis in pregnancy is penicillin. The type, route, interval, and duration of treat varies with the type of syphilis present. Penicillin is the only therapy shown to effectively treat and prevent fetal disease, and thus is called for in all cases of infection in pregnancy. Even patients with severe allergy to penicillin should be desensitized and then treated with penicillin for this reason. Congenital syphilis can have devastating consequences for the fetus/newborn. The clinical spectrum of congenital syphilis includes stillbirth, neonatal death, nonimmune hydrops, and neonatal hepatosplenomegaly, characteristic skin rash, condyloma lata, snuffles, jaundice, pseudoparalysis, anemia, thrombocytopenia, and edema. Stigmata in children older than 2 years of age include interstitial keratitis, nerve deafness, anterior bowing of shins, frontal bossing, mulberry molars, Hutchinson teeth, saddle nose, rhagades, and Clutton joints.

QUESTIONS

1. At 24-year-old G2P1001 presents for her initial prenatal care at 12 weeks of gestation. She reports that her current sexual partner tested positive for gonorrhea. She would like to be tested. What is the most appropriate test to order at this time?
   a. Nucleic acid amplification for *Neisseria gonorrhea*
   b. Nucleic acid amplification for *N. gonorrhea* and *Chlamydia trachomatis*
   c. Culture for *N. gonorrhea*
   d. Culture for *N. gonorrhea* and *C. trachomatis*
   e. Nucleic acid amplification for *N. gonorrhea* and culture for *C. trachomatis*

2. She tests positive. What is the most appropriate treatment for her?
   a. Ceftriaxone IM
   b. Doxycycline PO
   c. Ceftriaxone IM and doxycycline PO
   d. Cetriaxone IM and azithromycin PO
   e. Doxycycline and azithromycin PO

3. The patient is concerned about what, if any, effects this infection may have on her infant. You reassure her that all infants are treated with antibiotics after birth to prevent which of the following neonatal gonococcal infection?
   a. Cellulitis
   b. Pharyngitis
   c. Conjunctivitis
   d. Pneumonia
   e. Encephalitis

4. A 28-year-old G1P0 presents at 28 weeks with pain and burning of the vulva. Physical examination shows vesicles on the labia minora bilaterally but none on the vagina or cervix. You suspect an HSV infection. What is the best test to determine the etiology of this infection?
   a. HSV viral culture of vesicular swab
   b. HSV polymerase chain reaction of vesicular swab
   c. Tzank smear of vesicular swab
   d. HSV serologies of maternal serum
   e. HSV polymerase chain reaction of maternal serum

5. She is confirmed to have an active HSV-2 infection. Her serologies show IgG for HSV-1, but they are negative for HSV-2. What type of HSV infection does she have?
   a. First-episode primary genital herpes
   b. First-episode nonprimary genital herpes
   c. Second-episode primary genital herpes
   d. Second-episode nonprimary genital herpes
   e. Recurrent genital herpes

6. What is the most appropriate treatment for the patient's genital herpes infection?
   a. Acyclovir PO for 5 days
   b. Acyclovir PO for 7–10 days
   c. Gancyclovir PO for 5 days
   d. Valacyclovir IV for 5 days
   e. Valacyclovir IV for 7–10 days

7. She presents to Labor & Delivery triage at term for decreased fetal movement and has a biophysical profile of 6/10. The decision is made to proceed with delivery. She reports vulvar burning and tingling. What is the most appropriate mode of delivery for her?
   a. Cesarean delivery only if herpes lesions on the vulva are present
   b. Cesarean delivery only if herpes lesions on the vaginal or cervix are present
   c. Cesarean delivery regardless of the presence of genital herpes lesions
   d. Induction of labor if she has no genital herpes lesions
   e. Induction of labor regardless of the presence of genital herpes lesions

8. She is concerned about the risks of her neonate becoming infected. Which of the following is the most significant manifestation of neonatal herpes infection?
   a. Cellulitis
   b. Pharyngitis
   c. Conjunctivitis
   d. Pneumonia
   e. Encephalitis

9. A 32-year-old G2P0101 presents for prenatal care for the first time at 28 weeks. She had a positive RPR with a titer of 1:32 on her routine prenatal labs. What is the most appropriate confirmatory test for syphilis?
   a. Darkfield microscopy of maternal blood
   b. *Trepona palladium* culture of cervical secretions
   c. Fluorescent treponemal antibody absorption test
   d. Treponemal serologies of maternal blood
   e. Cervical cytology

10. Review of her prenatal records reveals that her RPR was negative 10 months ago during her last pregnancy. What type of syphilis does she have?
    a. Primary
    b. Secondary
    c. Early latent
    d. Late latent
    e. Tertiary

11. What is the most appropriate treatment for her at this time?
    a. Benzathine penicillin IM for a single dose
    b. Benzathine penicillin IM weekly for 3 doses
    c. Benzatheine penicillin IM daily for 10–14 days
    d. Aqueous crystalline penicillin IV for 10–14 days
    e. Procaine penicillin plus probenecid PO for 10–14 days

12. If she were allergic to penicillin, what would be the most appropriate treatment?
    a. Doxycycline PO twice daily for 14 days
    b. Ceftriaxone IV daily for 10–14 days
    c. Tetracycline PO 4 times daily for 14 days
    d. Amoxicillin plus probenecid PO twice daily for 14 days
    e. Benzathine penicillin IM after penicillin desensitization

13. She returns after delivery, now 6 months from her initial positive RPR test of 1:32. The repeat value from 2 days ago is 1:16. What is the most appropriate treatment for her at this time provided she is not penicillin allergic?
    a. Repeat RPR in another 6 months
    b. Benzathine penicillin IM
    c. Doxycycline PO
    d. Ceftriaxone IV
    e. Amoxicillin plus probenecid PO

14. Which of the following infections is NOT associated with preterm delivery?
    a. Trichomoniasis
    b. Bacterial vaginosis
    c. Vulvovaginal candidiasis
    d. Chlamydial cervicitis
    e. Gonorrhea cervicitis

15. Which of the following is the most serious neonatal infection caused by *C. trachomatis*?
    a. Cellulitis
    b. Pharyngitis
    c. Conjunctivitis
    d. Pneumonia
    e. Encephalitis

16. Which of the following topical therapies can be used to treat genital warts in pregnancy?
    a. Podophyllin resin
    b. Podofilox
    c. Imiquomod
    d. Tricholoracetic acid
    e. Gentian violet

51

Maternal-Fetal Infections

RICHARD BEIGI | CHRISTINA J. MEGLI

(see *Creasy and Resnik's Maternal-Fetal Medicine, 9e: Ch 51*)

Summary

Infections of the mother have the capability to be transmitted across the placenta-to the fetus. These infections can cause disease in both maternal and fetal hosts. The placenta is a major barrier to most infections. Infections that cause disease at the maternal-fetal interface can be teratogenic, interfere with placental function, and cause stillbirth and fetal inflammatory responses.

Cytomegalovirus (CMV) is a DNA herpesvirus and is the most common congenitally acquired viral pathogen. Transmission is predominantly transplacental, and maternal infection is largely subclinical. Primary infection has the greatest risk for vertical transmission. Infection at earlier gestational ages causes more severe disease in the fetus. Congenital CMV can also be acquired with reinfection of a new strain and reactivation. These cause the majority of neonatal cases but are often milder in clinical presentation. Polymerase chain reaction or culture of amniotic fluid is the gold standard for diagnosis. There is no treatment for congenital CMV infection.

Toxoplasma gondii is a protozoan parasite that can be transmitted vertically. Maternal infection is through ingestion of contaminated food containing the oocytes of the parasite. Screening is not universal in the United States, and diagnosis is typically made by a known exposure of history. *T. gondii* is one of the few vertical infections that can be treated. Treatment regimens are based on gestational age. In the first trimester spiramycin is used, but after 18 weeks pyrimethamine, folinic acid, and sulfadiazine are used. Pediatric consultation is important for neonatal treatment. Prevention is through avoiding uncooked meat and contact with cat litter.

Zika virus (ZIKV) is an RNA flavivirus associated with Congenital Zika syndrome. ZIKV is transmitted to the maternal host through vector-dependent (mosquito) and vector-independent mechanisms (sexual contact). Infection is typically symptomatic, and symptoms include rash, fever, arthralgias, and conjunctivitis. Vertical transmission causing Congenital Zika syndrome occurs in <10% of maternal cases. Congenital Zika syndrome includes microcephaly, subcortical abnormalities, ocular abnormalities, contractures, and motor defects. Non−nervous system findings have been reported as well. Diagnosis is through molecular testing, and only those with symptoms or ongoing exposure to an area of actively circulating ZIKV should be tested. Congenital diagnosis is based on clinical examination and detection of ZIKV. There is no treatment for ZIKV. Prevention is using mosquito repellant in endemic areas.

Rubella is caused by Rubella virus infection. Immunity is lifelong, and vaccination has reduced the incidence of rubella. Maternal presentation is subclinical but can lead to congenital rubella syndrome with transplacental transmission. Vertical transmission occurs before 18 weeks and results in deafness, cataracts, central nervous system defects, and cardiac malformations. There is no treatment, and prevention is through vaccination.

Parvovirus B19 is a DNA virus that is transmitted through respiratory droplets. Maternal clinical presentation is subclinical or through known exposure to an infected child. Serologic immunity is protective from vertical transmission. In the absence of immunity there is a risk of fetal transmission that can cause fetal anemia, thrombocytopenia, hydrops, and stillbirth. The risk of hydrops is dependent on gestational age at presentation, but patients should be monitored for 8 weeks after exposure/infection. Treatment of the virus is supportive. In the setting of hydrops, the cause is severe anemia and bone marrow suppression, so intrauterine transfusion (IUT) can be used for treatment.

Listeria monocytogenes is a gram-positive bacterium that can cause maternal and fetal disease called listeriosis. Transmission is through contaminated food, and pregnancy is a risk factor for maternal and fetal illness. The incubation period is up to 28 days and can be mild in clinical presentation. Adverse neonatal outcomes are high and include stillbirth, preterm birth, and miscarriage. Diagnosis is through a positive blood culture, and treatment is recommended with ampicillin.

Streptococcus agalactiae, also known as Group B Streptococcus (GBS), is a gram-positive bacterium and a major obstetric pathogen. GBS colonizes the genital and gastrointestinal tract in approximately 20% of women. GBS can ascend the genital tract and is associated with preterm birth, chorioamnionitis, and early-onset sepsis (EOS) in neonates and maternal sepsis. The pathogenesis of the bacteria switching from a commensal to a virulent organism is not understood. Thus, the approach to reduce disease has been to undertake universal intrapartum prophylaxis. GBS screening occurs between 36 and 37 weeks. If positive, intrapartum treatment is indicated with penicillin or ampicillin. In the setting of delivery before 37 weeks, GBS prophylaxis is indicated unless negative. Non−beta-lactam antibiotics are limited by lack of study and rising GBS resistance.

QUESTIONS

1. Second infections of which of the following are not associated with clinical disease?
   a. Rubella
   b. *Treponema pallidum*
   c. *T. gondii*
   d. CMV
   e. GBS

2. In which of the following scenarios is IgG avidity testing for CMV infection recommended to counsel on risk of transmission of congenital CMV?
   a. IgM unknown IgG negative
   b. IgM negative IgG positive
   c. IgM negative IgG negative
   d. IgM positive IgG negative
   e. IgM positive IgG positive

3. Which of the following is the optimal time to begin treatment for toxoplasmosis after seroconversion?
   a. 1 week
   b. 10 weeks
   c. 4 weeks
   d. It doesn't matter

4. Which of the following determines correct treatment for toxoplasmosis?
   a. Gestational age of diagnosis
   b. Site of primary infection
   c. Mechanism of transmission
   d. Parasitemia
   e. Amniocentesis

5. Which of the following best describes the incidence of congenital Zika syndrome with ZIKV infection in pregnancy?
   a. 10%−15%
   b. 5%−10%
   c. <5%
   d. 25%
   e. >25%

6. Which of the following infections contain pathogens that are latent?
   a. ZIKV, toxoplasmosis, listeria
   b. Human immunodeficiency virus (HIV), syphilis, chlamydia
   c. VZV, herpes simplex virus (HSV), CMV
   d. HIV, syphilis, herpesviruses, GBS
   e. None of the above

7. Primary CMV is best diagnosed by which of the following?
   a. IgG positive, IgG high avidity
   b. IgM positive IgG positive IgG low avidity
   c. Polymerase chain reaction (PCR) serum positive
   d. PCR from amniocentesis positive
   e. IgG negative, IgG low avidity
   f. IgM positive, IgG positive IgG high avidity
   g. IgM negative IgG positive

8. Which of the following vaccines is not recommended in pregnancy?
   a. Influenza
   b. Hepatitis B
   c. Yellow fever
   d. Measles, mumps, rubella
   e. TdaP
   f. Sudden acute respiratory syndrome−coronavirus 2 messenger RNA vaccine

9. Which of the following includes pathogens that can be transmitted through parturition and the maternal fetal interface?
   a. GBS, HSV, ZIKV, parvovirus B19
   b. CMV, *T. gondii*, ZIKV
   c. GBS, HSV, listeria, CMV
   d. Listeria, GBS, *T. gondii*
   e. VZV, listeria, HSV

10. Which of the following is the parvovirus B19 VP2 capsid binding site?
    a. Globoside or the P antigen on cells
    b. Trophoblasts, decidual cells, and endothelium
    c. Osteoclasts
    d. Leukocytes
    e. Platelets and Hofbauer cells

11. Which of the following pathogens can cause hydrops?
    a. Parvovirus B-19
    b. GBS
    c. *Escherichia coli*
    d. *L. monocytogenes*
    e. Varicella

12. Inflammasome activation is important for defense against which of the following infections?
    a. GBS
    b. *T. pallidum*
    c. *L. monocytogenes*
    d. Parvovirus B-19
    e. CMV

13. Which of the following is the best way to determine severity of fetal disease from parvovirus B19 infection?
    a. Umbilical cord Dopplers
    b. Umbilical artery Dopplers
    c. Viremia
    d. IgG avidity
    e. Thrombocytopenia in percutaneous umbilical cord blood sampling (PUBS) specimen

14. Which of the following is the most common cause of early-onset sepsis (EOS)?
    a. GBS
    b. *L. monocytogenes*
    c. *H. influenza*
    d. *E. coli*
    e. HSV

15. Which of the following pathogens is <u>not</u> considered a teratogen?
    a. CMV
    b. HSV
    c. *L. monocytogenes*
    d. *T. gondii*
    e. ZIKV

16. Which of the following pathogens are typed in transplant donors and recipients due to the risks of congenital disease?
    a. Toxoplasmosis, CMV, *L. monocytogenes*
    b. HSV, *T. pallidum*
    c. CMV, *T. gondii*
    d. HIV, hepatitis C virus, CMV
    e. HSV, varicella zoster virus, CMV

17. Which of the following is the classic pathologic finding of listeriosis in the placenta?
    a. Owl-eye inclusions
    b. Microthrombus development
    c. Histiocytic infiltrate
    d. Microabscess and macroabscess development
    e. Disruption in the syncytial layer

18. A teacher presents for consultation at 16 weeks after a child in her class was diagnosed with Fifth disease. You order serologies and she is negative for parvovirus IgG. Her IgM is pending. Which of the following is the best next step?
    a. Repeat serologies in 8 weeks
    b. Amniocentesis for diagnosis of congenital infection
    c. Cordocentesis to evaluate for fetal anemia
    d. Ultrasound with middle cerebral artery (MCA) Dopplers

19. Proper food preparation decreases the risk of congenital infection of which of the following pathogens?
    a. GBS
    b. *L. monocytogenes*
    c. CMV
    d. ZIKV

20. A woman presents at 36 weeks for routine prenatal care with a history of childhood penicillin allergy. The patient has had no obstetric complications and has no complaints. What is the next step in management?
    a. Test for penicillin allergy.
    b. Send a GBS culture.
    c. Send a PCR for GBS.
    d. Counsel her on intrapartum prophylaxis with vancomycin.
    e. Treat her with clindamycin to decrease colony count before delivery.

21. Which of the following is the best recommendation for a patient at 19 weeks with recent travel to Brazil who is concerned about Zika infection?
    a. It is recommended that she is tested with an immunoassay or PCR.
    b. She should have an ultrasound to screen for Congenital Zika syndrome.
    c. Amniocentesis is recommended for testing.
    d. The likelihood of a positive result is low, followed by a detailed discussion regarding risks and benefits.
    e. The likelihood of a positive result is high, followed by pregnancy options counseling.

22. Which of the following is the best advice for a patient with repeated work trips during pregnancy to a Zika-endemic area?
    a. It is recommended that she is tested with an immunoassay or PCR.
    b. She should have an ultrasound to screen for Congenital Zika syndrome.
    c. Amniocentesis is recommended for testing.
    d. The likelihood of a positive result is low, followed by a detailed discussion regarding risks and benefits.
    e. The likelihood of a positive result is high, followed by pregnancy options counseling.

23. Which of the following is the most common infectious cause of fetal growth restriction in a daycare worker whose fetus also has echogenic bowel, concern for a small head circumference, and ventriculomegaly?
    a. Toxoplasmosis
    b. Parvovirus
    c. CMV
    d. ZIKV
    e. GBS

Cardiac Diseases

DANIEL G. BLANCHARD | LORI B. DANIELS | LAITH ALSHAWABKEH

(see *Creasy and Resnik's Maternal-Fetal Medicine*, 9e: Ch 52)

Summary

Pregnant women with heart disease are at higher risk for cardiovascular complications during pregnancy and also have a higher incidence of neonatal complications. However, the significant hemodynamic changes that accompany pregnancy make the diagnosis of certain forms of cardiovascular disease difficult. During normal, uncomplicated pregnancies, women frequently experience dyspnea, orthopnea, easy fatigability, dizzy spells, and occasionally even syncope.

Nevertheless, certain findings indicate heart disease in pregnancy and should suggest the presence of a significant cardiovascular abnormality. These symptoms include severe dyspnea, syncope with exertion, hemoptysis, paroxysmal nocturnal dyspnea, and chest pain related to exertion. Physical signs of organic heart disease include a fourth heart sound (S_4 gallop), cyanosis, clubbing, diastolic murmurs, sustained cardiac arrhythmias, and loud, harsh systolic murmurs.

During prepregnancy counseling, the physician should describe the nature of heart disease in terms comprehensible to prospective parents. The risk to the woman, which can vary from negligible to prohibitive, should be spelled out as clearly as possible. On this basis, the patient may be advised that the contemplated pregnancy would be one of the following: safe, uncomfortable and necessitate treatment, at significantly increased risk, or extremely dangerous and prohibited.

Some cardiac disorders are so serious in nature that the physiologic changes of a superimposed pregnancy pose prohibitive risks to the mother; they carry such a high maternal mortality risk that pregnancy is contraindicated. Examples include the following:

- Dilated cardiomyopathy or left ventricular dysfunction (ejection fraction <40%–45%) of any cause
- Severe pulmonary hypertension of any cause
- Marfan syndrome, especially with aortic root dilation (diameter >4 cm)
- Severe symptomatic aortic stenosis, mitral stenosis, or aortic regurgitation

The most serious of these cardiac disorders are those involving pulmonary hypertension, particularly those associated with a right-to-left shunt in cardiac blood flow (Eisenmenger syndrome). Severe idiopathic ("primary") pulmonary arterial hypertension carries a high risk in pregnancy. Pregnancy is not advised in women with this condition because the mortality rate is in the range of 30%.

Valvular heart disease is also relatively common in pregnant women, including bicuspid aortic valve with stenosis, mitral regurgitation, and mitral stenosis. If aortic stenosis is severe and causes symptoms, the woman should be advised against becoming pregnant until the valve is replaced. Maternal mortality rates as high as 17% in women with severe aortic stenosis have been reported.

Severe mitral stenosis is also not well tolerated, and symptoms of heart failure may occur. Moderate to severe mitral regurgitation is generally well tolerated, assuming left ventricular systolic function is preserved.

Because premenopausal women enjoy substantial protection against coronary atherosclerosis, ischemic heart disease is rarely relevant to obstetric practice. However, coronary artery disease (CAD) may be found in women of childbearing age when other risk factors, such as diabetes mellitus, smoking, or severe dyslipidemia, overwhelm the natural protection they should normally enjoy. Lupus erythematosus, especially when treated with steroidal agents, may also precipitate premature CAD. Coronary atherosclerosis appears in a significant proportion of patients who have received a cardiac transplant and may be observed in cases with familial hypercholesterolemia.

Spontaneous coronary artery dissection (SCAD) was considered to be rare and confined mostly to women soon after pregnancy. However, recent improvements in imaging and diagnostic techniques have shown that SCAD is not an infrequent occurrence but is an important cause of acute coronary syndromes, particularly in young women. Treatment has included placement of a stent, emergency coronary bypass operation, and thrombolysis.

This chapter discusses in detail these and other cardiac conditions that can adversely affect outcomes in pregnancy.

QUESTIONS

1. A 26-year-old G1P0 at 24 weeks' gestation with a recent history of palpitations returns for a follow-up appointment. A Holter monitor has shown occasional premature atrial contractions but no atrial fibrillation. An electrocardiogram (ECG) shows a leftward axis, which is new compared with an ECG early in pregnancy. Which of the following is the best next step in management?
   a. Continued cardiac monitoring for 1 month
   b. Echocardiographic examination to evaluate for cardiac structural disease
   c. Discontinuation of caffeine-containing drinks
   d. Reassurance, with routine follow-up visit and examination
   e. Treatment with low-dose metoprolol

2. A 28-year-old nulliparous woman with a history of sudden death in several family members presents for preconceptional counseling. She has had no palpitations, chest pain, or exertional dyspnea. Physical examination is normal except for a II/VI systolic ejection murmur, which increases to III/VI with Valsalva maneuver. Echocardiography confirms the finding of obstructive hypertrophic cardiomyopathy. Which of the following is NOT correct?
   a. The patient should have genetic testing to help assess long-term cardiac risk.
   b. If the patient becomes pregnant, elective cesarean delivery should be performed when labor begins.
   c. Beta-blockers should be continued during pregnancy to prevent tachycardia.
   d. IV beta-blocker (esmolol) can be used during labor to prevent tachycardia.

3. A young woman from Southeast Asia presents during early (and her first) pregnancy. She has had little medical care during her life but has noted mild dyspnea on exertion during her pregnancy so far. On examination, she has a continuous cardiac murmur, which peaks during systole. Echocardiogram shows a moderate-sized patent ductus arteriosus (PDA) with no evidence of right-to-left flow from the pulmonary artery to the aorta. What is the best next step in management?
   a. Immediate surgical correction of the PDA
   b. Immediate placement of percutaneous closure device
   c. Placement of percutaneous PDA closure device after delivery
   d. Use of arterial vasodilators to decrease left-to-right flow through the PDA

4. Of the following congenital shunts of the same size, which confers the lowest risk for fixed pulmonary hypertension and Eisenmenger physiology in young women?
   a. Patent ductus arteriosus
   b. Atrial septal defect (ASD)
   c. Ventricular septal defect

5. A young woman with a normal BMI presents for preconceptional counseling. Her vital signs are normal, but she has a II/VI systolic murmur. A screening echocardiogram shows a thickened aortic valve without regurgitation. The aortic root is moderately increased in diameter. The patient's screening echocardiogram images are suspicious for bicuspid aortic valve. Which one of these tests would you NOT perform?
   a. Genetic evaluation for Marfan disease
   b. Chest computed tomography (CT) scan to evaluate ascending aorta
   c. Echo evaluation of aortic valve area
   d. Evaluation of ascending aortic diameter

6. Which of the following is associated with an increase neonatal morbidity in women with heart disease?
   a. Left heart obstruction
   b. Maternal smoking during pregnancy
   c. Multiple gestation
   d. Mechanical heart valve
   e. All of the above

7. A woman who is 16 weeks pregnant and has a bileaflet mechanical valve in the aortic position presents for evaluation. She is eager to stop warfarin, as she has heard this can cause fetal abnormalities. What is the best next step in management?
   a. Continue warfarin and start apixaban.
   b. Stop warfarin and start aspirin plus clopidogrel.
   c. Continue warfarin.
   d. Stop warfarin and start subcutaneous enoxaparin.

8. A 40-year-old G2P1001 at 8 weeks' gestation and chronic hypertension presents for initiation of care. Which ONE of the following medications can be continued?
   a. Enalapril
   b. Hydrochlorothiazide
   c. Spironolactone
   d. Losartan

9. Which of the following valvular conditions is LEAST well tolerated during pregnancy?
   a. Moderate to severe mitral stenosis
   b. Moderate to severe pulmonic valve stenosis
   c. Moderate to severe aortic stenosis
   d. Moderate to severe coarctation of the aorta

10. A 35-year-old woman with polycystic kidney disease (serum creatinine of 2.0) and familial hypercholesterolemia presents for preconception counseling. She has a family history of coronary disease and has occasional episodes of chest pain (both at rest and with exertion). What is the best next step in evaluation?
    a. Coronary CT scan
    b. Invasive coronary angiography
    c. Exercise ECG test
    d. Exercise echo or nuclear scan

11. A 30-year-old pregnant woman presents with new-onset chest pain early in her third trimester. She has no risk factors for premature CAD. However, her ECG shows anterior ST elevation, consistent with an anterior wall myocardial infarction. The pain has improved with intravenous nitroglycerin. What is the most appropriate diagnostic test?
    a. Nuclear perfusion study of the heart
    b. Coronary angiography
    c. Coronary CT angiogram
    d. Echocardiography (cardiac ultrasound)

12. A pregnant woman comes to her doctor with worsening dyspnea. An echocardiogram shows moderate (and global) left ventricular systolic dysfunction. Peripartum cardiomyopathy (PPCM) is suspected. Which of the following does NOT increase the risk of PPCM?
    a. Maternal age <30 years
    b. African-American racial background
    c. Hypertension
    d. Preeclampsia

13. A 25-year-old nulliparous woman with Marfan syndrome comes in to discuss the risks of pregnancy. The diameter of her ascending aorta is 4.3 cm. Which of the following is NOT true?
    a. The risk of aortic rupture or dissection during pregnancy is ~5% (1 in 20).
    b. Beta blockers should be prescribed throughout the entire pregnancy.
    c. Cesarean delivery is recommended in women with Marfan syndrome and aortic root enlargement.
    d. Aortic valve replacement is indicated if aortic regurgitation gradually becomes moderate to severe.

Coagulation Disorders in Pregnancy

ROBERT M. SILVER | MING Y. LIM

Summary

The coagulation system consists of a remarkable set of factors that allow a delicate balance between cessation of bleeding after tissue injury and maintenance of the integrity of vascular blood flow. Abnormalities in this system can lead to increased risk of both hemorrhage and thrombosis. Pregnancy poses markedly elevated risk for both pathologies, making an understanding of coagulation imperative for obstetricians. After vascular injury, activation of the coagulation cascade and simultaneous platelet adhesion, activation, and aggregation are required to form the optimal fibrin-platelet plug to avoid or stop bleeding. The system is held in check by several factors. The endothelial cell lining covers a thrombogenic subendothelium and is vasodilatory. It is an active participant in preventing inappropriate platelet activation, as well as the anticoagulant and fibrinolytic systems. The hemostatic system is controlled by a potent series of circulating anticoagulant proteins and a highly regulated fibrinolytic system.

On balance, the maternal hemostatic system has evolved to be prothrombotic, likely as protection against obstetrical hemorrhage. The causal link between pregnancy and venous thromboembolism (VTE) is best explained by the Virchow triad, a framework that categorizes elements of the pathophysiology of VTE as venous stasis, vascular damage, and hypercoagulability.

Numerous conditions, termed *thrombophilias*, may further predispose individuals to VTE during pregnancy. The most common acquired thrombophilia is antiphospholipid syndrome (APS). APS requires the presence of at least one clinical criterion (i.e., confirmed thrombosis or pregnancy morbidity) and one laboratory criterion (i.e., lupus anticoagulant, anticardiolipin antibodies, or anti–β_2-glycoprotein-1 antibody). In addition to VTE, people with APS are at increased risk for placental-mediated obstetric complications such as pregnancy loss, preeclampsia, and fetal growth restriction. Treatment with heparin and low-dose aspirin appears to reduce the risk of VTE and improve pregnancy outcomes.

Heritable thrombophilias involve mutations leading to decreased amounts or function of anticoagulant proteins or increased amounts or function of procoagulant proteins. The factor V Leiden mutation and deficiencies of antithrombin III, protein C, and protein S involve abnormalities of anticoagulant proteins. The prothrombin gene mutation is characterized by an increase in the procoagulant factor II. Depending on factors such as the thrombogenicity of the thrombophilia, coexisting obesity, personal history of VTE, family history of VTE, cesarean delivery, and personal preference, prophylactic or therapeutic anticoagulation during pregnancy and/or postpartum may be appropriate. Although heritable thrombophilias had been associated with adverse obstetric outcomes in the past, the association has not held in prospective studies and anticoagulant therapy does not improve pregnancy outcomes.

The most common cause of maternal thrombocytopenia ($<100,000/\mu L$) is gestational thrombocytopenia. This is typically mild ($>70,000/\mu L$), asymptomatic, and incidentally diagnosed. No treatment or intervention is required. Primary immune thrombocytopenia (ITP) is the most common pathologic cause of maternal thrombocytopenia. Treatment is initiated if there is bleeding, platelets are $<20,000/\mu L$, or platelets are $<50,000/\mu L$ in the third trimester or at the time of delivery. Common therapies include corticosteroids and/or intravenous immunoglobulin (IVIG). Platelet transfusion is reserved for bleeding, surgery, or neuraxial anesthesia. Fetal and neonatal thrombocytopenia may occur with ITP. However, serious problems are rare, and in most cases intrapartum care should be routine.

Fetal or neonatal alloimmune thrombocytopenia (AIT) is the most frequent cause of serious fetal and neonatal thrombocytopenia. In contrast with ITP, maternal antibodies are directed against fetal but not maternal platelets. It is usually diagnosed after birth in an infant with unexplained severe thrombocytopenia, often associated with ecchymoses or petechiae. The most serious bleeding complication is intracranial hemorrhage (ICH), which occurs in 10% to 20% of infants with AIT, and rarely it can occur in utero. Confirmation of diagnosis requires assessment of platelet antigen incompatibility and demonstration of specific antiplatelet antibodies that is best accomplished in specialty laboratories. Treatment in subsequent pregnancies includes IVIG and/or steroids, and dosing is based on disease severity. Delivery is typically by cesarean, although vaginal delivery is reasonable if fetal platelet count is $>50,000/\mu L$.

Thrombotic thrombocytopenic purpura (TTP) and atypical hemolytic uremic syndrome (aHUS) are thrombotic microangiopathies that are characterized by thrombocytopenia, hemolytic anemia, and organ dysfunction. Both TTP and aHUS are hard to distinguish from each other, as well as from preeclampsia/eclampsia or hemolysis, elevated liver enzyme levels, and low platelet (HELLP) syndrome. Testing for ADAM metallopeptidase with thrombospondin type 1 motif 13 (ADAMT13) activity is the most reliable method of diagnosing TTP and should be ordered for any pregnancy-associated thrombotic microangiopathies. The diagnosis of aHUS is made by exclusion once all other diagnoses (including TTP) have been ruled out, as there is no reliable diagnostic test for aHUS. Treatment is primarily supportive; treatment with plasmapheresis and steroids (for TTP) or anti-C5 antibody (for aHUS) may also be useful. Delivery of the fetus should be considered in refractory cases, especially at later gestations.

Several bleeding disorders may complicate pregnancy. The most common is von Willebrand disease, which may occur in up to 1% of individuals. There are several subtypes, and treatments consist of von Willebrand factor replacement and, in some cases, desamino D-arginine vasopressin. In most cases, care of women with bleeding disorders is best coordinated among experts in hematology, anesthesia, and obstetrics.

QUESTIONS

1. Which components of Virchow's triad increase the risk for VTE during pregnancy?
   a. 1
   b. 2
   c. 3

2. Which of the following is most true for lower extremity deep vein thrombosis during pregnancy?
   a. They occur on the right and left sides with equal frequency.
   b. They occur about 65% of the time on the left side.
   c. They occur about 85% of the time on the left side.
   d. They occur about 65% of the time on the right side.
   e. They occur about 85% of the time on the right side.

3. Procoagulant activity is increased during pregnancy through higher levels of which clotting factors?
   a. Factors VII, VII and X
   b. Fibrinogen and von Willebrand factor
   c. both a and b

4. Anticoagulant activity is decreased during pregnancy primarily through _____.
   a. Reduced Antithrombin activity
   b. Increased PAI-1 activity
   c. Increased activity of Protein C
   d. Increased resistance to activated protein C

5. What are the laboratory features of APS?
   a. Finding of Lupus anticoagulant activity and moderate-high positive IgG or IgM anticardiololipin antibodies and again 6 weeks later.
   b. Finding of Lupus anticoagulant activity and moderate-high positive IgG or IgM anticardiololipin antibodies or moderate-high levels of anti-beta-2-glycoportein-1 antibodies on two occasions 12 weeks apart.
   c. Finding of Lupus anticoagulant activity and moderate-high positive IgG or IgM anticardiololipin antibodies and again 12 weeks later.
   d. Finding of Lupus anticoagulant activity and moderate-high positive IgG or IgM anticardiololipin antibodies or moderate-high levels of anti-beta-2-glycoportein-1 antibodies on two occasions 6 weeks apart.

6. What is the appropriate treatment during pregnancy for someone with two pregnancy losses at 8 weeks' gestation and moderate positive levels of IgM anticardiolipin antibodies?
   a. No treatment
   b. Low molecular weight heparin
   c. Low dose aspirin
   d. Low molecular weight heparin and low dose aspirin

7. What is the appropriate treatment during pregnancy for someone with APS and prior pulmonary embolus?
   a. Prophylactic (low dose) low molecular weight heparin through pregnancy and the puerperium.
   b. Prophylactic (low dose) low molecular weight heparin and low dose aspirin through pregnancy and the puerperium.
   c. Full dose low molecular weight heparin through pregnancy and the puerperium.
   d. Full dose low molecular weight heparin and low dose aspirin through pregnancy and the puerperium.

8. The most common heritable thrombophilia in the United States is:
   a. Factor V Leiden mutation
   b. Prothrombin gene mutation
   c. Antithrombin III deficiency
   d. Protein C deficiency
   e. Protein S deficiency

9. The most thrombogenic heritable thrombophilia is:
   a. Factor V Leiden mutation
   b. Prothrombin gene mutation
   c. Antithrombin III deficiency
   d. Protein C deficiency
   e. Protein S deficiency

10. It is not appropriate to treat patients with low risk thrombophilia and no prior VTE or adverse pregnancy outcome with low molecular weight heparin.
    a. True
    b. False

11. What is the most common cause of maternal thrombocytopenia?
    a. Autoimmune thrombocytopenia
    b. Alloimmune thrombocytopenia
    c. Incidental thrombocyyopenia
    d. Thrombotic thrombocytopenia

12. What are possible treatments for ITP in pregnancy?
    a. Corticosteroids and IVIG
    b. Platelet transfusions for bleeding, surgery and neuroaxial anesthesia.
    c. Splenectomy or biologics for refractory cases.
    d. All of the above

13. How is the diagnosis of thrombotic thrombocytopenic purpura (TTP) made?
    a. Bone marrow biopsy
    b. Platelet aggregation studies
    c. ADAMTTS13 activity
    d. Beta-thromboglobulin levels

14. What is appropriate treatment for TTP?
    a. Platelet transfusion
    b. IVIG
    c. Plasmaphoresis
    d. Corticosteroids

Thromboembolic Disease in Pregnancy

STEPHANIE T. ROS

(see *Creasy and Resnik's Maternal-Fetal Medicine, 9e: Ch 3*)

Summary

Venous thromboembolism is among the top causes of pregnancy-related death in the United States. The prevalence is reported to be 1 per 1627 births, 77% of which include deep venous thrombosis (DVT), and the remaining 23% include pulmonary embolism (PE). Rapid diagnosis is essential; in nonpregnant adults who have a fatal PE, death occurs within 1 hour of symptom onset in 65% of patients.

The most likely location for a DVT in a pregnant patient is the lower extremity (98.4%), with the left leg more commonly affected (80%). Onset is most likely in the antepartum period compared with postpartum (74% vs. 26%). However, when compared with nonpregnant women not on contraceptives, the risk of VTE rises throughout pregnancy and peaks in the peripartum and early postpartum period. Most pregnant patients with PE are diagnosed postpartum (60.5%), and this is strongly associated with cesarean delivery.

RISK FACTORS

The changes to various coagulation factors during pregnancy lead to increased thrombin-generating potential, decreased endogenous anticoagulant effects, and impaired fibrinolysis. There are also anatomic changes due to uterine compression and progesterone-mediated increase in venous capacitance. Pregnant people are more likely to have other risk factors such as hospitalization and infection. All of this results in a sixfold increase in risk of VTE in pregnant patients compared with nonpregnant women younger than 40 years of age.

Cesarean delivery is an established risk factor for VTE, particularly PE. This is further increased in patients 35 years of age or older and in obese patients. Inherited and acquired thrombophilias also contribute to VTE risk in pregnancy and the puerperium.

DIAGNOSIS OF VENOUS THROMBOEMBOLISM IN PREGNANCY

Diagnosis of VTE in pregnancy and postpartum can be challenging. Most symptoms associated with VTE are also common in normal pregnancy (unilateral or bilateral lower extremity edema, pain, warmth, tenderness), and many of those with VTE in pregnancy or postpartum do not present with the typical features. There is no validated risk-assessment model for VTE in pregnancy.

Imaging to evaluate for DVT should begin with compression ultrasound (CUS) with color Doppler. Magnetic resonance imaging venography without contrast can be considered for additional assessment of pelvic veins. The role of D dimer is uncertain in the evaluation of pregnant patients for VTE. There is a known elevation in D dimer in pregnancy, unrelated to thrombosis; levels are not expected to normalize until 6 weeks postpartum. A negative D-dimer test does not rule out thrombosis.

The most effective diagnostic schemes combine multiple testing modalities.

ACUTE PULMONARY EMBOLISM

Clinical findings of acute PE include chest pain and dyspnea; these are seen in 61%–81% of pregnant and 55%–69% of postpartum patients ultimately confirmed to have a PE. In terms of initial diagnostic studies, chest radiography is the best first step in evaluation; this allows for ruling out other conditions such as pneumonia or pneumothorax and also better differentiation of patients who would benefit from a ventilation-perfusion (V/Q) scan. Those with a normal chest radiograph are more likely to obtain a diagnostic result with a V/Q scan than computed tomographic pulmonary angiography (CTPA) (94% vs. 70%). If the chest radiograph is abnormal, the V/Q scan is more likely to be nondiagnostic than a CTPA. Other tests are available, but their utility is hampered by pregnancy and its accompanying physiologic adaptations. Electrocardiography (ECG) can be considered as part of the evaluation; however, the interpretation is complicated by changes on the ECG noted with physiologic changes of pregnancy such as physiologic Q waves in leads 3 and aVF. Similarly, oxygen saturation and arterial blood gas assessment is clouded by normal physiologic changes of pregnancy with a normal increase in PO_2. Only 30%–40% of nonpregnant patients with acute PE have echocardiographic abnormalities (right ventricular hypokinesis and dilation, abnormal motion of the interventricular septum).

In terms of diagnostic testing, V/Q scanning can be considered in those with a normal chest radiograph. There is a lower radiation dose to the pregnant patient compared with CTPA, but data are lacking regarding comparative radiation exposure for the fetus with these two tests. Experts agree that with either of these studies, the measured radiation to the fetus is low. One systematic review found a sensitivity of 100% for V/Q scanning for VTE. CTPA is considered the first-line test for those who are not pregnant; systematic reviews have similarly found a 100%

sensitivity for CTPA for VTE. Magnetic resonance imaging can also be used to image the pulmonary vasculature. However, the contrast agent used is gadolinium and studies have demonstrated teratogenicity. Therefore, even though magnetic resonance imaging eliminates the radiation concerns of both CTPA and V/Q scan, it is considered contraindicated in pregnancy.

In order to avoid radiation exposure, many algorithms for diagnosis of PE begin with CUS of the lower extremities. However, it has been shown that the number of patients needed to screen with CUS to find a clot and thus avoid further workup is more than 50, making this a less effective strategy. The challenges with using D dimer are discussed earlier; in the evaluation for PE, there are some data demonstrating that in those who have none of the YEARS criteria (signs of DVT, hemoptysis, and PE as the most likely diagnosis), a D-dimer level of <1000 μg/L or one or more YEARS criteria and a D dimer <500 μg/L can be followed clinically without additional imaging. Other studies have shown that this strategy results in too many patients with PE not receiving necessary imaging. Therefore, utility of D dimer in this context also remains uncertain. One algorithm that has been adopted by multiple specialty societies is shown in Figure 54.7.

TREATMENT OF VTE IN PREGNANCY

Any pregnant patient who has a new VTE should be treated with therapeutic anticoagulation for 3−6 months and the first 6 weeks after delivery. Low-molecular-weight heparin (LMWH) and unfractionated heparin (UFH) are preferred during pregnancy because they do not cross the placenta. Postpartum warfarin may be used. Direct oral anticoagulants have limited data in pregnancy and therefore are not recommended.

There are data demonstrating the superiority of LMWH over UFH in the nonpregnant population, but that research is lacking in pregnancy. LMWH has a low risk of heparin-induced thrombocytopenia (HIT), osteoporosis, and bleeding. The dosing is weight based at 1 mg/kg twice daily; it is not clear if monitoring anti-factor Xa levels in order to adjust dose is beneficial. Unfractionated heparin can be administered intravenously in the acute phase, with the dose modified to meet aPTT goals. Determination of intramuscular dosing is more challenging. It can be started at 10,000 units every 12 hours and then titrated depending on the aPTT.

In the postpartum setting, anticoagulation can be resumed 4−6 hours after a vaginal delivery or 6−12 hours after cesarean delivery; if a patient requires therapeutic dosing, consider delaying for 24 hours after a spinal anesthetic.

Warfarin is a vitamin K antagonist. It takes approximately 6 days to reach antithrombotic effects, during which time patients should be treated with heparin to avoid paradoxical thrombosis. Warfarin can interact with other medications and dietary factors to alter its effectiveness. Dosing is titrated to an international normalized ratio between 2.0 and 3.0.

Heparin-induced thrombocytopenia (HIT) is a potential complication of treatment with UFH or, less commonly, with LMWH. In a patient diagnosed with HIT, an alternative anticoagulant to consider is fondaparinux.

Patients with mechanical heart valves present a complex circumstance for anticoagulation during pregnancy. Warfarin has been used in this setting, despite the risk of teratogenicity and the risks of fetal and placental hemorrhage, because of the risk of valvular thrombosis. The American College of Chest Physicians endorses one of three options for therapy in this group: (1) adjusted-dose LMWH, (2) adjusted-dose UFH, or (3) UFH or LMWH until the 13th week of pregnancy, then warfarin until 36 weeks, then return to UFH or LMWH. The latter strategy avoids the teratogenic effects of warfarin, but using heparin does increase the risk of valve thrombosis.

Antithrombin deficiency is another special situation where multidisciplinary care is required and may include not only anticoagulation but also utilization of antithrombin replacement.

Use of thrombolytic therapy in pregnancy is rare due to risk of abruption and puerperal hemorrhage, but it may be considered in cases of hemodynamic instability.

PREVENTION OF VENOUS THROMBOEMBOLISM IN PREGNANCY

Graduated compression stockings in patients in whom immobilization is anticipated reduces occurrence of VTE. Intermittent pneumatic compression devices also decrease relative risk of DVT compared with placebo and are recommended for use in all women undergoing cesarean in the perioperative and postoperative periods.

NEURAXIAL ANESTHETIC CONSIDERATIONS

The Society for Obstetric Anesthesia and Perinatology guidelines provide considerations for neuraxial anesthesia in patients receiving thromboprophylaxis. Typically, holding prophylactic UFH or LMWH for 12 hours and adjusted-dose UFH or LMWH for 24 hours before neuraxial anesthesia is sufficient, checking coagulation status first for those taking UFH. Prophylactic UFH should be restarted no sooner than 1 hour after catheter removal; low-dose LMWH 12 hours after neuraxial blockage and 4 hours after catheter removal; for those on intermediate or adjusted dose LMWH, 24 hours after blockade and 4 hours after catheter removal is prudent.

QUESTIONS

1. Pregnancy is associated with which of the following changes?
   a. Decreased levels of factor VIII
   b. Decreased levels of fibrinopeptide A
   c. Decreased levels of plasminogen activator inhibitor (PAI)-1
   d. Decreased activity of protein S
   e. Decreased resistance to activated protein C

2. A 39-year-old pregnant patient is admitted to the hospital with pyelonephritis. Her fever resolves after initiation of antipyretics and antibiotics. She receives antiemetics and is able to tolerate meals and oral hydration. On hospital day 2 she is diagnosed with a left lower extremity deep venous thrombus. Which of the following risk factors is most likely to contribute to her development of DVT?
   a. Maternal age >35
   b. Nausea and vomiting
   c. Pyelonephritis
   d. Hospitalization
   e. Administration of antibiotics

3. Which of the following patient scenarios represents the highest risk of VTE in pregnancy?
   a. A patient with a prior VTE diagnosed at the time of a humerus fracture
   b. A patient who is heterozygous for factor V Leiden mutation
   c. A patient who has a sister with VTE and is heterozygous for prothrombin G20210A mutation
   d. A patient with a grandmother with VTE and no inherited thrombophilia

4. A patient reports new onset of right lower extremity edema, warmth, and pain. On examination, her right lower extremity is erythematous and the site is tender to touch. In a patient with this presentation, what is the likelihood that she will have a DVT on imaging?
   a. <10%
   b. About 25%
   c. About 40%
   d. About 60%
   e. >70%

5. Which of the following is the most important component of venous ultrasound for detection of deep venous thrombosis?
   a. Visualization of the popliteal vein
   b. Thorough visualization of distal calf veins
   c. Demonstration of compressibility of the venous lumen in transverse plane
   d. Echogenic material in the venous lumen
   e. Loss of normal phasic flow pattern

6. In which of the following conditions would a D-dimer test be most likely to provide a reliable assessment of VTE risk in a patient who reports chest pain and dyspnea?
   a. A pregnant person at 7 weeks' gestation
   b. A patient at 4 days' postpartum
   c. A pregnant person at 37 weeks' gestation
   d. A patient on the day of delivery
   e. A patient at 10 weeks' postpartum

7. A 37-year-old pregnant person at 19 weeks presents with chest pain, dyspnea, and tachycardia. She has an elevated D dimer and a nondiagnostic venous ultrasound because the calf veins were not clearly visualized. She has a chest radiograph that demonstrates some atelectasis. What is the next best step in evaluation or management?
   a. Computed tomographic pulmonary angiography
   b. Ventilation-perfusion scan
   c. Expectant management
   d. Empiric therapy with therapeutic-dose heparin
   e. Empiric therapy with prophylactic-dose heparin

8. A patient is diagnosed with a DVT after a car accident, at which time she is also incidentally discovered to be 6 weeks' pregnant. She has a negative workup for inherited or acquired thrombophilia and no family history of VTE. Which of the following is the most appropriate management?
   a. Initiate prophylactic dose UFH through 6 weeks' postpartum.
   b. Initiate therapeutic dose LMWH for 1 year.
   c. Initiate therapeutic dose LMWH for 3 months and then reduce to prophylactic dose until delivery. Resume therapeutic dose anticoagulation for 6 weeks postpartum.
   d. Initiate therapeutic-dose LMWH until 12 weeks and then transition to warfarin. Resume LMWH at 36 weeks until delivery and through 6 weeks postpartum.

9. A patient presents for prenatal care and reports that she has a history of pulmonary embolism at age 18. She is found to be homozygous for factor V Leiden. She has two family members with VTE. She recalls that at the time she was started on "an injection" but because of subsequent development of a new blood clot in her leg and a change in her "lab work" (she is unsure which), she was switched to a different medicine. Records cannot be obtained. What is the next best step in management?
   a. Treat with fondaparinux.
   b. Treat with prophylactic dose LMWH.
   c. Manage expectantly.
   d. Treat with therapeutic dose UFH.
   e. Treat with daily low-dose aspirin.

10. A patient with a DVT diagnosed at 32 weeks undergoes vaginal delivery with an epidural. What is the recommendation for removal of her epidural catheter and resumption of her anticoagulation?
    a. Wait 1 hour after catheter removal before beginning LMWH.
    b. Wait 4 hours after catheter removal before beginning LMWH.
    c. Wait 12 hours after catheter removal before beginning LMWH.
    d. Wait 24 hours after catheter removal before beginning LMWH.

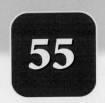

55

Anemia in Pregnancy

SUMIRE KITAHARA | SARAH J. KILPATRICK

(see Creasy and Resnik's Maternal-Fetal Medicine, 9e: Ch 55)

Summary

EVALUATION OF ANEMIA AND MORPHOLOGIC CLASSIFICATION OF ANEMIA (MICROCYTIC ANEMIA, NORMOCYTIC ANEMIA, MACROCYTIC ANEMIA)

Nutritional etiologies of anemia can be suggested by evaluating red blood cell (RBC) size, or mean corpuscular volume (MCV). Low or normal MCV should prompt investigation of iron deficiency. High MCV should prompt investigation of folate and/or vitamin B_{12} deficiencies. Investigation of iron deficiency anemia includes serum iron studies (iron, iron-binding capacity, and % iron saturation) and serum ferritin. Serum ferritin is an indirect indicator of body iron stores but may be increased by inflammatory processes and anemia of chronic disease. Increased levels of soluble transferrin receptor may elucidate masked iron deficiency. Serum folate and vitamin B_{12} levels are good tests to evaluate macrocytic anemia. Additional tests include RBC folate when there is concern that vitamin B_{12} deficiency may be masking folate deficiency by falsely normalizing or elevating serum folate and elevated methylmalonic acid to diagnose mild vitamin B_{12} deficiency. A peripheral blood smear review will provide additional morphologic clues in evaluation of anemia to guide additional diagnostic testing, such as hemoglobin (Hb) high-performance liquid chromatography (HPLC) for thalassemias and hemoglobinopathies; hemolysis labs (lactate dehydrogenase, haptoglobin, Coombs, bilirubin); flow cytometry for inherited RBC membrane defects; and acquired paroxysmal nocturnal hemoglobinuria (PNH).

SPECIFIC ANEMIAS (IRON DEFICIENCY ANEMIA, MEGALOBLASTIC ANEMIA, HEREDITARY SPHEROCYTOSIS/HEREDITARY ELLIPTOCYTOSIS, ACQUIRED AUTOIMMUNE HEMOLYTIC ANEMIA, GLUCOSE-6-PHOSPHATE DEHYDROGENASE DEFICIENCY, APLASTIC ANEMIA, PNH, ALPHA/BETA THALASSEMIAS, SICKLE CELL ANEMIA, HEMOGLOBIN SC, HEMOGLOBIN S/BETA THALASSEMIA, HEMOGLOBIN C TRAIT/DISEASE, HEMOGLOBIN E/E, SYSTEMIC DISEASE)

Complete blood cell (CBC) count and blood smear findings with personal and family history of hemolytic anemia can allow presumptive diagnosis of hereditary spherocytosis and hereditary elliptocytosis, which can be confirmed by flow cytometric analysis specific for RBC membrane defects. When hemolytic anemia due to glucose-6-phosphate dehydrogenase (G6PD) deficiency is suspected, the screening assay should be performed after acute hemolytic event has resolved. Hemoglobin HPLC can identify thalassemias and hemoglobinopathies. Characteristic abnormal RBC indices suggest thalassemia including disproportionately decreased MCV relative to degree of decrease in hemoglobin, normal to increased RBC count. Characteristic abnormal RBC morphologies suggest some hemoglobinopathies (sickle cells, HbS/HbC poikilocytes, hemoglobin C crystals, target cells), prompting hemoglobin HPLC to further characterize the variant hemoglobin. Molecular testing to further evaluate thalassemias may be valuable when genetic counseling is indicated.

IRON KINETICS

There are high rates of iron deficiency in reproductive-age women with one third of pregnant women having a ferritin level of <20 µg/L and 15% with severe iron depletion with ferritin value <12 µg/L. The average requirement of daily iron intake in pregnant women is $22-23$ mg/day of iron, but median intake is 15 mg. Maternal iron is transferred to the fetus via serum transferrin, which binds to receptors on the syncytiotrophoblast, where the iron is released and binds to ferritin in placenta cells. The folate requirement is 400 µg/day for a nonpregnant woman and 600 µg/day during pregnancy. Because adequate folate intake before and during the first weeks of pregnancy reduces occurrence of neural tube defects, all women considering pregnancy should consume 600 µg of folate daily.

EFFECT OF MATERNAL ANEMIA ON MATERNAL AND FETAL OUTCOMES

Although profound maternal anemia can have adverse effects on the mother (preterm birth, postpartum hemorrhage, maternal death) and fetus (stillbirth, small for gestational age), the margin of safety appears to be large. It may be that the prevalence of severe anemia is too low in industrialized countries to see consistent associations with poor fetal or maternal outcomes. Recent data suggest that there may be long-term neonatal neurologic adverse outcomes associated with decreased cord blood transferrin, which warrants more evaluation.

IRON DEFICIENCY ANEMIA

Iron deficiency is the cause of 75% of all anemias in pregnancy, and its prevalence may be as high as 47%. Treatment with oral iron, such as ferrous sulfate, 325 mg one to three times daily and Hb can rise by as much as 1 g/week in severely anemic individuals. Parenteral iron is approved for use and is being used more commonly. Dosing is based on weight and Hb deficit, and there are several formulations routinely available.

AUTOIMMUNE HEMOLYTIC ANEMIA

The two major types of antibodies responsible for autoimmune hemolytic anemia are warm-reactive and cold-reactive antibodies, and diagnosis is suspected when a hyperproliferative, macrocytic anemia is identified. The critical study to confirm the diagnosis is a positive direct Coombs test. Treatment of acquired autoimmune hemolytic anemia is directed toward both the hemolytic process and underlying disease.

APLASTIC AND HYPOPLASTIC ANEMIA

Aplastic anemia is characterized by pancytopenia and hypoproliferative reticulocyte count in the presence of a hypocellular bone marrow and is of an immune-mediated attack on hematopoietic stem cells. Treatment in pregnancy consists of maintenance of Hb levels, prevention and treatment of infection, stimulation of hematopoiesis with androgens, splenectomy, intravenous immune globulin, and intravenous steroids.

HEMOGLOBINOPATHIES

Hemoglobinopathies can be divided into two general types: thalassemia syndromes or structural hemoglobinopathies (see next section). In thalassemias, a reduced amount of one or more of the globin subunits of normal Hbs is produced. The structural hemoglobinopathies occur because of a specific change in amino acid content of Hb. The thalassemia syndromes are named and classified by the type of chain that is inadequately produced. In the homozygous stage of alpha thalassemia, all four genes are deleted and no chains are produced, resulting in inability to synthesize normal HbF or any adult hemoglobins (Hb Bart hydrops fetalis), high-output cardiac failure, and stillbirth. HbH disease (deletion of three alpha genes) results in severe hemolytic anemia. In α-thalassemia minor (two genes deleted), this results in a mild hypochromic, microcytic anemia that must be differentiated from iron deficiency. β-thalassemia is an autosomal recessive disorder β-thalassemia major (homozygous form) is associated with severe childhood anemia requiring transfusions for life. β-thalassemia minor is not associated with adverse pregnancy outcomes.

SICKLE CELL TRAIT AND DISEASE

The frequency of sickle cell trait, sickle cell anemia (SCA), and compound HbS/HbC disease are approximately 8%, 0.2%, and 0.2%, respectively, in pregnant black women. Women with SCA had a significantly higher prevalence of deep vein thrombosis, pulmonary embolus, obstetric shock, pneumonia, sepsis, chorioamnionitis, endometritis, and transfusions. It is not known whether the frequency of painful crises in women with SCA changes with pregnancy. Major objectives of treatment are to end a painful crisis and to combat infection with hydration, oxygen therapy, and pain management. Acute chest syndrome is one of the most severe complications of SCA and can occur in up to 20% of pregnancies. There continues to be an increased risk for prematurity and fetal growth restriction in women with SCA. Prenatal vitamins without iron should be given to women who receive multiple transfusions, all women with SCA should have folic acid supplement of 4 mg/day, and pneumococcal vaccine should be given if the patient has not had it within a year.

HEMOGLOBIN SC DISEASE, HEMOGLOBIN E DISEASE

SC disease occurs among those who are doubly heterozygous for both Hb S and Hb C genes. It is present in <0.2% of pregnant African-American women. During pregnancy, up to 60% of patients with Hb SC disease present as if they had SCA. Except for the frequently experienced rapid and severe anemic crises resulting from splenic sequestration, clinical manifestations of Hb SC disease are similar to those of SCA but milder, and management of symptomatic patients is identical. Although perinatal outcomes with SC disease are better than with SCA, rates of painful crises, acute chest syndrome, and urinary tract infections were similar for women with Hb SC disease and those with SCA.

Hb E is a variant Hb caused by a mutation in the β globin gene. Patients who are compound heterozygotes for Hb E and thalassemia have a greater degree of microcytosis, are frequently anemic, and can be transfusion dependent.

QUESTIONS

1. Which of the following reflects the most common laboratory results in iron deficiency anemia?
   a. Decreased serum iron, increased iron binding capacity, decreased % saturation, increased soluble transferrin receptor
   b. Decreased serum iron, increased iron binding capacity, decreased % saturation, increased hepcidin
   c. Decreased serum iron, decreased iron binding capacity, decreased % saturation, increased soluble transferrin receptor
   d. Decreased serum iron, decreased iron binding capacity, decreased % saturation, increased ferritin

2. Laboratory results from a 26-year-old pregnant female in the second trimester are hemoglobin 10.1 g/dL, mean corpuscular volume 106 fL, vitamin B_{12} level 185 pg/mL, serum folate level 240 µg/L. Which additional laboratory results would be consistent with vitamin B_{12} deficiency and warrant further evaluation?
   a. Decreased methylmalonic acid, normal red cell folate
   b. Decreased methylmalonic acid, decreased red cell folate
   c. Elevated methylmalonic acid, normal to decreased red cell folate
   d. Elevated methylmalonic acid, elevated red cell folate

3. Which of the following is least informative in establishing a diagnosis of hemolytic anemia?
   a. Lactate dehydrogenase
   b. Haptoglobin
   c. Flow cytometry
   d. Serum ferritin
   e. Coombs test

4. Complete blood cell count RBC parameter abnormalities that suggest possible underlying thalassemia minor/trait include:
   a. Low RBC, low Hb, low MCV, high RDW
   b. High RBC, low-normal hemoglobin, low MCV, low RDW
   c. Low RBC, low Hb, high MCV, high RDW
   d. High RBC, low Hb, high MCV, low RDW

5. In which of the following clinical scenarios is there the highest chance of a pregnancy occurring with a fetus that has the severest form of alpha thalassemia?
   a. Parent A: silent carrier × Parent B: trait in cis
   b. Parent A: trait in cis × Parent B: trait in cis
   c. Parent A: trait in trans × Parent B: trait in trans
   d. Parent A: silent carrier × Parent B: trait in trans
   e. Parent A: trait in cis × Parent B: trait in trans

6. In which population is hemoglobin E disorders most prevalent?
   a. Northern European
   b. Southeast Asian
   c. Chinese
   d. African American
   e. Hispanic

7. Which of the following is not a feature of folate deficiency?
   a. Macrocytic anemia
   b. Fatigue
   c. Glossitis
   d. Dyserythropoietic changes in bone marrow
   e. Neurologic deficits

8. All of the following have a rising incidence in the United States because of Asian immigration, except:
   a. alpha thalassemias
   b. beta thalassemias
   c. Hb E disorders
   d. Hb C disorders

9. The treatment of a pregnant woman with paroxysmal nocturnal hemoglobinuria could include all of the following except:
   a. iron supplementation
   b. transfusion
   c. thromboprophylaxis
   d. corticosteroids
   e. bone marrow transplantation

10. Splenomegaly may be a feature in all of the following except:
    a. Hb E/E
    b. Hb E/β^+
    c. Hb E/β^0
    d. Hb S/β^+
    e. Hb S/C

11. In the United States, the most commonly used parenteral iron is:
    a. ferric gluconate
    b. low-molecular-weight iron dextran
    c. iron sucrose
    d. iron isomaltoside
    e. ferumoxytol

12. Iron deficiency anemia in pregnancy has been associated all of following utcomes except:
    a. postpartum hemorrhage
    b. preterm birth
    c. worldwide maternal mortality
    d. preeclampsia
    e. perinatal mortality

13. In a patient with microcytic anemia, an initial test to rule in iron deficiency anemia is:
    a. ferritin
    b. total iron binding capacity
    c. peripheral blood smear
    d. % iron saturation
    e. serum iron

14. All of the following are consistent with Beta-thalassemia except:
    a. MCV <80 μm^3
    b. Hb A2 <3.1%
    c. Hb <11 g/dL
    d. normal iron studies
    e. autosomal recessive disorder

15. The frequency of sickle cell trait in African-Americans is approximately:
    a. 1/10
    b. 1/100
    c. 1/200
    d. 1/500
    e. 1/1000

16. It is recommended that pregnant patients with SCA should receive all of the following except:
    a. prenatal vitamins with iron
    b. 4 mg/day of folic acid
    c. pneumococcal vaccine
    d. prenatal vitamins without iron
    e. baseline type and screen

17. SCA is associated in pregnancy with increased risks of all except:
    a. preeclampsia
    b. preterm birth
    c. pulmonary embolus
    d. sepsis
    e. postpartum hemorrhage

18. Which statement below is true about hemoglobin SC disease in pregnancy?
    a. Hemoglobin SC disease is more common than SCA.
    b. It is uncommon for patients with hemoglobin SC disease to have a pain crisis in pregnancy.
    c. Patients with hemoglobin SC disease do not have an increased risk for preterm delivery compared with patients without hemoglobinopathy.
    d. The peripheral smear characteristics that are consistent with hemoglobin SC disease include target cells and rare sickle cells.

19. Treatment for hemolytic anemia in pregnancy is least likely to include:
    a. splenectomy
    b. corticosteroids
    c. blood transfusion
    d. plasmapheresis
    e. immunosuppression

20. Pregnant patients with sickle cell trait may be at increased risk for pyelonephritis.
    a. True
    b. False

Malignancy in Pregnancy

DAVID E. COHN | BHUVANESWARI RAMASWAMY |
BETH CHRISTIAN | KRISTIN BIXEL

(see *Creasy and Resnik's Maternal-Fetal Medicine, 9e: Ch 56*)

Summary

- Although relatively rare when diagnosed during pregnancy, gestation-associated cancer is a complicated situation that requires expert multidisciplinary care to achieve optimal maternal and fetal outcomes.
- Cancer treatment can have a long-standing impact on the health of mother and fetus and impacts the perinatal management of the maternal-fetal unit.
- Pregnancy itself may impact cancer treatment recommendations compared with those for a nonpregnant patient but does not seem to impact cancer incidence or prognosis.

QUESTIONS

1. A 26-year-old G1P0 presents for her new prenatal appointment at 8 weeks' gestation by last menstrual period. Ultrasound confirms an intrauterine pregnancy concordant with dates provided. Ultrasound also demonstrates a 12-cm complex adnexal mass. This mass is palpable on examination and mobile. She does not have any current symptoms other than mild bloating and pelvic pressure. Which of the following would NOT be an appropriate next step?
   a. Obtain a magnetic resonance imaging (MRI) scan.
   b. Schedule her for interventional radiology–guided biopsy of the mass.
   c. Plan for surgical intervention at 14 weeks' gestational age.
   d. Obtain tumor markers including CA 125, lactate dehydrogenase, and inhibins.

2. What is the most common ovarian germ cell tumor diagnosed in pregnancy?
   a. Dysgerminoma
   b. Granulosa cell tumor
   c. Serous adenocarcinoma
   d. Clear cell carcinoma

3. A 32-year-old women presents for prenatal care at 18 weeks' gestational age. She reports a history of abnormal Pap tests, though her last cytologic examination was 3 years prior (atypical squamous cells of undetermined significance). On pelvic examination, you note a friable and raised lesion on her anterior cervix. What is your next step?
   a. Pap test
   b. MRI
   c. Cervical conization
   d. Cervical biopsy

4. A 32-year-old woman presents for prenatal care at 14 weeks' gestational age. She reports a history of abnormal Pap tests, though she does not know when her last Pap test was. On pelvic examination you note a friable and slightly raised lesion on her anterior cervix that measures 2.5 cm. Biopsy confirms moderately differentiated squamous cell carcinoma (SCC). MRI of the abdomen and pelvis demonstrates a 3.5-cm mass confined to the cervix without evidence of parametrial or vaginal involvement and no enlarged lymph nodes. This is consistent with stage IB2 SCC of the cervix. What would you recommend assuming this is a desired pregnancy?
   a. Level II ultrasound and aneuploidy screening
   b. Consultation with maternal fetal medicine
   c. Induction of labor at 36 weeks followed by definitive therapy 6–8 weeks later
   d. Neoadjuvant chemotherapy with cesarean radical hysterectomy and pelvic lymphadenectomy at term gestation
   e. Counsel patient that continuation of pregnancy greatly increases her risk of death from her cancer. Recommend immediate radical hysterectomy with fetus in situ, bilateral salpingectomy, and pelvic lymphadenectomy
   f. a, b, and d

5. Administration of chemotherapy (carboplatin and paclitaxel) in the second trimester is most commonly associated with what complication?
   a. Cardiac anomaly
   b. Fetal growth restriction
   c. Oligohydramnios
   d. Neurocognitive delay
   e. Limb defects

6. Your patient needs surgery for choledocolithiasis/cholecystitis at 18 weeks' gestation. You recommend all of the following except:
   a. Minimally invasive surgical approach with open entry technique
   b. Set intraperitoneal pressure to 12 mm Hg
   c. Prophylactic tocolytics
   d. Check fetal heart rate before and after the procedure

7. A 40-year-old G2P1 at 17 weeks' gestation notes a breast mass. She presents to the office for evaluation, and you note a 2-cm firm, mobile mass in the left lateral breast. What is your next step?
   a. Imaging with ultrasound
   b. Fine-needle aspiration
   c. Excisional biopsy
   d. Serial examinations
   e. Defer evaluation until after delivery

8. A 40-year-old G2P1 at 20 weeks' gestation notes a breast mass. She presents to the office for evaluation, and you note a 1.5-cm firm, mobile mass in the left lateral breast. Ultrasound confirms a solid breast mass. Core-needle biopsy demonstrates poorly differentiated infiltrating ductal carcinoma. She undergoes lumpectomy with ipsilateral axillary dissection. Unfortunately, she is found to have metastatic disease in her axillary lymph nodes, and adjuvant chemotherapy is recommended. All of the following are important considerations except:
   a. Fetal growth should be monitored regularly.
   b. Chemotherapy should be held 3−4 weeks' before planned delivery to avoid significant myelosuppression in mother/neonate.
   c. Breastfeeding is contraindicated while receiving chemotherapy.
   d. Induction of labor or cesarean delivery at 36 weeks is recommended to avoid unplanned labor and prolonged delays in treatment.

9. The most common malignancy to metastasize to the placenta is:
   a. Melanoma
   b. Breast
   c. Ovarian
   d. Cervical
   e. Colon

10. A 31-year-old G2P1 at 14 weeks' gestational age presented with painless hematochezia and change in stool caliber. She has a family history notable for Lynch syndrome, though she has not undergone testing herself. You recommend
    a. Rectal suppositories/stool softeners as you suspect hemorrhoids
    b. Magnetic resonance enterography
    c. Colonoscopy as soon as possible
    d. Colonoscopy after delivery

11. A 31-year-old G2P1 at 14 weeks' gestational age presented with hematochezia. Colonoscopy reveals an apple core lesion approximately 20 cm from the anus. Biopsy confirms adenocarcinoma. MRI reveals a 4-cm lesion in the sigmoid colon without discernable lymphadenopathy. What is the most appropriate next step?
    a. Order a positron emission tomography/computed tomography (CT) scan.
    b. Defer additional workup or management until fetus is viable.
    c. Refer for surgical resection.
    d. Start neoadjuvant chemotherapy.

12. A 24-year-old woman, gravida 4, para 2 comes to the office with a mass in her left neck. She is currently 9 weeks' pregnant. On physical examination, there is a 3×2 cm mass in her left neck, which is firm and immobile. She undergoes a fine-needle aspirate, which shows no evidence of malignancy. Which of the following is the most appropriate next step in management?
    a. Follow-up imaging with CT neck after delivery.
    b. Refer for an excisional or core biopsy.
    c. Order a positron emission tomography/CT scan.
    d. Start antibiotics with amoxicillin and clavulanate for 14 days.

13. A 24-year-old woman, gravida 2, para 1 comes to the office with a mass in her left neck. She is currently 9 weeks' pregnant. On physical examination, there is a 3×2 cm mass in her left neck, which is firm and immobile. She undergoes an excisional biopsy that demonstrates classical Hodgkin lymphoma, nodular sclerosis subtype. After appropriate counseling regarding the risks and benefits of imaging in the setting of pregnancy, she completes a staging CT neck and chest and an MRI of the abdomen/pelvis, which show no other areas of involvement with lymphoma. A bone marrow biopsy shows no evidence of involvement with lymphoma. Which of the following is the most appropriate next step in her treatment?
    a. Involved site radiation therapy to the left cervical lymph node.
    b. Initiate treatment with doxorubicin (Adriamycin), bleomycin, vinblastine, dacarbazine (ABVD) chemotherapy.
    c. Wait until the second trimester, and then initiate treatment with ABVD chemotherapy.
    d. Initiate treatment with ABVD chemotherapy in the second trimester with a reduced dose of Adriamycin.

14. A 32-year-old woman, gravida 2, para 1 has been diagnosed with stage III diffuse large B-cell lymphoma. She is currently 20 weeks' pregnant. She will be starting treatment with rituximab and CHOP chemotherapy. Which of the following conditions is the most likely fetal complication resulting from treatment with rituximab?
    a. B lymphocyte depletion lasting for months after delivery
    b. Patent ductus arteriosus
    c. Spina bifida
    d. Renal agenesis/dysgenesis

15. A 29-year-old woman with a diagnosis of chronic myeloid leukemia in chronic phase is currently on treatment with nilotinib. She achieved a major molecular response, which has been sustained for 36 months. She plans to become pregnant. This patient should be advised to do which of the following?
    a. Continue nilotinib during pregnancy.
    b. Change treatment to imatinib.
    c. Hold therapy with nilotinib and monitor closely.
    d. Change treatment to interferon alpha.

57

Renal Disorders in Pregnancy

RAVI I. THADHANI | BRETT C. YOUNG

(see Creasy and Resnik's Maternal-Fetal Medicine, 9e: Ch 57)

Summary

Although women with preexisting chronic kidney disease typically have stable or transient worsening of their kidney function during pregnancy, pregnancy-related conditions may occasionally induce irreversible worsening of kidney function. Pregnant patients with chronic renal disease often have a higher risk for associated obstetric comorbidities.

ACUTE RENAL FAILURE SECONDARY TO OBSTETRIC ETIOLOGIES

Preeclampsia: Preeclampsia is a systemic syndrome of pregnancy characterized by new-onset hypertension and proteinuria after 20 weeks' gestation. Both glomerular filtration rate (GFR) and effective renal plasma flow decrease in preeclampsia. Although functional decrements are usually mild or moderate and reverse rapidly after delivery, an occasional preeclamptic patient may progress to acute renal failure. For patients with preeclampsia with severe features causing acute renal failure, delivery is recommended.

Hemolytic Uremic Syndrome and Thrombotic Thrombocytopenic Purpura: Two other entities that may result in acute renal failure in pregnancy include hemolytic uremic syndrome (HUS) and thrombotic thrombocytopenic purpura (TTP). HUS and TTP are important causes of acute kidney injury characterized by thrombocytopenia and microangiopathic hemolytic anemia. Distinguishing TTP/HUS from preeclampsia with severe features or hemolysis, elevated liver enzyme levels, and lowered platelets (HELLP) syndrome can be difficult. Thrombocytopenia, microangiopathic hemolytic anemia, acute kidney injury, proteinuria, and hypertension occur in both TTP-HUS and HELLP, although elevated liver enzymes are more common in HELLP syndrome. Although many of the laboratory findings in preeclampsia and HUS/TTP overlap, the degree of renal impairment is worse in HUS/TTP and will not typically improve after delivery. The mainstay of treatment for TTP is plasmapheresis.

Acute fatty liver of pregnancy (AFLP): AFLP is an extremely rare complication that is estimated to occur in about 1 in 10,000 pregnancies. These patients present typically in the third trimester with nausea and vomiting, jaundice, and abdominal pain with elevated creatinine, bilirubin, transaminitis, thrombocytopenia, hypofibrinogenemia, and an elevated INR. Management of AFLP includes early recognition, aggressive management of the coagulopathy, correction of any hypoglycemia, and prompt delivery. The syndrome typically remits after the birth with no residual hepatic or renal impairment.

CHRONIC KIDNEY DISEASE AND PREGNANCY

GFR increases during pregnancy as a normal physiologic change in gravidas. Chronic kidney disease (CKD) has classically been divided into five stages on the basis of the GFR. Perinatal complications such as preterm labor, preeclampsia, small-for-gestational-age (SGA) infants, and stillbirths are increased for all five stages of CKD, with risks increasing in parallel with the worsening degree of CKD. Women with stages 1 and 2 CKD, in general, have successful pregnancies and do not have an altered long-term renal prognosis, assuming blood pressure is well controlled and proteinuria is minimal (<1 g per 24 hours). Women with moderate to severe kidney disease have increased risks for preeclampsia (>70%), moderate to severe anemia (>60%), and SGA neonates (>50%). The rates of prematurity were increased given these aforementioned risks, with 6% of pregnancies delivered before 28 weeks, 24% of pregnancies delivered before 34 weeks, and 76% of pregnancies delivered before full term at 37 weeks' gestation.

Preexisting Chronic Kidney Diseases: Our chapter reviews select conditions including glomerulonephritis, nephrotic syndrome, diabetic nephropathy, lupus nephritis, granulomatosis with polyangiitis, polyarteritis nodosa, systemic sclerosis, reflux nephropathy, autosomal dominant polycystic kidney disease, urolithiasis, and solitary kidney.

Renal Transplant: More patients are becoming pregnant after successful treatment of end-stage renal disease (ESRD) with a renal transplant and immunosuppression treatment. For patients with a renal transplant, there is an increased likelihood of adverse maternal and fetal outcomes including preeclampsia and fetal growth restriction. Close collaboration with a multidisciplinary team and adherence to a selected immunosuppression regimen in pregnancy are paramount to optimize outcomes.

End-Stage Renal Disease: Patients with ESRD who require dialysis during pregnancy or who become pregnant while on dialysis have an increased likelihood for adverse maternal and fetal outcomes including up to 80% likelihood of preeclampsia. However, despite the known high risk of perinatal complications, successful pregnancies on chronic hemodialysis or peritoneal dialysis are becoming more common. During pregnancy, careful attention to frequency and duration of dialysis, fluid balance, treatment of anemia, treatment of hypertension, and assessment of obstetric complications including preeclampsia, abruption, fetal growth restriction are paramount.

QUESTIONS

1. Which of the following conditions is most likely to be associated with acute renal failure in pregnancy?
   a. Ovarian hyperstimulation syndrome
   b. Polyarteritis nodosa
   c. Autosomal dominant polycystic kidney disease
   d. Solitary kidney

2. A patient who has donated a kidney subsequently becomes pregnant 6 months later. In the first trimester, her creatinine is 0.7 mg/dL. What is the most likely outcome of the pregnancy?
   a. Preeclampsia
   b. Term delivery with SGA infant
   c. Renal insufficiency above her baseline creatinine
   d. Unremarkable pregnancy course

3. A patient with a renal transplant becomes pregnant. Which of the following immunosuppression medications is associated with teratogenic effects?
   a. Azathioprine
   b. Cyclosporine
   c. Tacrolimus
   d. Mycophenolate mofetil
   e. Prednisone

4. A patient is considering pregnancy after a renal transplant; she is on immunosuppression treatment. Which of the following factors is associated with the best pregnancy outcomes for the patient?
   a. Absence of rejection episodes in the past 12 months
   b. Absence of proteinuria
   c. Waiting 24 months since the transplant
   d. Serum creatinine is under 2 mg/dL

5. A patient with end-stage renal disease on dialysis is awaiting transplant and becomes pregnant. Which of the following is the most likely pregnancy outcome?
   a. Large-for-gestational-age neonate
   b. Preterm delivery
   c. Diminished need of antihypertensive medications
   d. Decrease erythropoietin dosage

6. A patient with known nephrolithiasis develops severe acute-onset right flank pain radiating to her groin. She is diagnosed with urolithiasis of a 5-mm stone on the basis of imaging. She is initiated on treatment with oral and intravenous hydration and narcotic pain management. The most likely outcome is which of the following?
   a. Cystoscopy with stent placement
   b. Nephrostomy tube placement
   c. Lithotripsy
   d. Spontaneous stone passage

7. A fetus is noted to have bilateral enlarged, echogenic kidneys on ultrasound in the third trimester. The most likely paternal condition is which of the following?
   a. Autosomal recessive polycystic kidney disease
   b. Systemic sclerosis
   c. Polyarteritis nodosa
   d. Lupus nephritis
   e. Autosomal dominant polycystic kidney disease

8. A patient with type 1 diabetes with diabetic nephropathy is most likely to develop which of the following conditions in pregnancy?
   a. Nephrolithiasis
   b. Preeclampsia
   c. End-stage renal disease
   d. Pyelonephritis

9. A patient develops acute renal failure, thrombocytopenia, and mildly elevated blood pressures. A diagnosis of TTP is suspected and subsequently confirmed when a depressed level of ADAMTS13 is documented. What is the best next step in management?
   a. Peritoneal dialysis
   b. Blood pressure control
   c. Plasmapheresis
   d. Termination of the pregnancy
   e. Eculizumab

10. A patient is in the first trimester of pregnancy and has chronic renal disease with a creatinine of 1.1 mg/dL. Which of the following is the best next step for pre-eclampsia prophylaxis?
    a. Low-dose acetaminophen
    b. Low-dose aspirin
    c. Calcium supplement
    d. Vitamin C ascorbic acid
    e. Atorvastatin

11. A patient at 29 weeks with preeclampsia develops acute renal insufficiency with a creatinine of 1.3 mg/dL. Her blood pressure is controlled with labetalol and nifedipine. What is the most appropriate treatment at this time?
    a. Delivery
    b. Plasmapheresis
    c. Increase aspirin dosing
    d. Hydration
    e. Furosemide administration

12. In pregnancy, a patient has stage 2 chronic renal disease secondary to glomerulonephritis. Which of the following is the most likely outcome in the late third trimester?
    a. Transient improvement of kidney function
    b. Stable kidney function
    c. Significant worsening of kidney function
    d. End-stage renal disease

58

Respiratory Diseases in Pregnancy

KELLY S. GIBSON | JESSICA L. PIPPEN

(see *Creasy and Resnik's Maternal-Fetal Medicine, 9e: Ch 58*)

Summary

Respiratory disease in pregnancy has the potential for significant adverse maternal and fetal outcomes. However, with modern diagnostic and therapeutic techniques, the pregnancy outcome for women with infectious or chronic diseases including pneumonia, tuberculosis, influenza, severe acute respiratory syndrome−coronavirus 2, asthma, and cystic fibrosis can be significantly improved. Most of the diagnostic and therapeutic modalities used in the nonpregnant woman can be used safely in pregnancy. Most medications used to treat respiratory disease in pregnancy are also well tolerated by the fetus. With few exceptions, the diagnostic and treatment algorithms for respiratory disease in a pregnant woman closely resemble those used for a nonpregnant woman.

To accommodate both the increased metabolic demands of pregnancy and the physical changes from a gravid uterus, the respiratory system adapts with a higher minute ventilation to increase the availability of oxygen to tissues. There is no increase in respiratory rate, so the increase in maternal minute ventilation results from an increase in tidal volume with a decrease in the functional residual capacity. The resulting hyperventilation of pregnancy results in a compensated respiratory alkalosis (i.e., arterial partial pressure of carbon dioxide [$Paco_2$] ≤30 mm Hg) and a modest increase in arterial oxygenation tension (i.e., 101 to 104 mm Hg). The decrease in $Paco_2$ is matched by an equivalent increase in renal excretion of bicarbonate with a resulting decrease in plasma bicarbonate concentration to maintain the arterial pH near the normal nonpregnant level of about 7.4. The vital capacity does not change in pregnancy. The level of the diaphragm rises by about 4 cm, and the transverse diameter of the chest increases by 2 cm.

The physiologic anemia of pregnancy results in a reduction in the hemoglobin concentration and arterial oxygen carrying capacity and content. Despite this hemodilution, oxygen delivery is maintained at or above normal because of the 50% increase in cardiac output. Oxygen consumption increases steadily throughout pregnancy and is greatest at term, reaching an average of 331 mL/min at rest and 1167 mL/min with exercise. During labor, oxygen consumption increases by 40% to 60% and cardiac output increases by about 22%.

Pneumonia is the most common nonobstetric infection to cause maternal mortality. It can complicate pregnancy at any time during gestation and may be associated with preterm birth, poor fetal growth, and perinatal loss. Pneumonia, especially severe cases, must be promptly evaluated and treated to reduce maternal and neonatal morbidity and mortality. The true incidences of viral, *Legionella*, and *Mycoplasma* pneumonia in pregnancy are difficult to estimate; however, pneumococcus and *Haemophilus influenzae* remain the most common identifiable causes. Influenza A has a higher mortality rate among pregnant women than among nonpregnant patients.

Normal physiologic changes in the respiratory system associated with pregnancy result in a loss of ventilatory reserve. Coupled with the functionally altered immune response of pregnancy, this puts the mother and fetus at great risk from respiratory infection. The workup should include a physical examination, arterial blood gas determinations, a chest radiograph, sputum Gram stain and culture, and blood cultures. In addition to antibiotic therapy, oxygen supplementation should be given if needed. Hospital admission for all pregnant women with pneumonia is recommended for initial evaluation and management. Vaccination against pneumococcus, influenza, severe acute respiratory syndrome−coronavirus 2, and other pathogens is recommended in pregnancy for the prevention of severe disease and should be administered to all high-risk gravidas.

The varicella-zoster virus is a DNA virus that can cause viral pneumonia in pregnancy. Varicella pneumonia occurs most often in the third trimester, and the infection is likely to be severe. Gravidas with varicella pneumonia should be treated with antiviral therapy and admitted to the intensive care unit. Varicella vaccine is not recommended for use in pregnancy.

Infection with the HIV virus significantly increases the risk for pulmonary infection. *Streptococcus pneumoniae* and *H. influenzae* are the most commonly isolated organisms. A high index of suspicion is necessary when gravidas at risk for HIV infection present with symptoms such as weight loss, fatigue, fever, tachypnea, dyspnea, and nonproductive cough. The onset of disease can be insidious, including normal radiographic findings, and it can then proceed to rapid deterioration. Therapy for *Pneumocystis jirovecii pneumonia* in pregnancy includes trimethoprim-sulfamethoxazole.

Tuberculosis kills more than 1 million women per year worldwide. The rate of tuberculosis in pregnancy is rising in the United States. There is an increased risk of severe preeclampsia, eclampsia, placenta previa, postpartum hemorrhage, sepsis, and anemia in those women with active TB compared with those without. High-risk gravidas should be screened for tuberculosis and treated appropriately for latent tuberculosis infection without overt disease and with antituberculosis therapy (isoniazid, rifampin, ethambutol) for active disease. The newborn also should be screened for evidence of tuberculosis. Proper screening and therapy will lead to a good outcome for the mother and infant in most cases.

Asthma may be the most common potentially serious medical condition to complicate pregnancy. It is characterized by chronic airway inflammation with increased airway responsiveness to a variety of stimuli and airway obstruction that is partially or completely reversible. Factors that may lead to worsening asthma during pregnancy include pregnancy-associated changes in levels of sex hormones, psychosocial stress, nonadherence, and respiratory infections. Insight into the pathogenesis of asthma has changed with the recognition that airway inflammation occurs in almost all cases. The primary goal of asthma management during pregnancy is to maintain adequate oxygenation of the fetus by preventing hypoxic episodes in the mother. It is safer for pregnant women to be treated with asthma medications than it is for them to have asthma symptoms and exacerbations. Asthma should be treated in a step-wise fashion based on symptoms and pulmonary function testing.

The literature on restrictive lung disease in pregnancy is limited, but most patients with restrictive lung disease complicating pregnancy, including those with pulmonary sarcoidosis, can have a favorable pregnancy outcome. Patients with restrictive lung disease can have worsening of their clinical condition with a potential for both maternal and fetal morbidity and possibly mortality. Depending on the location of the lesions, patients with restrictive lung disease may have pulmonary hypertension, which can be associated with a mortality rate as high as 50% during gestation.

Cystic fibrosis (CF) is an autosomal recessive disease that involves the exocrine glands and epithelial tissues of the pancreas, sweat glands, and mucous glands in the respiratory, digestive, and reproductive tracts. Chronic obstructive pulmonary disease, pancreatic exocrine insufficiency, and elevated levels of sweat electrolytes are present. From 2000 to 2010, there was a significant linear increase in the prevalence of CF in pregnancy. The latest treatment option, cystic fibrosis transmembrane conductance regulator (CFTR) modulators, have limited data in pregnancy, do cross the placenta, and have been associated with neonatal cataracts. Pregnant women with CF are more likely to die, require mechanical ventilation, and have infectious complications compared with women without CF, although the absolute risks are low and these events are relatively rare. Factors that may predict poor outcome include prepregnancy evidence of poor nutritional status, significant pulmonary disease with hypoxemia, and pulmonary hypertension. Care of the gravida with CF should be a coordinated multidisciplinary team effort.

QUESTIONS

1. Which of the following meets criteria for severe pneumonia?
   a. Respiratory rate $\geq$ 30 breaths/min
   b. Platelet count <100,000/μL
   c. PaO_2/FiO_2 ratio $\leq$ 250
   d. All of the above

2. What is the most likely identifiable pathogen in pregnant women with pneumonia?
   a. Hemophilus pneumoniae
   b. Mycoplasma
   c. Varicella
   d. Influenza A

3. Viral pneumonias are more virulent in pregnancy because of:
   a. increased helper T cell
   b. decreased helper T cell
   c. enhanced lymphocyte proliferative response
   d. increased cell-mediated lymphocyte toxicity

4. A 23-year-old G1P0 patient presents with a 3-day history of productive cough and dyspnea. The patient has a temperature of 38.5°C and has a chest radiograph that shows a left lower lobe consolidation. Initiation of antibiotics in what time frame has been shown to reduce morbidity and mortality?
   a. 10 hours
   b. 2 hours
   c. 24 hours
   d. 4 hours

5. Compared with the general population, pregnant women are at higher risk for developing influenza pneumonia after infection with influenza. Which condition has the least increase in risk for pulmonary complications with influenza infections?
   a. Cystic fibrosis
   b. Asthma
   c. Chronic obstructive pulmonary disease
   d. Anemia

6. Pneumocystis pneumonia is treated with the following antibiotic:
   a. Doxycycline
   b. Bactrim
   c. Azithromycin
   d. Ceftriaxone

7. The following antituberculosis agents are safe in pregnancy EXCEPT:
   a. Ethambutol
   b. Isoniazid
   c. Streptomycin
   d. Rifampin

8. A 40-year-old G6P5005 patient at 12 weeks and 3 days presents with hemoptysis, fever, malaise, and 20-lb weight loss. You suspect active tuberculosis. Which of the following confirms the diagnosis?
   a. Sputum positive for acid-fast bacilli
   b. Positive interferon gamma release assay
   c. Chest radiograph with evidence of cavitation
   d. Purified protein derivative > 15 mm

9. Pneumocystis pneumonia prophylaxis should be initiated in HIV-positive patients with the which of the following findings?
   a. Genital candidiasis
   b. RNA viral load >1000
   c. CD4 count <100 cells/mm³
   d. CD4 count <200 cells/mm³

10. Pregnant patients with varicella are more likely to have infection complicated by pneumonia. Which of the following reflects the mortality rate of varicella pneumonia?
    a. 11%−15%
    b. 20%
    c. 75%
    d. 35%–40%

11. To accommodate both the increased metabolic demands of pregnancy and physical changes from a gravid uterus, the respiratory system adapts in which way?
    a. A higher minute ventilation
    b. An increase in respiratory rate
    c. A decrease in tidal volume
    d. An increase in the functional residual capacity

12. Physiologic changes during pregnancy result in all of the following EXCEPT:
    a. a compensated respiratory alkalosis
    b. a modest increase in arterial oxygenation tension
    c. an increase in the $Paco_2$ early in pregnancy
    d. an increase in renal excretion of bicarbonate with a resulting decrease in plasma bicarbonate concentration

13. Respiratory changes of pregnancy are due in part to the role of _____ acting as a respiratory stimulant and lowering the carbon dioxide threshold of the respiratory center.
    a. carbonic anhydrase B
    b. progesterone
    c. estrogen
    d. prolactin

14. Select the TRUE statement regarding respiratory changes in pregnancy:
    a. Because there are increases in respiratory rate, minute ventilation does not change.
    b. The physiologic dead space is increased by about 60 mL in pregnancy. This may result from dilation of the small airways.
    c. Residual volume is increased by about 20%, from 1000 to 1200 mL.
    d. Vital capacity, which is the maximum volume of gas that can be expired after a maximum inspiration, increases in pregnacy.

15. At 28.2 weeks' gestation your patient is noted to have anemia with a hemoglobin of 10.2 g/dL. This anemia results in a reduction in the hemoglobin concentration and arterial oxygen-carrying capacity and content. Which of the following is FALSE regarding oxygen delivery during pregnancy?
    a. The pregnant patient depends on cardiac output for maintenance of oxygen delivery more than the nonpregnant patient.
    b. Oxygen consumption increases steadily throughout pregnancy and is greatest at term.
    c. During labor, oxygen consumption increases by 40% to 60%.
    d. When a pregnant patient has low oxygen delivery, she can usually compensate well during labor without fetal compromise.

16. Approximately 5%–8% of pregnancies are complicated by asthma. Factors that may lead to worsening asthma during pregnancy include all of the following EXCEPT:
    a. changes in levels of sex hormones
    b. decreased tissue responsiveness to medications
    c. nonadherence
    d. respiratory infections

17. A 27-year-old G0 presents for preconception counseling. The patient has a history of severe persistent asthma and is concerned about asthma control during pregnancy. You inform that patient:
    a. Even if the asthma is well controlled, the chances for a successful pregnancy are low.
    b. A significant relationship has been reported between lower FEV_1 during pregnancy and decreased risk for low birth weight and prematurity.
    c. Optimization of asthma control should be achieved before conception.
    d. The primary goal of asthma management during pregnancy is to avoid medication exposure.

18. When managing a patient with asthma during pregnancy, which of the following is FALSE?
    a. Using the peak expiratory flow rate is more sensitive than the FEV_1 value after a maximal inspiration for pulmonary function assessment.
    b. The typical peak expiratory flow rate should be 380 to 550 L/min during pregnancy.
    c. Trigger avoidance should be a mainstay of therapy as 75% to 85% of patients with asthma have positive skin test results for common allergens.
    d. The reduction in bronchospasm can be achieved with a step-care approach.

19. A 31-year-old G4P2103 at 11.2 weeks' gestation presents with a complain of worsening asthma. The patient reports using albuterol five times a day. You recommend:
    a. Stop smoking and add a medium-dose inhaled corticosteroid plus a long-acting beta agonist.
    b. Stop smoking and add a low-dose inhaled corticosteroid and theophylline.
    c. Stop smoking and add a low-dose inhaled corticosteroid and a short course of oral steroids.
    d. Stop smoking and see pulmonologist for complete pulmonary function testing to confirm the diagnosis of asthma.

20. You see a patient with CF for a preconception consult. You advise the patient that the following risks are increased in pregnancy:
    a. macrosomia
    b. post-date pregnancy
    c. maternal death
    d. cardiac hypertrophy

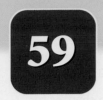

59

Diabetes in Pregnancy

THOMAS R. MOORE | CAMILLE ELISE POWE | PATRICK CATALANO

(see *Creasy and Resnik's Maternal-Fetal Medicine, 9e: Ch 59*)

Summary

The epidemic of diabetes continues to sweep the globe with the total affected population predicted to rise by 50% to 700 million by 2045. In the United States, approximately 34 million persons with diabetes account for more than 10% of the population.

Classification of Diabetes Mellitus

Categories of diabetes include:
1. Type 1 diabetes mellitus (T1DM): due to autoimmune beta cell destruction, usually leading to absolute insulin deficiency
2. Type 2 diabetes mellitus (T2DM): due to a progressive loss of beta cell insulin secretion, frequently on the background of insulin resistance
3. Gestational diabetes mellitus (GDM): diabetes diagnosed in pregnancy
4. Diabetes due to other causes, such as maturity-onset diabetes of the young, cystic fibrosis, and drug-induced diabetes

GESTATIONAL DIABETES TESTING

GDM is diagnosed with either a one-step or two-step testing regimen performed near the end of the second trimester. The American College of Obstetricians and Gynecologists (ACOG) currently recommends using the two-step procedure: a 50-g glucose challenge test, which, if abnormal, is followed by 100-g, 3-hour oral glucose tolerance test (OGTT) (with two abnormal values diagnostic of GDM). Globally, the International Association of Diabetes and Pregnancy Study Groups and the World Health Organization recommend a one-step 75-g, 2-hour OGTT for which a single abnormal value diagnoses GDM.

PREGNANCY COMPLICATIONS WITH DIABETES

Fetal Congenital Anomalies

While the incidence of congenital anomalies in normoglycemic pregnancies is 3–4%, fetal malformations occur in more than 20% when first trimester Hb A_{1c} is above 8.5%. Because the critical period for teratogenesis is at 5 to 8 weeks of gestation, metabolic care must be optimized preconceptionally to reduce the rate of fetal malformations.

Fetal Macrosomia

Macrosomia is typically defined as birthweight >90th percentile for gestational age or birthweight >4000 g at term. Because 70% of fetal growth occurs in the third trimester (~1000 g at 28 weeks to ~3500 g at term), glycemic control after 20 weeks is critical in the prevention of macrosomia. Increased growth in the infants of mothers with diabetes (IDM) involves insulin-sensitive tissues such as subcutaneous fat in the abdomen, with 95% of the variance in abdominal circumference accounted for by subcutaneous fat rather than intraabdominal structures such as liver size. Birthweight in IDM correlates strongly with second- and third-trimester postprandial glucose measurements with mean 2-hour postprandial glucose 120 mg/dL or less. Approximately 20% of infants are macrosomic, but when average 2-hour postprandial glucose values measure ≥160 mg/dL, the rate of macrosomia is above 35%.

Birth Injury

Birth injury is more common among IDM, with macrosomic fetuses at the highest risk for brachial plexus palsy, facial nerve injury, fractures of the humerus or clavicle, and cephalohematoma. Although the incidence of shoulder dystocia is 5%–7% among infants of nondiabetic pregnancies weighing greater than 4000 g, with IDM the shoulder dystocia risk is increased fivefold.

Neonatal Hypoglycemia

Approximately 15% to 25% of IDM develop hypoglycemia during the immediate newborn period, but neonatal hypoglycemia is less common when tight glycemic control is maintained during the third trimester and in labor. Because undertreated neonatal hypoglycemia may lead to seizures, coma, and brain damage, it is important that the obstetric team optimize maternal glucose levels during labor/delivery and for the neonatal team to perform frequent postnatal glucose monitoring until infant metabolic stability is established. There are potential long-term neurodevelopmental consequences of neonatal hypoglycemia.

Respiratory Distress Syndrome (RDS)

Respiratory morbidity is 10-fold more frequent in IDM than in those whose mothers have normoglycemia (22.2% vs. 2.7%). This is likely related to delayed fetal lung maturity in pregnancies affected by diabetes (typically 38–39 weeks vs. 34–35 weeks with normal glycemia).

MATERNAL HYPERTENSION AND PREECLAMPSIA

Women with pregestational diabetes account for about 2% of deliveries but have significantly increased incidence of hypertension (OR = 14.2), preeclampsia (OR = 3.4), cesarean delivery (OR = 11.3), and preterm birth (OR = 4.4). Use of low-dose aspirin (81 mg) from 16 weeks of gestation lowers the preeclampsia risk in high-risk pregnancies generally, though evidence specifically in women with diabetes is lacking.

Glucose Management

Glycemic Goals. ACOG and the American Diabetes Association (ADA) recommend the following:
- Fasting 70–95 mg/dL (3.9–5.3 mmol/L)
- One-hour postprandial 110–140 mg/dL (6.1–7.8 mmol/L) *or*
- Two-hour postprandial 100–120 mg/dL (5.6–6.7 mmol/L)

Oral Hypoglycemic Agents

Despite the lack evidence of teratogenicity for most of hypoglycemic agents, only metformin and glyburide are recommended for limited use in pregnancy. The ADA and ACOG caution that oral hypoglycemics should be avoided because of uncertainty of transplacental fetal effects.

Metformin readily crosses the placenta, with fetal blood levels similar to those in the maternal circulation. Regarding fetal teratogenesis, first-trimester metformin treatment has been associated with a statistically significant 57% reduction in birth defects. Metformin-treated women achieve significantly better third-trimester glycemic control than placebo-treated women, have 23% less maternal weight gain and 15% lower cesarean delivery rate. Metformin-exposed infants have 7% lower mean birthweight, and 40% fewer have weight above the 97th centile. Metformin exposure in utero may increase childhood body weight, but additional studies are needed.

Use of glyburide has become widespread because of its ability to enhance pancreatic insulin secretion. The safety of glyburide in pregnancy compared with insulin, assessed in eight randomized clinical trials, found similar maternal glycemic control levels and cesarean delivery rates, with an average 95-g lower infant birthweight, which was not statistically significant. Several more recent observational studies, as well as a 2018 randomized control trial, suggested inferior perinatal outcomes with glyburide compared to insulin.

Insulin

Compared with preconception levels, total daily insulin dosages in the first trimester typically decline by 15% at 10 weeks' gestation and then rise linearly through the second and third trimesters, almost tripling (+280%) by 34 weeks. Fasting insulin doses rise modestly into the third trimester (50% increase), whereas premeal bolus insulin doses escalate markedly (400% increase). A mixture of short-acting and intermediate- or long-acting insulins is typically employed with weekly or biweekly glucose level reviews.

PREGNANCY MANAGEMENT

Assessing Fetal Size and Risk of Injury with Delivery

Newborns weighing more than 4000 g are responsible for 42% to 74% of shoulder dystocia cases and 56% to 76% of all brachial plexus injuries, even though they comprise only 6% of births. In pregnancies complicated by diabetes, ~20% of fetuses from diabetic pregnancy weighing 4500 g or more at birth have shoulder dystocia; ~20% of these have recognizable brachial plexus injury, and ~10% of those injuries result in permanent deficit. Since the risk of birth injury is proportional to birthweight, much effort has been focused on sonographic estimated fetal weight (EFW) using measurements of head, abdomen, and femur. Using an EFW target of 4000 g for risk of birth injury at ~36 weeks of gestation, sensitivity values of ~40%

and positive predictive values of ~80% have been achieved. However, since only approximately 20% of those estimated 4000-g fetuses will experience shoulder dystocia, and less than half of those will experience injury, the yield in preventing fetal injury with antepartum sonography is low. Thus, there is currently no method of reliably identifying the fetus who is likely to experience shoulder dystocia and injury during birth without a significantly high false-positive rate. Therefore, ACOG recommends discussing the risks and benefits of scheduled cesarean delivery in mothers with diabetes if the fetal weight is estimated to exceed 4500 g.

Delivery Timing

Because of the significant rise in risk of stillbirth and shoulder dystocia in pregnancies complicated by diabetes after 40 weeks, delivery is often timed between 37 and 39 weeks despite the associated risk of failed induction and cesarean delivery. One randomized clinical trial was performed to assess whether the cesarean rate could be reduced by expectant management versus routine induction at 38 weeks' gestation in women with diabetes. Although there was a significant increase in large-for-gestational-age infants (23% vs. 10%) in those expectantly managed, there was no difference in the cesarean delivery rate, suggesting that intervention in pregnancy complicated with diabetes could be delayed until 39+ weeks' gestation. In another study that compared pregnancies associated with diabetes undergoing induction of labor (IOL) at 38 or 39 weeks with those laboring spontaneously, the 38-week IOL group had a 27% lower risk of cesarean delivery but 36% higher admission rate to neonatal intensive care unit. Women in the 39-week IOL group, compared with those in the 39-week expectant group, also had a 27% lower risk of cesarean delivery but with no difference in rate of neonatal intensive care unit admission.

An additional concern is the rate of fetal death, perinatal asphyxia, and neonatal death, which rises with advancing gestation. A retrospective cohort study of women with GDM delivering at 36 to 42 weeks' gestation in California calculated the stillbirth risk during each week of continuing pregnancy versus the infant mortality risk at the gestational age 1 week hence. With GDM, the mortality rate with expectant management was lower than the risk with delivery at 36 weeks (17.4 vs. 19.3 per 10,000), but at 39 weeks, the mortality risk of expectant management exceeded that of delivery (RR = 1.8; 95% CI, 1.2−2.6).

When all these factors are considered, the optimal time for delivery of most pregnancies complicated by diabetes is between 39 and 40 weeks of gestation. However, coexisting maternal hypertension, suboptimal glucose control, or suspicious fetal biophysical testing results are important cofactors that may influence decisions regarding delivery timing. Because of the delay in fetal lung maturity in diabetic pregnancies, delivery before 39 weeks' gestation should be performed only for compelling maternal or fetal concerns.

QUESTIONS

1. Pregnancy and carbohydrate metabolism. In addition to the effect of pregnancy on insulin resistance, what other "independent" effect does pregnancy have on maternal carbohydrate metabolism?
   a. Increases insulin response in early pregnancy
   b. Increases insulin response in late pregnancy
   c. Decreases fasting hepatic glucose production, resulting in decreased fasting glucose concentrations with advancing gestation
   d. Decreases maternal appetite in midpregnancy

2. GDM newborn fat mass. Increased birthweight in newborns of mothers with GDM includes an increase in:
   a. lean body mass (e.g., for length)
   b. head circumference
   c. fat mass
   d. subcutaneous edema

3. Insulin resistance mechanism. Increased peripheral insulin resistance during pregnancy (skeletal muscle) is related to:
   a. a decrease in peripheral insulin receptors
   b. a decrease in postreceptor insulin signaling cascade
   c. a decrease in Glut 4
   d. increased fat mass in late pregnancy

4. Type 2 diabetes testing. A 38-year-old G1P0 patient attends her first prenatal visit at 9 weeks of gestation. She has a strong family history of diabetes, and her body mass index is 32. Which of the following is **the least accurate test** recommended by ACOG to diagnose diabetes mellitus in the first trimester of pregnancy?
   a. Fasting blood glucose followed by a 75-g glucose load and a 2-hour plasma glucose measurement
   b. Two-step 50-g OGTT
   c. One-step 75-g OGTT
   d. Random HbA1c

5. 3 hr versus 2 hr GTT. Two tests for GDM are currently used: one-step 75-g OGTT and two-step OGTT. The ACOG recommends using the two-step test for the following reasons **except**:
   a. the first step, drinking 50 g glucose nonfasting, is more efficient
   b. requiring two abnormal values on the 100-g, 3-hour test lowers the false-positive rates and improves predictive values
   c. the one-step 75-g OGTT has been shown to increase significantly the numbers diagnosed with GDM without demonstrating improved pregnancy outcomes
   d. the two-step OGTT has reduced the percentage of macrosomic infants delivered from GDM pregnancies compared with the one-step OGTT

6. Insulin resistance in pregnancy. Maternal insulin resistance rises in all trimesters of pregnancy **except**:
   a. first trimester and postpartum
   b. first and second trimesters
   c. second and third trimesters
   d. third trimester and postpartum

7. Preeclampsia risk reduction with low-dose aspirin (LDASA). LDASA is recommended in pregnant women with diabetes to reduce risk of preeclampsia. According to ACOG recommendations, for optimal effect, LDASA should be started
   a. during pregnancy planning
   b. when human chorionic gonadotropin is positive
   c. between 12 and 16 weeks of gestation
   d. before 28 weeks of gestation

8. Macrosomia on 36-week scan. A 24-year-old nulliparous patient with GDM on insulin therapy undergoes a 32-week "growth ultrasound," which documents:
   • Head circumference: 30 cm, 53rd percentile
   • Abdominal circumference: 30 cm, 93rd percentile
   • Femur length: 5.8 cm, 20th percentile
   • Estimated fetal weight: 2280 g, 92nd percentile
   The best option for the next step is:
   a. Schedule cesarean delivery at 36 weeks of gestation.
   b. Schedule cesarean delivery at 37 weeks of gestation.
   c. Schedule labor induction at 36 weeks of gestation.
   d. Schedule labor induction at 37 weeks of gestation.
   e. Schedule repeat growth imaging at 36 weeks of gestation.

9. Metformin and GDM. A 33-year-old patient at 29 weeks of gestation with type 2 diabetes is taking Humulin (NPH; intermediate-acting insulin) at 10 p.m. to control her fasting (6 a.m.) glucose levels, which have remained in the 110−130 mg/dL range over the past 4 weeks despite progressive Humulin dosage increases. Also, recently she has been awakening at 4 a.m. with hypoglycemia (glucose level 55−65 mg/dL) and must drink 6−8 oz of fruit juice. Which of the options below is the optimal next step?
   a. Add metformin 500 mg at bedtime.
   b. Set an alarm and take Humulin at midnight.
   c. Discontinue the intermediate-acting Humulin and begin taking long-acting Lantus at 10 p.m.
   d. Eat a 700-kcal snack at midnight.

10. Nonmacrosomic DM induction timing. A 42-year-old G4 P0 patient with type 2 diabetes and 3 prior miscarriages is referred for advice regarding delivery timing, currently at 36 weeks of gestation. She is normotensive. A sonographic fetal weight estimate at 35 weeks was 2412 g, 70th percentile. Her recent HbA1c is 6.8. The patient seeks advice on the optimal route and timing for infant outcome, and your best recommendation is:
    a. Labor induction at 39 0/7 to 39 6/7 weeks
    b. Cesarean delivery at 39 0/7 to 39 6/7 weeks
    c. Labor induction at 38 0/7 to 38 6/7 weeks
    d. Cesarean delivery at 38 0/7 to 38 6/7 weeks
    e. At 37 weeks of gestation, another ultrasound EFW and cesarean if EFW >4000 g

11. GDM target glucose values. When reviewing finger-stick glucose results on a patient with newly diagnosed GDM, which of the following target values is **incorrect?**
    a. Fasting glucose <95 mg/dL (5.3 mmol/L)
    b. One-hour postprandial glucose <140 mg/dL (7.8 mmol/L) or
    c. Two-hour postprandial glucose <130 mg/dL (6.7 mmol/L)
    d. All glucose values ≥63 mg/dL

12. Postpregnancy follow-up of GDM. Your patient with diet-controlled GDM during pregnancy returns for postpartum visit. What further testing should be done?
    a. Perform 2-hour 75-g OGTT and refer to primary care as type 2 diabetes if fasting is above 125 mg/dl or 2-hour value is above 200 mg/dL.
    b. Perform 2-hour 75-g OGTT and refer to primary care as type 2 diabetes if fasting is above 125 mg/dL and 2-hour value is above 200 mg/dL.
    c. Obtain HbA1c and refer to primary care if above 5.8%.
    d. Review postpartum finger-stick glucose values and refer to endocrinology if abnormal.

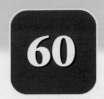

60

Pregnancy in Women With Obesity

MICHELLE A. KOMINIAREK | JORDAN STONE | DORA J. MELBER |
LAURYN C. GABBY

(see *Creasy and Resnik's Maternal-Fetal Medicine, 9e: Ch 60*)

Summary

Background: Obesity has reached epidemic proportions in the United States. A total of 36.5% of reproductive-age persons were overweight or obese in 2015−2016, translating to a high percentage of persons with obesity during a pregnancy. The risks of obesity are wide ranging and reach preconception, pregnancy, and postpartum periods. These risks are further amplified in a higher body mass index (i.e., BMI ≥50 kg/m²). Furthermore, obesity is cited as a contributing factor in more than 50% of maternal deaths. No organ system is spared from the effect of obesity in pregnancy. There are known changes in the cardiovascular, respiratory, endocrine, gastrointestinal, and coagulation systems related to obesity.

Associated risks: Prepregnancy obesity increases the risk of a variety of congenital anomalies, particularly open neural tube defects and cardiac defects. Obesity is also associated with increased risk of stillbirth, having pregestational diabetes mellitus and chronic hypertension, and developing preeclampsia and gestational diabetes. Pregnancy is an independent risk factor for obstructive sleep apnea, compounding the association with obesity. Associations between both preterm births and postdate gestations have been reported with obesity. Compared with persons with a normal body mass index (BMI), persons with obesity are two to three times more likely to need labor augmentation or induction and are at increased risk of cesarean delivery for obstructed or prolonged labor and postpartum hemorrhage due to atony. Persons with obesity are also at increased anesthetic risk, including multiple attempts at regional placement, failed regional anesthesia, and failed intubations.

Management: Given the increasing incidence of obesity and obesity-related complications, it is critical to identify opportunities to improve the safe delivery of care provided during pregnancy, delivery, and postpartum. Clinicians caring for persons with obesity may consider including in their counseling that obesity increases the risk of congenital anomalies and decreases the sensitivity of currently available genetic screening and ultrasound imaging options. Screening for gestational diabetes mellitus should be considered early in pregnancy. While obesity-related complications may be indications for scheduled induction, there is some evidence to support scheduled induction of labor due to obesity alone. Clinicians should also consider the physical capacity of hospital equipment (e.g., long laparotomy instruments, long safety belts, hospital beds, wheelchairs, toilets). Joint guidelines from several societies recommend 2 g of cefazolin for persons less than 120 kg and 3 g for persons 120 kg or greater as antibiotic prophylaxis for cesarean delivery. Decisions as to the type of skin incision should be made on the basis of body habitus distribution, access to the lower uterine segment, and patient and clinician preference. Clinicians should close subcutaneous adipose tissue when it measures greater than 2 cm and avoid placement of subcutaneous drains. Prophylactic negative pressure wound therapy in persons with obesity is not recommended. Either staples or subcuticular suture are reasonable options to consider for skin closure after a cesarean delivery. There is currently no consensus regarding the duration of medical thromboprophylaxis with heparin or low-molecular-weight heparin for optimal prevention of thromboembolism among persons with obesity. However, if clinicians determine that thromboprophylaxis is warranted, weight-based dosing is more effective (than empiric dosing) in achieving prophylactic target anti–factor Xa levels. Early postpartum surveillance for wound complications, postpartum depression, and breastfeeding difficulties can be considered. The postpartum visit is an opportunity to address postpartum weight retention and referral to medical and surgical obesity management programs.

Weight management: Approximately 60% of persons with obesity exceed weight gain goals, which are 5−9 kg. Excessive gestational weight gain is associated with large-for-gestational-age infants, cesarean delivery, postpartum weight retention, and increased prepregnancy BMI in the next pregnancy. Several studies, including large randomized controlled trials, have addressed behavioral interventions, such as diet modification and increasing exercise, among persons with obesity. While behavioral interventions appear to decrease gestational weight gain among persons with obesity by 1–2 kg, these interventions do not appear to consistently improve perinatal outcomes.

Bariatric surgery: Pregnancy outcomes in persons with prior bariatric surgery appear to be relatively good. Large cohort studies that matched for prepregnancy BMI and several meta-analyses report lower risks for hypertension, gestational diabetes, large-for-gestational-age infants, and macrosomia; however, there were increased risks for small-for-gestational-age infants in pregnancies that occurred after bariatric surgery. Some experts suggest delaying conception for 12−24 months given that most weight loss occurs within the first year and so that weight loss goals can be achieved. It is important for clinicians to be cognizant of the potential for surgical complications of bariatric surgery (e.g., internal hernias causing acute surgical emergencies). Nutritional deficiencies are common problems that occur primarily after Roux-en-Y procedures but can still occur after any type of bariatric procedure. Common deficiencies include iron, vitamin B₁₂, folate, and calcium. The recommendations for screening and supplementation are adapted from the general population of individuals having bariatric surgery.

QUESTIONS

1. A 31-year-old gravida 4, para 3 presents to your clinic for routine prenatal care. Your patient has chronic hypertension and the BMI was 46 kg/m² at the first prenatal visit. Which of the following statements are true about the prevalence of obesity in the United States?
   a. The prevalence of obesity decreases by age.
   b. The rate of obesity has decreased over the past 10 years.
   c. Prepregnancy obesity rates are highest among whites compared with other race/ethnicities.
   d. Persons without a college degree are more likely to have obesity before pregnancy.

2. A 32-year-old Hispanic gravida 2, para 1 presents to your clinic for a new obstetric visit. You calculate a BMI of 36 kg/m². On the basis of the World Health Organization and National Institutes of Health definitions of obesity, the appropriate category for this patient is:
   a. Normal weight
   b. Overweight
   c. Obesity class 1
   d. Obesity class 2
   e. Obesity class 3

3. A 35-year-old gravida 1, para 0 presents in active labor and requires an emergency cesarean delivery due to terminal fetal bradycardia. The decision is made to proceed with general anesthesia. The patient's BMI is 50 kg/m². Which of the following represent challenges to successful ventilation in this patient?
   a. Increased time before hypoxemia ensues after pre-oxygenation
   b. Ventilation-perfusion mismatch
   c. Increased chest wall compliance
   d. Decreased oxygen consumption

4. You are following a 27-year-old gravida 1, para 0 for routine prenatal care in your clinic. In the third trimester, you notice a weight gain of 50 lb (22.7 kg) since the first prenatal visit. You provide counseling that excessive gestational weight gain is a risk factor for:
   a. Small-for-gestational-age infant
   b. Postdate delivery
   c. Cesarean delivery
   d. Neonatal respiratory depression

5. You are finishing a routine scheduled cesarean delivery of a 21-year-old gravida 2, para 1 whose admission BMI was 48 kg/m². On the basis of available evidence, which of the following statements is true regarding Pfannenstiel incision closure after a cesarean delivery?
   a. A drain should be placed if subcutaneous adipose tissue measures greater than 2 cm.
   b. The subcutaneous tissue layer should be closed if adipose tissue measures greater than 2 cm.
   c. Prophylactic negative pressure wound therapy is routinely recommended for patients with obesity.
   d. For skin closure, staples should always be considered over subcuticular suture closure for patients with obesity.

6. An 18-year-old gravida 2, para 1 comes to the office for a first prenatal visit at 6 weeks' gestation. This is a strongly desired pregnancy. Your patient reports a 20-lb (9.1-kg) weight loss over the past year while taking orlistat. The BMI calculated in the clinic today is 35 kg/m². Which of the following are you most likely to recommend?
   a. Continue orlistat.
   b. Stop orlistat, and switch to phentermine-topiramate.
   c. Stop orlistat, and switch to metformin.
   d. Stop orlistat.

7. A 26-year-old gravida 0 comes to the office for a preconception visit. The BMI is currently 42 kg/m² and there are no other chronic medical conditions. Your patient is concerned about how obesity during pregnancy may impact the long-term health of future offspring. Which of the following is most correct about exposure to obesity during pregnancy?
   a. Obesity is associated with adverse cognitive and neurodevelopmental outcomes in offspring.
   b. Obesity is associated with type 1 diabetes in offspring.
   c. Obesity is associated with early childhood cancers in offspring.
   d. Obesity is associated with asthma and other chronic lung diseases in offspring.

8. A 37-year-old gravida 3, para 3 presents for a preconception consult to your outpatient office. Your patient had a sleeve gastrectomy 1 year ago and has lost 40 lb (18.1 kg). The BMI is now 32 kg/m² and your patient is interested in getting pregnant. Your patient reports gestational diabetes during the previous pregnancy. What is the first priority in caring for this patient?
   a. Counseling on delaying conception for 1−2 more years
   b. Counseling on the risks associated with advanced age
   c. Screening for diabetes
   d. Treatment with metformin to promote additional weight loss
   e. Screening for folate deficiency

9. A 25-year-old gravida 2, para 1 presents for a first prenatal visit at 14 weeks' gestation. There are no medical problems, but a prepregnancy BMI is 35 kg/m². You provide counseling on appropriate diet and exercise during pregnancy and the risks of obesity in pregnancy. What counseling do you provide about recommended weight changes during pregnancy?
   a. Weight loss until body mass index is <30 kg/m²
   b. Maintain current weight
   c. Gain 0-9 lb (0-4 kg)
   d. Gain 11-20 lb (5-9 kg)
   e. Gain 22-33 lb (10-15 kg)

10. A 43-year-old gravida 3, para 2 is having a third repeat cesarean delivery. The prepregnancy BMI is 50 kg/m^2 and there has been a 20-lb (9-kg) weight gain this pregnancy. After the second cesarean delivery, your patient had a wound separation and was treated with antibiotics for cellulitis. What is recommended to reduce the risk for surgical site infection?
    a. Vertical skin incision
    b. Drain placement in the subcutaneous tissue
    c. Closure of the subcutaneous tissue
    d. Prophylactic wound vacuum

11. A 39-year-old gravida 1 is currently 31 weeks' pregnant. Your patient reports having a Roux-en-Y gastric bypass procedure 3 years ago. Your patient is in the emergency department with a 1-day history of nausea, vomiting, and epigastric pain. The vitals are as follows: afebrile with a pulse of 110 bpm and a blood pressure of 100/50. The physical examination is notable for diffuse abdominal pain and distension. The cervix is closed, and there are no regular contractions. The hemoglobin is 11 g/dL, urine protein is negative, and liver function tests are normal. Which of the following diagnoses do you suspect?
    a. Hyperemesis gravidarum
    b. HELLP syndrome (hemolysis, elevated liver enzymes, and low platelet counts)
    c. Gastroesophageal reflux disease
    d. Internal herniation

12. You just completed a scheduled repeat cesarean delivery of a 27-year-old gravida 2, para 2 at 39 weeks' gestation. Medical problems include pregestational diabetes, hypothyroidism, and depression. The BMI at delivery was 50 kg/m^2. The surgery was uncomplicated, and the estimated blood loss was 600 mL. To optimally reduce the risk for venous thromboembolism, which of the following do you order?
    a. Enoxaparin 30 mg subcutaneously every 24 hours
    b. Enoxaparin 40 mg subcutaneously every 24 hours
    c. Enoxaparin 0.5 mg/kg subcutaneously every 12 hours
    d. Enoxaparin 1.0 mg/kg subcutaneously every 24 hours

13. You are seeing a 28-year-old gravida 1, para 0 at 34 weeks' and 4 days' gestation in the office for a return prenatal visit. Your patient self-identifies as Black, has a prepregnancy BMI of 43 kg/m^2, and has no other significant medical comorbidities. The ultrasound at 20 weeks' gestation demonstrated normal fetal anatomy. The estimated fetal weight was in the 30th percentile at a 32-week sonogram. How would you counsel the patient about the risk of stillbirth and the value of fetal surveillance as the pregnancy progresses?
    a. The risk of stillbirth is only marginally increased compared with a Black person with a nonobese BMI; however, it would be reasonable to start weekly fetal surveillance at 37 weeks' gestation.
    b. The risk of stillbirth is significantly higher than a person with obesity who identifies as White; however, there is limited evidence that fetal surveillance would decrease this risk.

c. The risk of stillbirth in all persons with class 3 obesity is approximately the same, and fetal surveillance is recommended starting at 36 weeks' gestation.
    d. The risk of stillbirth is significantly increased compared with a White person with obesity, and there is strong evidence to start fetal surveillance at 37 weeks' gestation.

14. A 31-year-old gravida 1, para 0 comes in for a return prenatal visit at 37 weeks' and 0 days' gestation. The prepregnancy BMI was 51 kg/m^2, and there has been a weight gain of 25 lb (11.3 kg) to date in this pregnancy. Your patient is planning a vaginal trial of labor and has several questions about the delivery. Which of the following is true regarding this patient's anticipated intrapartum course?
    a. A BMI greater than 50 is an indication for elective cesarean delivery and should be recommended.
    b. The duration of the active phase of labor is typically longer among persons with obesity compared with those without obesity.
    c. Class 3 obesity is a medical indication for induction of labor at 39 weeks' gestation and should be recommended.
    d. None of the above.

15. A 40-year-old gravida 2, para 1 is admitted at 38 weeks' and 3 days' gestation for an induction of labor due to preeclampsia without severe features. The prepregnancy BMI was 45 kg/m^2, and the weight on admission to labor and delivery is 298 lb (135 kg). Oxytocin is started, an amniotomy is performed, and the cervical examination progresses to 7 cm dilation. The cervical examination is unchanged after more than 6 hours, and a cesarean delivery is recommended for arrest of dilation. The anesthesiologist administers cefazolin 3 g IV and azithromycin 500 mg IV. Which of the following is true regarding this regimen for your patient?
    a. There is level 1 evidence that adjunctive preoperative azithromycin reduces surgical site infection for nonelective cesarean delivery.
    b. There is level 1 evidence that preoperative cefazolin 3 g is superior to cefazolin 2 g at preventing surgical site infection in persons with class 3 obesity undergoing nonelective cesarean delivery.
    c. Per the American Society of Health-System Pharmacists guidelines, persons with class 3 obesity should receive azithromycin 100 mg IV at the time of nonelective cesarean delivery.
    d. Azithromycin is only indicated as adjunctive preoperative antibiotic prophylaxis for persons undergoing cesarean delivery for arrest of descent.

16. A 32-year-old gravida 5, para 4 presents to the office at 37 weeks' gestation. The prepregnancy BMI was 42 kg/m^2, and there has been a weight loss of 3 lb (1.4 kg) during this pregnancy. What counseling would you provide regarding your patient's weight?
    a. There are no known risks to inadequate weight gain or weight loss in pregnancy.
    b. Your patient is at increased risk of a small-for-gestational-age infant.
    c. Your patient is at increased risk of cesarean delivery.
    d. The weight loss is within the recommended guidelines for the prepregnancy BMI.

17. A 32-year-old gravida 0 presents to the office for evaluation of infertility. The BMI is currently 39 kg/m^2. Your patient reports having timed, unprotected intercourse for the past 2 years and now desires referral to an infertility specialist. How do you counsel your patient regarding obesity and fertility treatments?
    a. Ovulation induction with medication is equally successful in persons with and without obesity.
    b. Intrauterine sperm injection is equally successful in persons with and without obesity.
    c. Weight loss improves response to infertility treatments.
    d. After successful implantation via in vitro fertilization, the risk of pregnancy loss is similar in persons with and without obesity.

18. A 28-year-old gravida 0 and a 29-year-old male partner present for a preconception visit. Your patient's BMI is 42 kg/m^2, and the partner's BMI is 46 kg/m^2. After discussing the risks of obesity in pregnancy, they inquire about the risks of obesity in the male partner. You counsel the couple that obesity is associated with decreased male fertility, as well as what other findings?
    a. Reduced live birth per cycle of assisted reproductive technology
    b. Birth defects
    c. Preterm delivery
    d. Preeclampsia

19. A 24-year-old gravida 1 presents for an ultrasound at 18 weeks' gestation. The BMI is 52 kg/m^2, and the visualization of fetal anatomy is limited. Which of the following is a true statement regarding the diagnosis of congenital anomalies in persons with obesity?
    a. The absolute value of alpha fetoprotein is a reliable predictor of neural tube defects in persons with and without obesity.
    b. Obesity is associated with a decreased fetal fraction of cell-free DNA.
    c. The American Institute of Ultrasound in Medicine endorses a detailed anatomy ultrasound in persons with a BMI ≥40 kg/m^2.
    d. Obesity does not substantially increase the risk of fetal anomalies.

20. A 34-year-old gravida 3, para 2 presents to your office to establish prenatal care at 12 weeks' gestation. The current BMI is 44 kg/m^2. In addition to screening for diabetes and hypertension, what other screening would you consider to assess the risk for complications?
    a. Fasting total cholesterol
    b. Transthoracic echocardiogram
    c. Sleep apnea
    d. Pulmonary function tests

21. A 29-year-old gravida 3, para 2 is postpartum day 3 following an uncomplicated vaginal delivery. The BMI is 43 kg/m^2, and the recovery is going well, except for difficulty with breastfeeding. The baby is latching well, but the milk supply is limited. There are no other comorbidities. Your patient asks if obesity may be related to issues with breastfeeding. What counseling do you provide?
    a. Obesity is not associated with breastfeeding success.
    b. Obesity is associated with decreased nutrients in the breast milk.
    c. More in-hospital assistance for breastfeeding is provided to persons with obesity.
    d. Obesity is associated with delayed lactogenesis.

61

Thyroid Disease in Pregnancy

LINDA ANNE BARBOUR | AMY MIYOSHI VALENT

(see Creasy and Resnik's Maternal-Fetal Medicine, 9e: Ch 61)

Summary

Thyroid disease in pregnancy has major implications for both maternal and offspring health, but interpretation of thyroid functions due to changes in physiology and test performance can be confusing. Robust treatment trials, which begin early in pregnancy, are limited. Major physiologic changes include thyroid stimulation by human chorionic gonadotropin (hCG), estrogen-induced rise in thyroxine-binding globulin (TBG), changes in clearance of thyroid hormone (TH), increased iodine metabolism, and placental activity of type 1 and type 2 deiodinases. The thyroid gland increases slightly in size, but in iodine-deficient areas the gland may increase 20%–50%, also known as the *thyroid goiter* of pregnancy. Iodine requirements increase in pregnancy, and TH synthesis typically increases by 25%–30%. The fetus is dependent on maternal T4 until 18 weeks of pregnancy for normal early neurologic development. Pregnant persons with normal thyroid function can adapt appropriately to these alterations, but those with decreased thyroid reserve from Hashimoto thyroiditis, ablation, or partial thyroidectomy may not be able to adequately increase TH production to meet the demands of pregnancy. Thyroid-stimulating hormone (TSH) levels are lower in pregnancy due to high levels of hCG, which have thyrotrophic action, and TT4 and TT3 increase by ~50% by 16 weeks due to the marked increase in estrogen-induced stimulation of TBG.

Physiologic changes of pregnancy influence TH metabolism and thyroid function tests. TSH is the most sensitive marker of primary thyroid dysfunction, has a short half-life of ~1 hour, and should be used as the first-line test except in pituitary-hypothalamic disorders; nonthyroidal illnesses; clinical conditions with high levels of dopamine, glucocorticoids, or somatostatin analogs; and mild iodine deficiency. T4 has a half-life of 5–7 days. Its assessment is required in the previously mentioned conditions, and it should be used to determine the degree of overt hypothyroidism and hyperthyroidism and to titrate antithyroid therapy in hyperthyroidism. T3 is the active hormone, but its production by the thyroid gland is only about 1/12th of T4, requiring availability through peripheral conversion of T4 by tissue-specific deiodinases. It has a shorter half-life of ~1 day and poorly crosses the placenta. The early fetal brain has predominately T4 receptors, strongly supporting the use of only levothyroxine (LT4) replacement in pregnancy. T3 should be checked in patients with hyperthyroidism because there are conditions in which its production may be higher than T4 (Graves disease and some autonomous nodules).

Patients with overt hypothyroidism (usually diagnosed as an elevated TSH and low free T4 [FT4] OR a TSH >10 mIU/L) should be started on an LT4 dose of 1.5 to 2.0 µg/kg/day. A full-replacement LT4 dose in pregnancy is estimated at ~2 µg/kg/day compared with outside of pregnancy, which is nearer to 1.6 µg/kg/day. Pregnant patients with subclinical hypothyroidism (SCH), usually caused by Hashimoto thyroiditis in the United States and accompanied by TPO antibodies, have partial thyroid dysfunction and are usually effectively treated with lower LT4 doses (50–75 µg/day) depending on the degree of TSH elevation and the patient's weight. Although there is a lack of consensus in the treatment of SCH due to the failure of randomized trails not to clearly show a benefit in maternal or infant outcomes, trials were limited by their late start in treatment (usually ~15-16 weeks), recruitment of patients with very mild SCH (mean TSH levels of only 4-6 IU/L), and variable assessment of thyroid peroxidase (TPO) antibodies, which may contribute to adverse outcomes from an autoimmune basis.

Overt hyperthyroidism, unless due to hCG-mediated gestational thyrotoxicosis, carries both maternal and fetal risks and should be treated, whereas subclinical hyperthyroidism should not. Furthermore, TSH-stimulating antibodies (thyroid-stimulating immunoglobulin [TSI] or TSH receptor antibody [TRAB]) at levels elevated threefold or greater carry risks for fetal and newborn Graves after 18 weeks. Antithyroid drugs (ATDs) reduce TH synthesis, and propylthiouracil (PTU) also inhibits deiodination of T_4 to T_3, which is why it is the preferred ATD for thyroid storm and primarily T_3 thyrotoxicosis; it is also preferred in the first trimester. The lowest ATD dose to maintain the FT4 at the upper reference range or TT4 at 1.5 times the upper nonpregnant reference range is recommended. Free T4 or TT4 (and often TT3) should be checked every 2–4 weeks during treatment since ATD requirements usually decrease with the immune suppression of pregnancy and overtreatment can cause fetal hypothyroidism.

Thyroid nodules are occasionally found in pregnancy, and the indications for fine-needle aspiration (FNA) are the same as outside of pregnancy and guided by sonographic characteristics. Thyroid cancer is not thought to behave more aggressively during pregnancy with respect to long-term survival.

QUESTIONS

1. A 30-year-old gravida 2, para 1 at 13 weeks' gestation is found at her first obstetrician appointment to have a TSH of 0.2 mIU/L (nonpregnant range 0.5–4.5) after being screened due to a family history of thyroid disease. Her family medicine provider adds a TT4 to her labs, which returns at 13 mcg/dL (nonpregnant normal range 4–12). On examination, her thyroid does not appear grossly enlarged but she has symptoms of fatigue, slight palpitations, and nausea. Heart rate is 110 bpm, and blood pressure is normal at 126/78 mm Hg. Which of the following is the most appropriate next step in management?
   a. Obtain a free T4 to determine if she is truly hyperthyroid.
   b. Obtain both a free T4 and a free T3 to determine her true thyroid status.
   c. Reassure her that no further evaluation or treatment is needed.
   d. Start treatment with a low dose of beta blocker for her palpitations and mild hyperthyroidism to avoid early antithyroid medication exposure to the fetus.
   e. Repeat TSH in midgestation.

2. A 26-year-old gravida 3, para 2 is screened at 10 weeks' gestation and found to have a TSH of 8.0 mIU/L. What further evaluation do you need?
   a. Check a free T4, since it is likely to be slightly low.
   b. Check both a free T4 and a TT3, since the free T4 may be normal but the TT3 is likely to be low.
   c. Check a free T4 to ensure a diagnosis of SCH.
   d. Check a free T4 to ensure a diagnosis of overt hypothyroidism.
   e. No clear reason to check any other labs but consider TPO antibodies.

3. A 26-year-old gravida 3, para 2 is screened at 10 weeks' gestation and found to have a TSH of 8.0 mIU/L and a normal FT4. She is asymptomatic. Her weight is 175 lbs. She strongly prefers not starting meds if this value is not considered to be critical. What are your options for management and treatment?
   a. Obtain TPO antibodies and, if positive, try to persuade her to start taking 150 mcg of LT4.
   b. Agree not to treat but repeat her TSH in 4 weeks and consider obtaining TPO antibodies.
   c. Tell her that not treating with at least 50 mcg has been shown in randomized trials to adversely affect offspring intelligence quotient.
   d. Check TPO antibodies and, if negative, tell her that she does not have SCH from Hashimoto and the TSH is likely a laboratory error.

4. A 38-year-old gravida 1, para 0 at 14 weeks' gestation presents to the emergency department with nausea, vomiting, a heart rate of 120 bpm, heat intolerance, and a 5-lb weight loss and is found to have a positive pregnancy test. A TSH is undetectable, and her free T4 is 2.6 ng/dL (nonpregnancy range 0.7–1.9) with a TT3 of 250 ng/dL (nonpregnancy range 90–180). You perform an ultrasound, which is consistent with a 13-week intrauterine pregnancy. On examination, the thyroid is not palpably enlarged, nor does she have evidence of exophthalmos. However, the patient does have a fine tremor on examination and increased reflexes, and she is diaphoretic. Which of the following is the most appropriate pharmacotherapy at this time?
   a. Begin treatment with PTU at 150 mg 3× per day given her symptomatology and signs.
   b. Begin intravenous fluids and consider a low-dose beta blocker while you send out TRAB and TSI levels.
   c. Begin treatment with PTU at 50 mg 3× per day, since her TT3 is disproportionly higher than the elevation of her FT4.
   d. Begin treatment with MMI 10 mg twice a day, since she is out of first trimester and she has an increased risk of hepatotoxicity to PTU.
   e. Begin MMI 10 mg twice a day and a low-dose beta blocker given her degree of hyperthyroidism and symptoms.

5. A 33-year-old gravida 3, para 2 at 8 weeks' gestation has a history of a near-complete thyroidectomy for Graves. The patient ran out of her Armour thyroid, which she was taking due to persistent hypothyroid symptoms on LT4 alone, in spite of a normal TSH. The patient weighs 112 kg at her OB intake visit with a nurse midwife, and she is found on her initial labs to have a TSH of 40 with a FT4 of 0.7 (nonpregnant normal range 0.8–1.8). She has a few 175 mcg tabs of LT4 at home leftover from before the switch to Armour thyroid. Which of the following is the most appropriate next step in management?
   a. Restart her previous dose of 175 mcg of LT4.
   b. Restart her previous dose of 175 mcg of LT4 every day but also add 2 tablets a week.
   c. Resume the Armour thyroid at the nonpregnancy dose.
   d. Replace the Armour thyroid with corresponding physiologic doses of 150 mcg daily of LT4 and 5 mcg twice a day of liothyronine (T3).
   e. Start 2 tabs every day of her previous dose (175 mcg) given how high her TSH is and fetal dependence of maternal thyroid hormone until 18 weeks.

6. A 21-year-old gravida 1 patient at 32 weeks' gestation presents in clinic with tachycardia, palpitations, diaphoresis, and weight loss with an undetectable TSH and FT4 of 5.3 ng/dL (nonpregnant normal range 0.7–1.9) and a TT3 of 900 ng/dL. Her TRAB and TSI are negative. She reports that she ran out of her PTU (150 mg 3× per day) that she took early in pregnancy about 6 weeks ago. Her liver function tests are slightly elevated with an alanine aminotransferase and AST ~1.5× normal. If untreated, this patient is at greatest immediate risk for which of the following disorders?
   a. High cardiac output failure
   b. Thyroid storm
   c. Preeclampsia
   d. Neonatal hyperthyroidism
   e. Fetal goiter

7. A 21-year-old gravida 1 patient at 32 weeks' gestation presents in the clinic with tachycardia, palpitations, diaphoresis, and weight loss with an undetectable TSH and FT4 of 5.3 ng/dL (nonpregnant normal range 0.7–1.9) and a TT3 of 900 ng/dL. She reports that she ran out of PTU (150 mg 3× per day), which she had been taking since early pregnancy about 6 weeks ago. Her liver function tests are slightly elevated with an alanine aminotransferase and aspartate transaminase ~1.5× normal. Which of the following is the most appropriate pharmacotherapy at this time?
   a. Beta blocker alone followed by plasmapheresis for possible hepatoxicity on PTU
   b. Beta blocker, cold iodide, and preparation for surgery, given she appears to have hepatotoxicity to PTU
   c. Beta blocker and low-dose MMI (5 mg twice a day), given her elevated liver function texts and concerns for hepatotoxicity
   d. Beta blocker with either PTU (150 mg every 8 hours) or MMI (12.5 mg every 12 hours)

8. A 34-year-old gravida 2, para 2 presents 1 month postpartum with a history of relapsing Graves disease that was treated with low-dose PTU in early pregnancy but was downtitrated and off medications by 24 weeks' gestation. The patient is breastfeeding but complaining of insomnia, nervousness, diaphoresis, and rapid weight loss. She recalls from her last pregnancy that she had a low TSH early postpartum but developed a high TSH transiently at ~6 months postpartum that resolved. Eventually she became hyperthyroid again before this pregnancy and had to be retreated with PTU in early pregnancy. The provider repeats a TSH, which is completely suppressed; FT4 is 2.2 ng/dL (nonpregnant normal range 0.7–1.9); and her TT3 is 160 ng/dL (nonpregnant normal range 90–180). On the basis of history, you obtain TPO antibodies, which are positive. Which of the following is the most likely explanation for these laboratory findings?
   a. Graves and Hashimoto mixed disease; hold off treatment at this time, with the possible exception of a low-dose beta blocker
   b. Graves and Hashimoto mixed disease; recommend an I-131 uptake and scan to determine if she has primarily Graves or postpartum thyroiditis
   c. Graves disease with stimulatory and inhibitory antibodies; begin low-dose PTU (50 mg twice a day)

   d. Rebound Graves disease; treat with PTU at 150 mg twice a day

9. A 40-year-old gravid 1 at 20 weeks' gestation is found on examination to have a 1- to 2-cm nodule. She has no symptoms of hoarseness or compression and otherwise feels well. There is a questionable family history of thyroid cancer in her father, who is now deceased, but the patient is unclear about any details. Which of the following is the most appropriate diagnostic or laboratory study at this time?
   a. Thyroid ultrasound
   b. FNA biopsy
   c. TSH
   d. Calcitonin level
   e. FNA with molecular markers to improve prediction of benignity or malignancy

10. A 32-year-old gravida 3, para 1 at 12 weeks' gestation presents with a history of Graves disease status post radioactive iodine ablation 2 years ago and on postprocedural levothyroxine replacement (150 mcg daily). TSH receptor antibody (TRAB) and TSI levels were 3× the normal range. Which of the following is the most appropriate next step in evaluation and management?
   a. Begin low-dose PTU along with 150 mcg LT4 to treat fetal hyperthyroidism but not render the patient hypothyroid (replace and treat strategy).
   b. Repeat TRAb or TSI at 20–24 weeks.
   c. Serial biometry starting at 24 weeks with antenatal fetal surveillance starting at 28–30 weeks.
   d. Repeat TSH at 20–24 weeks.
   e. Offer percutaneous umbilical sampling at 24–28 weeks to confirm fetal hyperthyroidism to guide treatment.

11. A 42-year-old gravida 2, para 0 at 10 weeks' gestation is referred for consultation regarding abnormal thyroid function labs with pregnancy complicated by in vitro fertilization, family history of cardiovascular disease, vegan status, and recent move from Algeria. Her primary provider screened for thyroid dysfunction with the patient's routine prenatal labs and ordered TSH (3.9 mIU/L) and FT4 (0.7 ng/dL; normal range 0.9–1.7). Thyroid function labs are repeated using equilibrium dialysis and have similar TSH and FT4 results. On examination, thyroid palpates with moderate enlargement but no difficulty breathing or swallowing. Which of the following is the most likely diagnosis?
   a. Lab error
   b. Isolated hypothyroxinemia of unclear etiology
   c. Isolated hypothyroxinemia secondary to iodine insufficiency
   d. Central hypothyroidism due to a pituitary abnormality
   e. Overt hypothyroidism

12. A 31-year-old gravida 4, para 0 presents at 6 weeks' gestation with history of papillary thyroid carcinoma that was treated with radioactive iodine 1 year ago. She has been followed with ultrasound and thyroglobulin (Tg) for surveillance and before conception was found to have a negative ultrasound but Tg at 5 ng/mL (normal range 3–40 ng/mL). Which of the following is the most appropriate pharmacotherapy and/or monitoring management?
    a. Molecular biomarkers for thyroid cancer recurrence
    b. Calcitonin levels
    c. Serial thyroid ultrasounds every 12 weeks
    d. Increase levothyroxine by 30% of prepregnancy dose, target a suppressed TSH and FT4 that is not elevated, and repeat Tg 6 months after last check
    e. Increase levothyroxine by 30% of prepregnancy dose, target a suppressed TSH and FT4 slightly above the upper limit of normal range, and repeat Tg 6 months after last check.

13. A 29-year-old gravida 1, para 0 at 17 weeks' gestation was transferred out of the intensive care unit for COVID-19 respiratory failure requiring intubation for 5 days and a course of corticosteroids. While in the intensive care unit (ICU), she had a suppressed TSH. She is improving now at 7 days after discharge from the ICU. The hospital team ordered thyroid function labs, which demonstrated a TSH 9 mIU/L and reflexed with a FT4 0.9 ng/dL (normal range 0.9–1.7). Which of the following is the most likely diagnosis?
    a. Subclinical hypothyroidism; start 50 mcg levothyroxine (LT4)
    b. Overt hypothyroidism; start weight-based LT4
    c. Hashimoto thyroiditis that was masked initially by the corticosteroids and severe acute illness while in the ICU; start 50 mcg LT4
    d. Non-thyroidal illness syndrome; no treatment at this time
    e. Non-thyroidal illness syndrome; begin 50 mcg LT4

14. A 36-year-old gravida 2, para 0 presents for preconception counseling with history complicated by secondary infertility and is working with reproductive endocrinologists for fertility options. During her workup, the patient was found to have a TSH of 1.9 mIU/L and was TPO positive. This patient should be advised to do which of the following during pregnancy?
    a. Start 50 mcg LT4 and follow TSH until 18 weeks' gestation.
    b. No treatment and follow TSH until 18 weeks' gestation and postpartum.
    c. No follow-up or treatment.
    d. Selenium.
    e. Start 100 ug of LT4 to try to better suppress the TPO antibodies.

15. A 34-year-old gravida 1 at 14 weeks' gestation and a history of overt hypothyroidism on an appropriate total replacement dose is found to have a TSH of 14 mIU/L. Pregnancy is complicated by a Roux-en-Y gastric bypass surgery 13 months before conception, and she still has problems with weight stabilization and digesting simple sugars. The patient appropriately increased her levothyroxine dose of 125 mcg daily to add 2 extra tablets per week on discovering a positive pregnancy test. She is taking ferrous sulfate, vitamin D, and calcium supplementation >4 hours from when she takes her levothyroxine. Which of the following is the most likely explanation for these laboratory findings?
    a. Drug interference with T4 absorption
    b. Drug compliance challenges
    c. Surgical malabsorption interfering with T4 absorption
    d. Physiologic pregnancy hormone changes

Other Endocrine Disorders of Pregnancy

DALAL S. ALI | KAREL DANDURAND | ALIYA A. KHAN

(see *Creasy and Resnik's Maternal-Fetal Medicine, 9e: Ch 62*)

Summary

CALCIUM HOMEOSTASIS DURING PREGNANCY

Calcium homeostasis is altered during pregnancy in order to meet the developing fetal requirements. Parathyroid hormone (PTH)-related peptide (PTHrP) rises as early as 3–13 weeks of pregnancy and results in enhanced conversion of 25 hydroxyvitamin D to 1,25 dihydroxyvitamin D. Increases in 1,25 dihydroxyvitamin D enhance calcium and phosphorus absorption from the maternal gut. This is associated with a reduction in PTH levels. The maternal breast and placenta are the primary sources of PTHrP during pregnancy (Figure 62.1). Calcitonin levels rise during pregnancy, and this may prevent excessive bone resorption and provide skeletal protection for the mother.

IMPACT OF PREGNANCY AND LACTATION ON MATERNAL SKELETON

The effect of pregnancy on bone turnover was previously evaluated and showed an increase of bone resorption markers by 14 weeks' gestation and further increases by 28 weeks, whereas markers of bone formation did not show a significant increase until 28 weeks' gestation. The effect of pregnancy on bone mineral density (BMD) is not well understood. Significant increases in estradiol may have a protective effect on the maternal skeleton during pregnancy. During lactation, however, reductions in BMD have been documented. Increased prolactin levels during breastfeeding reduce gonadotropin-releasing hormone (GnRH), resulting in decreases in estradiol levels with increases in RANKL expression and increases in osteoclast number and function. Adequate maternal calcium and vitamin D intake during pregnancy is important for maintaining skeletal health. PTHrP production from the lactating breast increases in response to high prolactin (Figure 62.2).

There is a synergistic effect of high PTHrP and low estradiol on increased bone resorption. This mechanism may lead to a progressive loss of 5%–10% of trabecular bone during the first 6 months of lactation, which recovers after weaning.

PRIMARY HYPERPARATHYROIDISM (PHPT)

PHPT is the most common cause of hypercalcemia in pregnancy and is diagnosed by the presence of hypercalcemia with an elevated or inappropriately normal PTH level. Symptoms are often nonspecific and may be overlooked as physiologic pregnancy manifestations. Gastrointestinal symptoms and hyperemesis gravidarum have been commonly described. Polyuria, polydipsia, renal colic, malaise, muscle weakness, fatigue, depression,

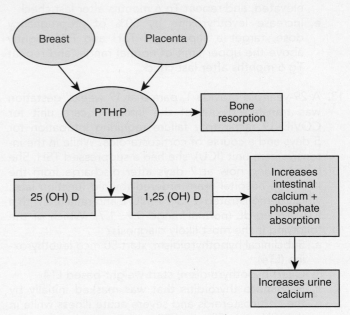

Figure 62.1 Calcium homeostasis during pregnancy.

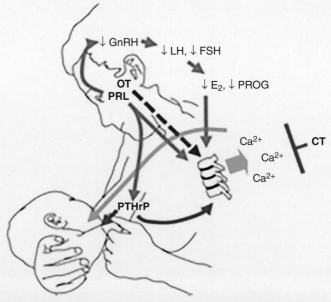

Figure 62.2 Impact of pregnancy and lactation on maternal skeleton.

and agitation have also been reported. Hereditary causes of PHPT must be considered in women of reproductive age, as they occur at a younger age in comparison with sporadic PHPT. These include multiple endocrine neoplasia syndromes type 1, 2A, and 4; hyperparathyroidism-jaw tumor syndrome; and familial isolated primary hyperparathyroidism. Familial hypocalciuric hypercalcemia (FHH) and use of lithium, thiazide diuretics, and calcium supplements need to be excluded before confirming the diagnosis of PHPT. Other conditions that can cause hypercalcemia, including malignancy, granulomatous disease, thyrotoxicosis, hypervitaminosis D or A, milk-alkali syndrome, immobilization, adrenal insufficiency, extrarenal calcitriol production, and rare inherited disorders of vitamin D metabolism, also need to be excluded. After confirming the diagnosis of PHPT in pregnancy, adequate hydration is advised. Medical treatment options are limited due to lack of long-term safety data. Calcitonin does not cross the placenta and has been used safely during pregnancy to acutely lower serum calcium. Cinacalcet (category C in pregnancy) has also been used in case reports. Bisphosphonates and denosumab should be avoided during pregnancy. In cases of severe hypercalcemia (corrected serum calcium ≥ 3 mmol/L), parathyroidectomy is advised, preferably in the second trimester. Preoperative imaging in pregnancy is limited to neck ultrasound. Maternal and fetal morbidities have been reported in cases with inadequately managed PHPT during pregnancy.

HYPOPARATHYROIDISM (HypoPT)

HypoPT is uncommon during pregnancy and is diagnosed in the presence of hypocalcemia with low or inappropriately normal PTH. The majority of cases are post neck surgery (75%). The remaining 25% of cases are caused by autoimmune disorders, inherited conditions, infiltrative diseases, radiation therapy, mineral deposition, magnesium abnormalities, or use of certain chemotherapeutic agents. Symptoms of hypocalcemia include paresthesia in the hands, face, and feet, as well as muscle cramps, brain fog, and confusion. In severe cases, hypocalcemia can result in bronchospasm, laryngospasm, seizures, cardiac arrhythmia, and congestive heart failure. Conventional therapy with elemental calcium, vitamin D, and active vitamin D analogs (calcitriol or alfacalcidol) is safe during pregnancy. The aim is to achieve eucalcemia with serum ionized calcium levels in the mid to low normal reference range and to avoid hypercalcemia and hypocalcemia. Maternal and fetal morbidity has been reported

in women with HypoPT. Reported fetal complications include neonatal hyperparathyroidism, which may lead to fetal skeletal demineralization and intrauterine fragility fractures. Severe maternal hypocalcemia may also result in miscarriage and preterm delivery secondary to premature uterine contractions.

Neonatal hypocalcemia, seizures, and tetany have also been reported with maternal hypercalcemia, as high maternal calcium can suppress the development of fetal parathyroid glands resulting in HypoPT.

PREGNANCY-RELATED OSTEOPOROSIS

A careful evaluation is required with exclusion of an underlying secondary cause of osteoporosis. These include, and are not strictly limited to, hypogonadism, PHPT, thyrotoxicosis, hypercortisolism, osteomalacia, osteogenesis imperfecta, malabsorptive state (e.g., celiac disease), eating disorders, inflammatory arthritis, and inflammatory bowel disease. Chronic use of medications like glucocorticoids, excessive thyroxine, anticonvulsants, GnRH analogs, selective serotonin reuptake inhibitor, and cytotoxic chemotherapeutic agents also needs to be excluded.

The physical examination includes assessment of body mass index (BMI) and evaluation of height loss, which may result from vertebral fractures. In the presence of height loss, spinal radiographs are advised following delivery with exclusion of vertebral compression fractures. Dual-energy x-ray absorptiometry (DXA) assessment can be completed postpartum and compared with prepregnancy values if available. Baseline biochemical assessment includes serum ionized calcium or serum calcium corrected for albumin, serum phosphorus, serum magnesium, serum alkaline phosphatase, 25 hydroxyvitamin D, creatinine, estimated glomerular filtration rate (eGFR), complete blood count, thyroid-stimulating hormone (TSH), PTH, serum immunoelectrophoresis, and 24-hour urine collection for calcium and creatinine. Screening for celiac disease should be considered if clinically indicated. Adequate calcium intake (1200 mg daily of elemental calcium from dietary and supplemental sources) and vitamin D intake should be ensured. In cases of severe osteoporosis, it is reasonable to discourage lactation. Use of calcitonin, bisphosphonates, teriparatide, vertebroplasty, and kyphoplasty to treat postpartum osteoporosis has been described in the literature. The benefit of such intervention is uncertain, given that most women who present with fractures during pregnancy or lactation experience a spontaneous increase in bone density after weaning.

QUESTIONS

1. A 26-year-old woman, gravida 2, para 1 presents to her family physician in the first trimester of pregnancy. She is healthy with no medical or surgical history. She takes a daily prenatal vitamin and maintains adequate dietary calcium intake of 1200 mg of elemental calcium daily. Physical examination is unremarkable. What are the hormonal changes in relation to calcium homeostasis you would anticipate in the first trimester?
   a. Increase in calcium and PTH, with no change in serum phosphorus, PTHrP, and 1,25 dihydroxyvitamin D
   b. Increase in PTHrP, 1,25 dihydroxyvitamin D and calcium, with decrease in phosphorus and PTH
   c. Decrease in PTH, increase in PTHrP and 1,25 dihydroxyvitamin D with no change in serum calcium and phosphorus
   d. No change to PTH, PTHrP, serum calcium, and phosphorus with marked increase in 1,25 dihydroxyvitamin D

2. A 21-year-old woman comes in for a preconception workup and assessment. She is healthy with no medical history apart from generalized fatigue and body aches. Her periods are regular. Physical examination is unremarkable.
   Laboratory investigation:

Hb	118 g/L (120–160)
Creatinine	68 umol/L (50–100)
TSH	1.78 mIU/L (0.32–4.0)
25 hydroxyvitamin D	39 nmol/L (desired 50–125)
Na	142 mmol/L (135–145)
K	4.6 mmol/L (3.5–5.0)
Corrected calcium	2.19 mmol/L (2.15–2.6)

   Following review of her laboratory investigations, what is the best next step in the management?
   a. Initiate vitamin D replacement with 1000–2000 IU daily and screen for iron deficiency anemia and celiac disease.
   b. Ask her to increase sun exposure.
   c. No intervention is required. Check iron study and B_{12}.
   d. Ask her to start prenatal vitamins and repeat laboratory tests when pregnancy is confirmed.

3. A 19-year-old gravida 1 presented to the acute medical unit with nausea, vomiting, and spasms in the hands and legs at 8 weeks' gestation. She has had recurrent oral candidiasis and was on fluconazole in a prior pregnancy. Physical examination reveals blood pressure 96/70 mm Hg and hyperpigmentation of the buccal mucosa. Cardiovascular, respiratory, and abdominal examinations are unremarkable.
   Laboratory Investigation:

Corrected calcium	1.89 mmol/L (2.15–2.6)
Phosphate	1.67 mmol/L (0.81–1.58)
PTH	0.4 pmol/L (1.6–9.3)
25 hydroxyvitamin D	55 nmol/L (desired >50)
Na	130 mmol/L (135–145)
K	5.0 mmol/L (3.5–5.0)

   On the basis of her clinical presentation and laboratory profile, which one of the following is the most likely diagnosis?
   a. DiGeorge syndrome
   b. Autoimmune polyglandular syndrome type 1
   c. Isolated hypoparathyroidism
   d. Barakat syndrome

4. A 36-year-old gravida 1 presents to the antenatal clinic at 11 weeks' gestation. Her medical history consists of hypothyroidism and hypoparathyroidism secondary to total thyroidectomy for papillary thyroid cancer 8 years before conception, with low risk of recurrence. Her medications include elemental calcium 1000 mg twice daily, calcitriol 0.25 mcg twice daily, L-thyroxine 88 mcg daily, magnesium 500 mg daily, vitamin D_3 1000 IU daily, and prenatal vitamins. She does not report symptoms of hypocalcemia. Physical examination is unremarkable. Chvostek and Trousseau signs are negative.
   Laboratory Investigation:

Corrected calcium	2.15 mmol/L (2.15–2.6)
Phosphate	1.59 mmol/L (0.81–1.58)
PTH	0.2 pmol/L (1.6–9.3)
25 hydroxyvitamin D	101 nmol/L (desired >50)
TSH	0.78 mIU/L (0.32–4.0)
FT4	18 pmol/L (9–19)

   After review of her laboratory results, what is the best advice for this patient?
   a. Take calcium supplements on an empty stomach for better absorption.
   b. Take calcium supplements with meals to act as a phosphate binder and avoid hyperphosphatemia. Also take L-thyroxine on an empty stomach and avoid taking it with calcium or other calcium containing vitamins.
   c. Increase calcitriol dose to 0.25 mcg three times daily.
   d. No need to continue vitamin D_3 supplements.

5. A 32-year-old gravida 2, para 1 presents to the emergency department with acute-onset sharp back pain of 2 days' duration. She is currently 4 weeks postpartum after an uncomplicated pregnancy and a vaginal delivery at 39 weeks' gestation. She is exclusively breastfeeding. Physical examination revealed tenderness on lumbar spine percussion, and there is a 2.5-cm height loss. Cardiovascular, respiratory, and abdominal examinations are unremarkable. Spine radiographs revealed grade 1 and 2 compression fractures at T12 and L1, respectively. Diagnosis of osteoporosis is suspected, and she was referred for BMD testing. Which of the following is the best next step?
   a. Manage conservatively with pain control pills and review again in 4 weeks.
   b. Further evaluate to exclude secondary causes of bone loss.
   c. Treat with oral bisphosphonate as she is young.
   d. Advise that pregnancy-related osteoporosis is a reversible condition, and no further investigation is required.

6. A 29-year-old primigravida is evaluated for intractable nausea and vomiting during her second trimester. Workup reveals a total corrected calcium for albumin of 2.74 mmol/L (N 2.15–2.60 mmol/L) and a PTH level of 15 pmol/L (N 1.6–6.9 pmol/L), PO_4 of 0.69 mmol/L (N 0.80–1.45 mmol/L) with a normal kidney function and vitamin D level. The calcium-to-creatinine clearance ratio is 0.026. Which of the following is the most common maternal complication of this patient's condition?
   a. Preeclampsia
   b. Pancreatitis
   c. Nephrolithiasis
   d. Fractures

7. A 24-year-old female, G2P1, is diagnosed with primary hyperparathyroidism during the third trimester of pregnancy as she is being investigated for an episode of nephrolithiasis. Her serum corrected calcium is 3.02 mmol/L (N 2.15–2.60 mmol/L) and is not responding to a conservative measure of intravenous hydration. Of the following pharmacologic interventions, which one is the safest to use during pregnancy in order to acutely lower her serum calcium level?
   a. Calcitonin
   b. Zoledronic acid
   c. Cinacalcet
   d. Denosumab

8. A primigravid 28-year-old woman at 20 weeks' gestation presents with hyperemesis gravidarum, and workup reveals hypercalcemia caused by primary hyperparathyroidism. Her serum corrected calcium is 3.10 mmol/L (N 2.15–2.60 mmol/L), and she is not responding to conservative measures, namely fluids and rehydration. As she is in her second trimester, a parathyroidectomy is planned to address her condition. Which of the following preoperative imaging is recommended to guide the parathyroidectomy?
   a. Sestamibi parathyroid scan
   b. Neck ultrasound
   c. Neck computed tomography with abdominal shielding
   d. Neck magnetic resonance imaging

9. Which of the following is true regarding pregnancy-related osteoporosis?
   a. Associated fractures have been shown to be associated with higher parity.
   b. A pregnancy-related osteoporosis fracture has a high risk of recurrence during subsequent pregnancies.
   c. The most frequent site of pregnancy-related osteoporosis fragility fracture is the wrist.
   d. Bone loss occurring during pregnancy and lactation spontaneously recovers in the following 6–12 months.

10. A 33-year-old female, G3P2, presents with spontaneous acute-onset back pain during her third trimester. A postpartum spinal radiograph reveals an L3 compression fracture with 50% vertebral body height loss that was not present prepregnancy. She is experiencing significant back pain from the fracture. Which of the following is the next best step?
    a. She should be treated with oral or intravenous bisphosphonate as soon as possible, as there is no concern regarding transplacental passage and harm to the fetus.
    b. The risk-benefit ratio of any active drug treatment should be discussed with the patient. Currently there are limited data regarding the benefits of teriparatide, calcitonin, or bisphosphonates.
    c. She should be offered raloxifene, as it has been proven to be an effective drug treatment in that specific patient population.
    d. She should be referred as soon as possible for vertebroplasty in order to avoid the use of any pharmacologic intervention.

63

Gastrointestinal Disorders of Pregnancy

THOMAS F. KELLY | THOMAS SAVIDES

(see *Creasy and Resnik's Maternal-Fetal Medicine, 9e: Ch 63*)

Summary

The anatomic and physiologic changes of the gastrointestinal tract during pregnancy may result in unfamiliar and unusual maternal symptoms in otherwise uncomplicated pregnancies. At times these symptoms may confuse patients and providers as well. Understanding the pregnancy-associated alterations in the gastrointestinal tract, as well as the risks and benefits of various diagnostic and therapeutic modalities, can help reduce unnecessary diagnostic delays and improve pregnancy outcomes.

Nausea and vomiting occur in the majority of pregnant women during first two trimesters but usually resolve before 20 weeks of gestation. Risk factors include first pregnancy, young age, fewer than 12 years of education, nonsmokers, and obesity. Vitamin B_6 is probably the best initial pharmacologic treatment, and the addition of doxylamine typically improves these symptoms. Ondansetron, the most frequently prescribed antiemetic in the United States, improves the nausea of early pregnancy but may carry a low risk for congenital anomalies.

Hyperemesis gravidarum occurs in about 0.5% live births but is the second most common cause of pregnancy-related hospitalizations. It is more likely to occur in gestational trophoblastic disease, hydrops, and fetal chromosomal abnormalities. Complications may include Wernicke encephalopathy and esophageal rupture. Management includes fluid resuscitation and electrolyte and thiamine replacement.

Gastrointestinal reflux disease is a common maternal complaint and increases with gestational age. It may be related to pregnancy hormone–induced smooth muscle relaxation of the lower esophageal sphincter, compounded by increasing intraabdominal pressure and delayed gastric emptying. Antacids relieve symptoms approximately in 30%–50% of cases. Diagnosis relies on clinical symptoms typically increasing with gestational age and occurring at night. Upper endoscopy should be reserved for cases refractory to medical management. Histamine receptor antagonists appear safe in pregnancy. Proton pump inhibitors, although more effective than H2 blockers, are less well studied. Treatments for peptic ulcer, an unusual complication, are similar to those for gastrointestinal reflux.

Appendicitis is one of the most common etiologies of an acute abdomen in pregnancy. While the incidence is not increased compared with that in nonpregnant individuals, appendiceal perforation rates are higher during gestation. This is likely due to diagnostic and therapeutic delays. Right lower quadrant pain is the most common symptom in the first trimester, but pain may focus higher in the right subcostal area in later pregnancy. Laboratory evaluation is useful primarily to exclude alternative diagnoses. Plain film and ultrasound imaging are often not helpful. Helical computed tomography (CT) is sensitive and specific in nonpregnant individuals, but experience in pregnancy remains limited. Magnetic resonance imaging (MRI) without contrast has no known adverse fetal effects and is considered a more appropriate imaging modality than CT with oral contrast for evaluation of significant abdominal pain in pregnant women. Prompt surgical intervention is the standard treatment. Laparoscopy has been performed with a good safety record.

Inflammatory bowel disease (IBD) refers to ulcerative colitis and Crohn disease. They differ in terms of intestinal wall layer involvement, anatomic location, and response to surgical resection. Both are treated with similar medications. There is an increased rate of preterm birth and low birth weights with IBD. Pregnancy does not appear to alter disease activity. Management includes antidiarrheal medications, sulfasalazine, 5-aminosalicylates, corticosteroids, azathioprine, and more recently antitumor necrosis factor medications.

Celiac disease is caused by an abnormal T-cell response to gluten in genetically predisposed individuals and is often underdiagnosed. Studies suggest that uncontrolled disease may be associated with adverse pregnancy outcomes, but whether this disorder is causative or merely an association is unknown. However, patients with anemia refractory to iron, hypokalemia, or hypocalcemia may benefit from evaluation for celiac disease. The most widely available screening test is the antiendomysial IgA. Instituting a gluten-free diet may reduce the negative effects of celiac disease.

Upper gastrointestinal endoscopy (esophagogastroduodenoscopy [EGD]) and colonoscopy are vital in the diagnosis and management of a variety of gastrointestinal disorders, but few pregnant patients require such procedures. While these procedures are often safe, complications are related to the endoscopy (perforation, bleeding, and infection) or sedation (cardiovascular events, aspiration, and fetal exposure). The American College of Obstetricians and Gynecologists has published guidelines related to endoscopy, including indications, during pregnancy.

QUESTIONS

1. A 20-year-old, G1 P0 at 12 weeks' gestation, during a routine prenatal visit, complains of constant nausea and vomits about three times daily. She has tried oral ginger without improvement. On examination the patient appears in no distress and is not dehydrated. Which of the following would be the most appropriate therapy?
   a. Ondansetron 4 mg orally every 8 hours
   b. Acupuncture twice weekly
   c. Vitamin B_6 25 mg orally every 8 hours
   d. Metoclopramide 10 mg every 8 hours
   e. Intravenous lactated Ringer infusion with multivitamins daily

2. A 35-year-old, G2 P1 at 15 weeks' gestation presents to the emergency department with nausea and vomiting for 8 weeks. She has a prior pregnancy complicated by hyperemesis gravidarum. On examination, she is dehydrated and mildly tachycardic but otherwise has no localizing signs suspicious for acute abdomen. Which of the following is the most appropriate initial concern that must be addressed?
   a. Hyperthyroidism
   b. *Helicobacter pylori* infection
   c. Hypoglycemia
   d. Thiamine deficiency
   e. Hypernatremia

3. A 26-year-old, G2 P1 at 20 weeks' gestation presents to the emergency department complaining of right-sided abdominal pain, fever, and nausea for 12 hours. She has been previously well, and the pregnancy has been uncomplicated. The emergency medicine attending is concerned about appendicitis and is asking for advice regarding further workup and management. Which of the following is the most appropriate statement?
   a. Abdominal ultrasound is the safest imaging modality and has the highest negative predictive value for ruling out appendicitis.
   b. Helical CT scanning is contraindicated in pregnancy given the fetal radiation exposure.
   c. Helical CT scanning is preferable to MRI.
   d. MRI using gadolinium contrast is preferred.
   e. An appendix diameter >6 cm suggests appendicitis regardless of imaging modality.

4. A 35-year-old, G1 P0 at 23 weeks' gestation presents to the emergency department complaining of right-sided abdominal pain. The subsequent evaluation suggests a high likelihood of appendicitis. A general surgeon who is consulted agrees with the diagnosis and plans to perform a laparoscopic evaluation and possible appendectomy. Which of the following statements is the most appropriate regarding laparoscopy in pregnancy?
   a. Laparoscopy should only be performed in the first and second trimesters.
   b. Laparoscopy often has longer operative times when compared with laparotomy.
   c. Verres needle entry is contraindicated during initial port placement.

   d. Limiting intraabdominal pressure to less than 12 mm Hg is advised.
   e. A cervical manipulator during laparoscopy is recommended.

5. A 26-year-old, G2 P1 at 18 weeks' gestation presents to you for consultation referred by her primary obstetrician. She has a 6-year history of ulcerative colitis with good control using infliximab and sulfasalazine. Which of the following is the most appropriate recommendation regarding her management?
   a. Discontinue sulfasalazine given the risks of teratogenicity.
   b. Discontinue infliximab as advised by consensus statements regarding IBD in pregnancy.
   c. Discontinue both medications and initiate a fluoroquinolone antibiotic.
   d. Continue both medications.

6. A 40-year-old, G1 P0 Ab1 presents for preconception counseling. She suspects that she recently developed celiac disease and is concerned about her pregnancy risks. She had a first-trimester miscarriage 5 years earlier. Which of the following statements is correct?
   a. The "gold standard" of diagnosis of celiac disease is the IgA antigliadin antibody level.
   b. The most widely available screening test is the anti-endomysial IgA test.
   c. There is a clear association with uncontrolled celiac disease and adverse pregnancy outcomes.
   d. Three quarters of patients with celiac disease are diagnosed after the age of 15.
   e. Celiac disease is often overdiagnosed.

7. A 25-year-old, G2 P1 at 8 weeks' gestation presents for a routine prenatal visit. She is complaining of new-onset substernal burning and regurgitation. An evaluation by her internist suspects gastrointestinal reflux disease. She has no evidence of intestinal bleeding. Which of the following is the appropriate next step in management?
   a. EGD
   b. Lifestyle and dietary changes
   c. Evaluation for *H. pylori* infection
   d. Initiate omeprazole

8. A 35-year-old, gravida 1 at 30 weeks' gestation presents for a routine prenatal visit. She is complaining of constipation with two bowel movements per week. Before pregnancy, the patient had problems of constipation and needed to resort to manual maneuvers to assist in defecation. Which of the following is the most appropriate next step in management?
   a. Attempt defecation in the evening or before meals.
   b. Reduce fluid and fiber intake.
   c. Initiate metoclopramide to improve intestinal transit.
   d. Avoid prolonged use of stimulant and hyperosmolar laxatives.
   e. Initiate caffeine intake in the morning.

9. A 28-year-old, G1 at 30 weeks' gestation presents to labor and delivery for rectal bleeding. She has a history of hemorrhoids when not pregnant. Anoscopy reveals the presence of internal hemorrhoids, one of which is bleeding, prolapsed but not incarcerated. She has not responded to conservative measures. Which of the following is the most appropriate next step in management?
   a. Sclerotherapy using 5% KCl injection
   b. Rubber band ligation
   c. Surgical hemorrhoidectomy
   d. Topical Monsel solution
   e. Interventional radiology with embolization

10. A 30-year-old, P1 at 27 weeks' gestation presents to labor and delivery for generalized upper abdominal pain. The workup reveals no obvious source, and the gastroenterology service is consulted. Which of the following is the most appropriate statement regarding upper GI endoscopy procedures in pregnancy?
   a. Wireless capsule endoscopy is the preferred modality in pregnancy.
   b. Endoscopic ultrasound is less sensitive than MRI looking for stones in the common bile duct.
   c. Gastrointestinal endoscopy in pregnancy has minimal risks, often unrelated to the procedure itself.
   d. Results from small studies suggest that endoscopy and colonoscopy are safe in pregnancy.
   e. No guidelines related to endoscopy in pregnant women exist.

Diseases of the Liver, Biliary System, and Pancreas

JOSE R. DUNCAN

(see *Creasy and Resnik's Maternal-Fetal Medicine, 9e: Ch 64*)

Summary

The obstetric provider should be familiar with the physiologic changes of pregnancy. Disorders that affect the liver, biliary system, and pancreas can occur during pregnancy, and the diagnosis may be delayed, as some of these symptoms are common in pregnancy. Ultrasound is the first imaging option to study the liver, pancreas, and biliary tract. However, when indicated, magnetic resonance, computed tomography, and cholangiopancreatography should not be withheld. And in some cases, a liver biopsy may be performed. We describe the most important illnesses during pregnancy.

INTRAHEPATIC CHOLESTASIS OF PREGNANCY

Intrahepatic cholestasis of pregnancy (ICP) occurs more often in the third trimester and is characterized by generalized pruritus that involves the palms and soles. The diagnosis is confirmed with elevated bile acid count, typically defined by levels greater than 10 μmol/L. Although the pathophysiology of this disease is not well understood, ICP is associated with adverse pregnancy, such as preterm birth, meconium aspiration, and even fetal demise. Ursodeoxycholic acid is the treatment of choice. Complications emerge more often with bile acid >40−100 μmol/L. Experts recommend delivery in the late preterm period when bile acids levels reach such values. But delivery can be undertaken at 37−39 weeks when bile acids are <40 μmol/L.

ACUTE FATTY LIVER OF PREGNANCY

Although rare, acute fatty liver of pregnancy (AFLP) increases the risk of maternal and perinatal mortality. Therefore, early diagnosis is of outmost importance. AFLP typically manifests in the third trimester with symptoms of nausea, malaise, pain, and anorexia. The diagnosis is made by the presence of six of the following criteria: vomiting, abdominal pain, polydipsia or polyuria, encephalopathy, hypoglycemia, hyperbilirubinemia, elevated urea, leukocytosis, elevated ammonia, elevated transaminases, ascites or echogenic liver on ultrasound, elevated creatinine, and microvascular steatosis. Correction of the coagulopathy and glycemic control with prompt delivery are recommended once this diagnosis is suspected.

HEMOLYSIS, ELEVATED LIVER ENZYME, LOW PLATELETS SYNDROME

Hemolysis, elevated liver enzyme, low platelets syndrome (HELLP) also occurs more often in the third trimester, and it is usually associated with hypertension. Specific laboratory findings of liver dysfunction such as hypoglycemia, high ammonia, and coagulopathy are usually not seen. Magnesium sulfate should be initiated, followed by delivery.

OTHER CONDITIONS THAT CAN OCCUR IN PREGNANCY

Individuals with chronic liver conditions such as Wilson disease, autoimmune hepatitis, Budd-Chiari syndrome, or cirrhosis may become pregnant, as well as those who have received a liver or pancreatic transplants. Therefore, providers should familiarize themselves with these conditions, their effect on pregnancy, and how pregnancy may affect these disorders.

Viral Hepatitis

Pregnancies can be complicated by viral hepatitis. The most common cause is hepatitis A virus, followed by hepatitis B and C viruses. However, it can be caused by other viruses.

All pregnant individuals should be screened for hepatitis B virus (HBV) as perinatal infection can potentially be prevented with antiviral medication like tenofovir in the third trimester when indicated (>6−8 log 10 copies/mL). Infants born from mothers with hepatitis B infection should receive immunoprophylaxis with immunoglobulin and vaccination within 12 hours of birth. Hepatitis B vaccination is recommended for all susceptible expectant mothers. Universal screening is also recommended for hepatitis C virus (HCV) with anti−hepatitis C virus antibodies. Perinatal transmission can occur, but in contrast with HBV, no preventative medication has been approved for this purpose in pregnancy. In pregnancies with HBV and HCV, interventions such as internal fetal monitoring, prolonged rupture of membranes, and episiotomy should be avoided when possible. Cesarean delivery should only be performed for usual obstetric indications, and breastfeeding should be encouraged.

Gallstones

Gallstones are common in pregnancy. If surgery is indicated, treatment should not be delayed because of pregnancy. When surgery is not immediately indicated, the surgery may be performed in the second trimester, a time of lower complications.

Pancreatitis

Pancreatitis is associated with an increased maternal morbidity and mortality. Therefore, management should be done in conjunction with experts on pancreatic disease and may require intensive care admission. The mainstay of treatment is bowel rest, intravenous fluid resuscitation, electrolyte replacement, and pain control.

Malignancies

When liver cancer is suspected, the diagnostic workup should not be delayed because of pregnancy, and the patient should be referred to oncology as soon as needed. Reproductive options such as termination of pregnancy should be discussed with the patient. If possible, chemotherapy should be avoided during the first trimester. Chemotherapy during the second and third trimester is considered relatively safe.

QUESTIONS

1. A 31-year-old G1P0 presents for her first prenatal visit at 8 weeks of gestation. She reports to the obstetrician that she had liver disease in childhood. Which of the following physiologic hepatic changes occur in pregnancy?
   a. Increased serum albumin
   b. Increased levels of factor VII and factor IX
   c. Decreased levels of factor VII and factor IX
   d. Decreased bile acid concentrations

2. A 24-year-old, primigravid woman at 36 weeks' gestation reports pruritus in her palms, soles, and entire body. She has tried Benadryl at home without success. You suspect ICP and order a bile acids serum count, as well as liver transaminases. What bile acids levels are associated with an increased rate of adverse outcomes?
   a. >10 μmol/L
   b. >25 μmol/L
   c. >35 μmol/L
   d. >40 μmol/L
   e. >15 μmol/L

3. A 28-year-old G5P3013 at 34 weeks' gestation is transferred to the emergency department somnolent. Her blood pressure is 130/85 and pulse is 110 beats per minute. She is afebrile with O_2 saturations of 96%. Her aspartate aminotransaminase (AST) is 1040 IU/L, and alanine aminotransaminase (ALT) is 1108 IU/L. Her creatinine is 1.5 mg/dL, the prothrombin time is mildly elevated, and platelets are 130,000 per μL. She is delivered and after delivery, her transaminases continue to increase. After administration of *N*-acetylcysteine, she dramatically improves. The most likely diagnosis is:
   a. HELLP syndrome
   b. Acetaminophen toxicity
   c. Alcohol poisoning
   d. Fatty liver of pregnancy
   e. Hemolytic uremic syndrome

4. An 18-year-old primigravida presents at 31 weeks' gestation to the emergency department complaining of decreased fetal movements. Her baby is placed on the electronic fetal monitor. Her blood pressure is 150/92 mm Hg. Her AST and ALT are 456 and 362 IU/L, respectively. A complete blood count demonstrated a hemoglobin of 11 g/dL and platelets of 45 000 per μL. The best next step is:
   a. Steroids for lung maturity and magnesium sulfate
   b. Cesarean delivery
   c. Epidural anesthesia and induction of labor
   d. IV antihypertensives and magnesium sulfate
   e. Discharge home

5. A 24-year-old G2P1001 at 32 weeks is transferred from another hospital due to worsening of her AST and ALT (both >1000 IU/L), nausea, vomiting, and altered mental status. Her total bilirubin is 1.5 mg/dL, Hb is 11.5 g/dL, platelets are 88,000 per μL, and glucose is 51 mg/dL. Her PT and PTT are elevated, and vital signs are stable. When she arrives at the hospital, you recommend admission to intensive care unit. What is the best next step in management?
   a. Steroids for lung maturity and magnesium sulfate
   b. Administer insulin
   c. Emergency cesarean delivery
   d. Correct coagulopathy and proceed with delivery
   e. Plasmapheresis

6. A 32-year-old woman with a history of chronic hepatitis B infection comes for her first prenatal visit. Her obstetrician orders a baseline laboratory evaluation. What laboratory test at 32 weeks of gestation will indicate a need for antiviral therapy to decrease the risk of perinatal transmission?
   a. RNA viral load >6−8 log 10 copies/mL
   b. DNA viral load >6−8 log 10 copies/mL
   c. AST >400 IU/L
   d. Positive hepatis B surface antigen
   e. Positive anti-core IgM for hepatitis B

7. A 34-year-old pregnant individual presents at 29 weeks with abdominal discomfort, nausea, jaundice, and pruritus. She has seen a hepatologist in the past who prescribed a medication that she stopped when she found out she was pregnant. Her liver enzymes are mildly elevated, and her bile acids are 43 μmol/L. You start her on ursodeoxycholic acid, and her symptoms improve. Her bile acid and transaminases improve also, and you note a positive antimitochondrial antibody test when reviewing her records. The most likely diagnosis is:
   a. Intrahepatic cholestasis of pregnancy
   b. Fatty liver of pregnancy
   c. Acute hepatitis
   d. Chronic hepatitis
   e. Primary biliary cirrhosis

8. A 42-year-old G5P3013 presents at 31 weeks of gestation with right upper quadrant abdominal pain that worsens with meals. Her transaminases are mildly elevated and bilirubins are normal. Her white blood cell count is normal. Her right upper quadrant sonogram shows multiple nonobstructive gallstones without thickening of the gallbladder wall. Her symptoms improve after treatment with pain medication, and you send her home. You inform her that in general the best time to perform a cholecystectomy in pregnancy is:
   a. Third trimester
   b. Second trimester
   c. First trimester
   d. Never

9. Unfortunately, the patient from question 8 returns 4 weeks later with worsening abdominal pain, nausea, and vomiting with jaundice. She appears ill. A repeat ultrasound shows multiple gallstones without gallbladder wall thickening and a negative Murphy sign. Her AST is 302 IU/L and serum glucose is 200 mg/dL. Her blood pressure is normal, there is leukocytosis, and platelets are normal. Amylase and lipase are six times normal values. The best next step in management is:
   a. Immediate delivery
   b. Antenatal corticosteroids and delivery
   c. Magnesium sulfate and delivery
   d. IV hydration, antibiotics, bowel rest, cholecystectomy
   e. Emergency cholecystectomy

10. A 33-year-old G2P1001 individual presents at 20 weeks of gestation to the emergency room complaining of abdominal pain, nausea, vomiting, jaundice, and dark urine. Her AST is 906 IU//L and her ALT is 865 IU/L. Lipase and amylase are normal. BP is 100/70 and pulse is 100. She is oriented and there is no rebound. Ultrasound shows an enlarged liver and a normal gallbladder. The most likely test to confirm the diagnosis is:
   a. Ceruloplasmin
   b. Hepatitis A IgG antibodies
   c. Hepatitis A IgM antibodies
   d. Hepatitis C IgM antibodies
   e. Hepatitis E IgM antibodies

11. A 27-year-old woman with HIV and chronic hepatitis B comes to your clinic for preconception consultation. She is concerned about perinatal transmission of both viruses. You recommend combined ART with tenofovir to decrease this risk, and you counsel her of the following:
   a. She will need a cesarean delivery.
   b. If HIV viral load is <1000 copies and hepatitis B is <6−8 log copies, the risk of perinatal transmission is impossible.
   c. Breastfeeding is always recommended with HIV and hepatis B co-infection.
   d. She does not need to worry about perinatal infection.
   e. Neonatal prophylaxis and vaccination for hepatitis B are recommended.

12. The following statement is true about expectant mothers with history of liver transplantation:
   a. There is no need to monitor levels of immunosuppressant agents.
   b. Potential adverse outcomes include preterm birth.
   c. Potential adverse outcomes include large-for-gestational-age infant.
   d. Pregnancy itself accelerates graft rejection.

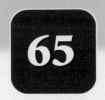

Pregnancy and Rheumatic Diseases

LISA R. SAMMARITANO | JANE E. SALMON | D. WARE BRANCH

(see Creasy and Resnik's Maternal-Fetal Medicine, 9e: Ch 65)

Summary

SYSTEMIC LUPUS ERYTHEMATOSUS

Systemic lupus erythematosus (SLE) is a systemic autoimmune disease with multiorgan involvement characterized by periods of remission and relapse. New classification criteria from the American College of Rheumatology (ACR) and European League Against Rheumatism (EULAR) were published in 2019 (Table 65.1). Therapy of SLE is dictated by both degree of disease activity and specific organ involvement; more serious and extensive inflammation is treated more aggressively. Unless contraindicated, all patients are treated with long-term antimalarial therapy, most commonly hydroxychloroquine, which should be continued in pregnancy.

Maternal and fetal pregnancy-related risks include an increased likelihood of gestational hypertensive disease, pregnancy loss, thromboembolic disease, iatrogenic preterm delivery, cesarean delivery, postpartum infection, and mortality. Unplanned pregnancy and active lupus, particularly active renal disease, predispose to complications; hence, preconception consultation and control of disease are strongly recommended. Severe SLE complications, including pulmonary arterial hypertension and moderate-to-severe renal disease, are contraindications to pregnancy. Stable SLE patients with low-level or inactive disease and with normal or near-normal renal function have a favorable pregnancy prognosis.

Preconception planning should include medication risk assessment and testing for renal function and antiphospholipid antibodies and anti–Ro/SSA and anti–La/SSB antibodies. Experts hold that those positive for anti–Ro/SSA and anti–La/SSB should undergo periodic fetal echocardiography from 16 to 26 weeks to detect early evidence of developing heart block. SLE patients are best managed during pregnancy via coordinated care among rheumatologists, maternal-fetal medicine specialists, and other medical specialists as required.

ANTIPHOSPHOLIPID SYNDROME

Antiphospholipid syndrome (APS) is an autoimmune condition characterized clinically by thrombosis (venous or arterial) and/or several adverse pregnancy outcomes. The diagnosis is confirmed by the presence of *repeatedly* positive, circulating antiphospholipid antibodies (aPL). The condition is associated with poor vascularization of the placenta, the downstream effects of which may include fetal death, preeclampsia, and placental insufficiency. The most serious thrombotic manifestation of APS is a thrombotic microangiopathy, catastrophic APS, a presentation that may initially mimic HELLP (Hemolysis, Elevated Liver enzyme levels, and Low Platelet levels) syndrome.

The ideal management regimen of APS during pregnancy minimizes the risk of adverse maternal and feta/neonatal outcomes. The conventional treatment used in APS pregnancy has been a combination of a heparin agent and low-dose aspirin (LDA), with the dose of heparin dependent on whether or not the patient has a history of thrombosis. In addition, the most up-to-date professional guidelines recommend considering the addition of hydroxychloroquine in patients not already on this agent. A summary of current treatment recommendations is shown in Table 65.3 of the textbook.

RHEUMATOID ARTHRITIS

Rheumatoid arthritis (RA) is an inflammatory disease marked predominantly by chronic symmetric inflammatory arthritis of small- and medium-size joints. In the nonpregnant population, the management of RA involves the use of disease-modifying antirheumatic drugs, or DMARDs, of which there are conventional (e.g., methotrexate, leflunomide), targeted (e.g., tofacitinib), and biologic (e.g., adalimumab, tocilizumab) agents, which have proven to significantly reduce long-term morbidity.

Preconception planning must include discontinuation of methotrexate or other agents contraindicated in pregnancy, with substitution of a pregnancy-compatible alternative. Pregnancy tends to have a beneficial effect on RA disease activity, with symptomatic improvement in at least 50% of affected women. Those that require ongoing treatment in pregnancy may be managed with low-dose glucocorticoids or anti-TNF agents. Current guidelines suggest avoiding the use of anti-TNF agents after the end of the second trimester or early third trimester; however, in practice, patients who require an anti-TNF agent may choose to continue the medication in the third trimester as a matter of benefits outweighing risks.

Pregnancy outcomes in patients with RA are generally favorable, though there may be a slightly increased risk of gestational hypertensive disease, small-for-gestational-age infants, preterm birth, and cesarean delivery. Most women with RA flare within the first 3 months postpartum; thus, postpartum care should be coordinated with the patient's rheumatologist.

SJÖGREN SYNDROME

Sjögren syndrome is characterized by keratoconjunctivitis and sicca, arthritis, and other symptoms. It is often secondary to another autoimmune disease such as SLE. Little is known about the interaction of pregnancy with the course of primary Sjögren syndrome. In the majority of cases, the most concerning possible adverse pregnancy outcome is neonatal lupus, including the possibility of fetoneonatal complete heart block secondary to most patients with the syndrome having anti–Ro/SSA and anti–La/SSB antibodies.

TABLE 65.1	Classification Criteria for Systemic Lupus Erythematosus

Entry Criterion

Antinuclear antibodies (ANAs) at a titer of ≥1:80 on Hep-2 cells or an equivalent positive test (ever)

If absent, do not classify as SLE
If present, apply additive criteria

Additive Criteria

Do not count a criterion if there is a more likely explanation than SLE.
Occurrence of a criterion on at least 1 occasion is sufficient.
SLE classification requires at least 1 clinical criterion and ≥10 points.
Criteria need not occur simultaneously.
With each domain, only the highest weighted criterion is counted toward the total score.*

Clinical domains and criteria	Weight	Immunology domains and criteria	Weight
Constitutional		*Antiphospholipid antibodies*	
Fever	2	Anti-cardiolipin antibodies OR Anti-β2GP1 antibodies OR Lupus anticoagulant	2
Hematologic		*Complement proteins*	
Leukopenia	3	Low C3 OR low C4	3
Thrombocytopenia	4	Low C3 AND C4	4
Autoimmune hemolysis	4		
Neuropsychiatric		*SLE-specific antibodies*	
Delirium	2	Anti-dsDNA antibody† OR Anti-Smith antibody	6
Psychosis	3		
Seizure	5		
Mucocutaneous			
Nonscarring alopecia	2		
Oral ulcers	2		
Subacute cutaneous OR discoid lupus	4		
Acute cutaneous lupus	6		
Serosal			
Pleural or pericardial effusion	5		
Acute pericarditis	6		
Musculoskeletal			
Joint involvement	6		
Renal			
Proteinuria >0.5 g/24 hr	4		
Renal biopsy class II or V lupus nephritis	8		
Renal biopsy class III or IV lupus nephritis	10		

Total score:

Classify as systemic lupus erythematosus with a score of 10 or more if entry criterion fulfilled.

*Additional criteria items within the same domain will not be counted.
†In an assay with ≥90% specificity against relevant disease controls.

SYSTEMIC SCLEROSIS

Systemic sclerosis (SSc), or scleroderma, is an uncommon condition characterized by thickened, hardened skin, characterized histologically by a marked increase in collagen in the dermis with hyalinization and often obliteration of small blood vessels. Raynaud phenomenon is a common feature. Systemic manifestations are diverse and largely caused by the progressive fibrosis of viscera that may involve multiple organ systems, including lungs, kidneys, heart, gastrointestinal tract, and musculoskeletal system. Data regarding pregnancy-related risks are limited, but pregnancy does not appear to exacerbate SSc. Life-threatening disease complications of SSc include interstitial lung disease, pulmonary arterial hypertension, and renal involvement, all of which should be assessed preconceptionally. Scleroderma renal crisis, with acute onset of severe hypertension, progressive renal insufficiency, microangiopathic hemolytic anemia, and thrombocytopenia, is a serious manifestation of SSc for which treatment with angiotensin-converting enzyme inhibitors may be lifesaving.

SYSTEMIC VASCULITIDES

The primary systemic vasculitides are a heterogeneous group of disorders classified on the basis of the predominant size of the vessels involved (large, medium, and small vessels). Vasculitis activity, end-organ damage from previous disease activity, and effects of immunosuppressive therapy are important considerations when approaching pregnancy. Data regarding pregnancy outcomes, neonatal outcomes, and effect of pregnancy on vasculitis disease activity are limited, though pregnancy outcomes in cohorts of patients with systemic vasculitides may include higher rates of pregnancy loss, preterm delivery, and delivery by cesarean section. The reported frequency of disease flares in case series is variable (20% to 40%).

Systemic vasculitides are generally characterized by relapsing disease courses, and pregnancy should be attempted when the disease is in a sustained remission (3−6 months). Inactive disease is associated with better maternal and neonatal outcomes. Immunosuppressive agents, such as cyclophosphamide, required to treat some systemic vasculitides, are teratogenic and should be discontinued before contemplation of pregnancy. Assessment of both vasculitis activity and end-organ damage should be performed before pregnancy and monitored throughout the peripartum period, with particular attention to hypertension and renal function. Specific vasculitides (Takayasu arteritis, polyarteritis nodosum, ANCA-associated vasculitis, and Behçet disease) are covered in the text of the chapter.

QUESTIONS

1. A 26-year-old G0 with SLE presents for preconception counseling. She is recently married, and she and her husband are planning for pregnancy. She was diagnosed with SLE at age 18, when she presented with fever, malar rash, arthritis, alopecia, and proteinuria. Renal biopsy showed diffuse proliferative lupus glomerulonephritis. Laboratory results at initial presentation were notable for positive ANA, positive double-stranded DNA, low complement levels, serum creatinine of 1.6, and urinary proteinuria of 4500 mg/24 hr. She was treated with high-dose corticosteroids, mycophenolate, hydroxychloroquine, and angiotensin-converting enzyme inhibitor therapy with resolution of lupus symptoms over 1 year. She has been maintained on hydroxychloroquine alone with no evidence of active lupus. Her physical examination is normal. Her laboratory results now show positive ANA, negative double-stranded DNA, normal complement levels, serum of creatinine 2.1, and urinary protein of 800 mg/24 hr. How do you advise this patient regarding best next steps for planning her family?
   a. Hydroxychloroquine is contraindicated during pregnancy; she should stop this and begin trying to conceive in 3 months.
   b. Her degree of kidney impairment precludes pregnancy due to maternal risk; she must adopt if she wants to have children.
   c. Her lupus is inactive at this time, with no clinical symptoms, normal dsDNA antibody, and normal complement levels; she can begin trying to conceive now.
   d. Though pregnancy is not absolutely contraindicated, the degree of renal impairment indicates a substantially increased risk of pregnancy complication requiring early delivery, with attendant neonatal risks of prematurity. Maternal risks include further renal impairment secondary to preeclampsia. Alternative options for this patient may include adoption or IVF with plans for a gestational carrier.

2. A 34-year-old G1P0 with SLE presents for evaluation at 8 weeks' gestation in an unplanned pregnancy. Her lupus was diagnosed at age 32, when she presented with lymphadenopathy, arthritis, and proteinuria. Renal biopsy showed membranous glomerulonephritis. Laboratory results at initial presentation were notable for positive ANA, positive double-stranded DNA, and low complement levels. She was treated with mycophenolate and rituximab and is currently maintained on hydroxychloroquine and prednisone 10 mg daily. She has had recent arthritis, malar rash, and low-grade fevers. Her current laboratory results show high double-stranded DNA antibody, low complement levels, stable creatinine of 1.0, and elevation in urine proteinuria since laboratory results 3 months ago, from 400 mg/24 hr to 2200 mg/24 hr. Her antiphospholipid antibodies are positive with high titer anticardiolipin and anti-beta2 glycoprotein I IgG and positive lupus anticoagulant. Her blood pressure today is 140/92. Which of the following factors does not increase this patient's risk for adverse pregnancy outcomes?
   a. Triple-positive antiphospholipid antibodies
   b. History of lupus nephritis
   c. Prior therapy with both rituximab and mycophenolate
   d. Current active lupus
   e. Unplanned pregnancy

3. A 30-year-old woman with SLE presents at 10 weeks' gestation with her first pregnancy. She initially presented at age 24 with arthritis, malar rash, oral ulcers, pleuritis, and dry eye and mouth symptoms. Laboratory results at that time showed positive ANA, positive double-stranded DNA, normal complement levels, and a positive anti-Ro/SS-A antibody. She has been reluctant to consider any medication for her SLE, since symptoms have been mild and intermittent. She was told by her new rheumatologist that her anti-Ro/SS-A antibody puts her at risk for having a child with neonatal lupus, including complete heart block. She asks for recommendations to improve fetal/neonatal outcome. You explain that although conclusive data are still limited, you suggest she consider which of the following
   a. Starting hydroxychloroquine now at a dose ≤5 mg/kg/day
   b. Starting dexamethasone now at a dose of 4−8 mg daily until 30 weeks' gestation
   c. Planning for serial fetal echocardiograms from weeks 20 through 30
   d. Starting IVIG infusions beginning at 12–14 weeks' gestation

4. A 26-year-old woman with SLE presents to discuss her current medications' safety for her planned pregnancy. She is now being treated with hydroxychloroquine, prednisone 5 mg daily, mycophenolate, and belimumab for symptoms of severe arthritis, alopecia, rash, and fatigue. The one medication that should be stopped at least 6 weeks before conception is
   a. Belimumab
   b. Hydroxychloroquine
   c. Mycophenolate
   d. Prednisone

5. An otherwise healthy 38-year-old, G2P0020 is referred to you for consultation regarding her history of two miscarriages occurring within the past 18 months. The prior miscarriages were at 6 weeks and 8 weeks, respectively. The couple has a negative evaluation for maternal endocrinopathies, uterine anomalies, and parental karyotype abnormalities. Genetic testing on abortus material was not done in either of her two miscarriages. The patient is negative for lupus anticoagulant (LA), IgG isotype anticardiolipin antibody (aCL), and anti-β2-glycoprotein-I (aβ2-GP-I) antibody. Her initial aCL IgM result was 28 MPL units, and repeat testing 3 months later showed 24 MPL units. The aβ2-GP-I IgM results were 21 and 24 SMU, respectively. Which of the following statements regarding this case is evidence based?
   a. The patient meets international criteria for definite antiphospholipid syndrome.
   b. Treatment during pregnancy with a heparin agent and low-dose aspirin is shown to improve pregnancy outcomes in patients such as this.
   c. The immunoassay results are in the low-positive range and are of uncertain significance with regard to autoimmune disease.
   d. Patients such as this are known to be at increased risk for preeclampsia relative to other 38-year-old nulliparas.
   e. The patient should be tested for other autoantibodies.

6. A 27-year-old G1P0101 seeks consultation regarding future pregnancies. Her only prior pregnancy was delivery for preeclampsia with severe features and fetal growth restriction with reversed umbilical artery end-diastolic flow at 26 weeks' gestation. She was tested for antiphospholipid antibodies and found to be positive for lupus anticoagulant (LA) and high-titer IgG isotype anticardiolipin (aCL) and anti-β2-glycoprotein-I (aβ2-GP-I) antibodies. Similar results were found on repeat testing several months later. She denies signs or symptoms of systemic lupus, has a normal serum creatinine, and has a recent urine protein-to-creatinine ratio result within the normal range. What should you tell her concerning another pregnancy?
   a. Her clinical history and antiphospholipid antibody profile place her at significant risk (>20%) for gestational hypertensive disease and placental insufficiency in her next pregnancy.
   b. Treatment during a next pregnancy with a heparin agent and low-dose aspirin will avoid adverse pregnancy outcomes with a high degree of certainty.
   c. Treatment with hydroxychloroquine during a next pregnancy has been shown in prospective trials to improve pregnancy outcomes.
   d. Treatment with hydroxychloroquine during a next pregnancy will reduce her risk of venous thromboembolism.
   e. Prospective trials have shown that intravenous immune globulin reduces the likelihood of fetal growth restriction in cases such as hers.

7. A 31-year-old nullipara seeks counsel about her RA management as she plans to undertake pregnancy. The patient describes mild wrist and proximal interphalangeal and metacarpal-phalangeal joint stiffness in spite of her current treatment with methotrexate (MTX) and nonsteroidal antiinflammatory drugs (NSAIDs). Concerning preconception- and pregnancy-related counseling and recommendations, which of the following is NOT true and/or NOT recommended?
   a. If the patient is positive for anti-SSA and/or anti-SSB antibodies, hydroxychloroquine is conditionally recommended for treatment during pregnancy.
   b. Methotrexate must be discontinued before conception, and the patient and her rheumatologist should establish control of her RA with pregnancy-compatible medications before conception.
   c. Repeat testing for rheumatoid factor and autoantibodies to citrullinated peptides (ACPAs) is required for disease-modifying drug adjustment during pregnancy.
   d. Half or more of patients with RA have symptomatic improvement during pregnancy.
   e. Though current guidelines suggest avoiding the use of anti-TNF agents after the end or the second trimester, patients who require an anti-TNF agent to control their disease may choose to continue the medication in the third trimester as a matter of benefits outweighing risks.

8. Regarding antirheumatic agents, which of the following is NOT true?
   a. Methotrexate and leflunomide are both known teratogens.
   b. All U.S. Food and Drug Administration–approved anti-TNF biologics are actively transported across the placenta via the neonatal Fc receptor.
   c. Cyclophosphamide and mycophenolate, both used in the treatment of lupus nephritis, should be discontinued before conception. If medications are required, they should be changed to azathioprine or tacrolimus.
   d. Since nearly all patients with RA experience relapse of their symptoms postpartum, coordinated care with a rheumatologic, usually with aggressive medical management, is recommended.
   e. Nonsteroidal antiinflammatory drugs are best avoided during pregnancy, particularly in the third trimester.

9. A 24-year-old primigravid woman with a history systemic sclerosis (scleroderma) comes in for her first prenatal visit. On physical examination the following are noted: blood pressure 140/80, diffuse skin thickening, and digital ulcers. Which of the following is NOT a potential medical complication associated with the diagnosis that may complicate her pregnancy?
   a. Worsening gastric reflux
   b. Gestational hypertension
   c. Autoimmune thrombocytopenia purpura
   d. Pulmonary hypertension

10. A 30-year-old woman, gravida 1, para 1 comes to the office for her 6-week postpartum visit. She tells you that she has dry eyes, dry mouth, and swollen glands. She was seen by a rheumatologist and told that she has Sjogren syndrome. Her evaluation for lupus and rheumatoid arthritis was negative. Which laboratory test should you order to guide your management?
    a. Anti-DNA antibody
    b. C-reactive protein
    c. Rheumatoid factor
    d. Antinuclear antibody
    e. Anti SS-A (anti-Ro) and anti-SS-B (La)

11. Pulmonary hypertension should be considered in prenatal counseling in women patients with all of the following diagnoses except:
    a. Systemic sclerosis
    b. Lupus
    c. Antiphospholipid syndrome
    d. Takaysu arteritis

12. A 26-year-old Turkish woman, gravida 1, para 1 comes to the office for her prenatal visit with worsening oral and genital ulcers. She tells you that she has had joint pain and swelling, as well as painful redness in her eyes in the past, which was from immunosuppressive drugs. On physical examination, she has superficial tender ulcers in her oral mucous membranes and vagina. Which of the following is the most likely underlying cause of this patient's condition?
    a. Rheumatoid arthritis
    b. Sjogren syndrome
    c. Bechet disease
    d. Systemic sclerosis (scleroderma)

66

Neurologic Disorders in Pregnancy

MICHAEL J. AMINOFF | VANJA C. DOUGLAS

(see *Creasy and Resnik's Maternal-Fetal Medicine*, 9e: Ch 66)

Summary

Women are as susceptible to neurologic disorders during gestation as at other times, and certain disorders may be aggravated or influenced by pregnancy. Investigation and management of many neurologic disorders may be complicated by the pregnancy and by concern about the safety of the developing fetus. This chapter describes some of the special problems posed by neurologic disorders during pregnancy, as well as problems posed by pregnancy in patients with neurologic disorders.

Approximately 0.5% of women have epilepsy, defined as the tendency for recurrent unprovoked seizures. Women with epilepsy should be advised about possible interactions between anticonvulsant drugs and oral contraceptive agents because certain anticonvulsants may interfere with the effectiveness of oral contraceptives and implanted progestins. Both epilepsy and some anticonvulsant drugs are associated with a higher risk of major congenital malformations and lower cognitive outcomes. To reduce these risks, women with epilepsy who are of child-bearing age should be treated with the smallest effective anticonvulsant dose possible, with monotherapy preferred to polytherapy. Folic acid supplementation should be provided, and certain anticonvulsant drugs such as valproic acid should be avoided. The effect of pregnancy on seizure frequency is variable. Seizure frequency increases in up to one-third of patients during pregnancy. Compliance with medication should be ensured. Because of accelerated metabolism of anticonvulsant drugs, dose adjustments are often necessary, and levels should be monitored before conception, throughout pregnancy, and in the postpartum period. Due to the risk seizures pose to the patient and fetus, anticonvulsant drugs are as necessary to epileptic patients during pregnancy as at other times.

Although most patients presenting with headache do not have severe underlying structural disease, head imaging and cerebrospinal fluid analysis should be considered in patients presenting with a new headache, neurologic signs or symptoms, fever, stiff neck, or rash during pregnancy. During pregnancy, cerebral venous sinus thrombosis and preeclampsia are important considerations. Magnetic resonance imaging (MRI) with venography can be performed without contrast to rule out the former and to identify mass lesions. Migraine is an important cause of headache among women of childbearing age. Combined oral contraceptives should be avoided due to an increased risk of stroke in the 20% of women with migraines in whom aura accompanies the headache. Progestin-only agents are considered safe. During pregnancy, most women experience a decrease in headache frequency after the first trimester, and migraine prevention should focus on avoidance of dietary and other precipitants of headache, since pharmacologic interventions may involve risk of fetal harm. Acetaminophen, metoclopramide, and caffeine after the first trimester are preferred options if drug treatment is required.

Pregnancy is a risk factor for ischemic stroke, with the greatest risk in the third trimester and postpartum. Pregnancy is not an absolute contraindication to thrombolytic agents, and intravenous tissue plasminogen activator improves functional outcomes when administered up to 4.5 hours after symptom onset. Mechanical embolectomy greatly improves outcomes in patients with stroke resulting from an accessible arterial occlusion when performed within 6 hours of onset and in select patients between 6 and 24 hours of onset. Noncontrast head computed tomography (CT), CT angiography, and CT perfusion are necessary to determine eligibility for these treatments. Although rare, intracranial hemorrhage (both intracerebral and subarachnoid) accounts for a disproportionate 4% to 7% of maternal mortality. Pregnancy-induced hypertension, preeclampsia, and eclampsia are risk factors for both ischemic and hemorrhagic stroke, and intracerebral hemorrhage is often caused by an arteriovenous malformation or aneurysm. Angiography is necessary to identify these vascular lesions, and treatment should not be delayed because of pregnancy.

Pregnancy may exacerbate certain neurologic conditions. Symptoms due to pituitary adenomas, meningiomas, neurofibromas, and hemangioblastomas may worsen during gestation, likely because these lesions have a tendency to increase in size with pregnancy. Vascular malformations including dural arteriovenous shunts in the skull or spine may present during pregnancy with symptoms of venous congestion in adjacent structures. Idiopathic intracranial hypertension is associated with pregnancy and use of oral contraceptive preparations. Other conditions may transiently improve during pregnancy. Multiple sclerosis, for example, tends to remit during pregnancy and relapse in the first 3 to 6 months after childbirth. Disease-modifying treatments for multiple sclerosis are usually suspended preconception and throughout pregnancy due to risk of fetal harm, although some medications may be considered on an individual basis if the potential maternal benefits are felt to outweigh the risk to the fetus. Exacerbations during pregnancy are treated with corticosteroids.

Patients with paraplegia (often traumatic) may deliver vaginally, but those with complete cord lesions above the fifth or sixth thoracic segment may develop autonomic hyperreflexia, and early consultation with an anesthesiologist before labor and delivery is recommended.

Neurologic infections that bear a special relationship to pregnancy include those to which a pregnant patient is more susceptible and those that may affect the nervous system of the developing fetus. Poliomyelitis is associated with fetal loss in the first trimester and may cause more severe neurologic involvement if it develops later in pregnancy. Tetanus, rarely encountered in developed countries with established vaccination programs, is an important cause of maternal morbidity and mortality after childbirth, surgery, or abortion in unvaccinated patients; neonates can also develop tetanus due to umbilical cord contamination during delivery. Infection with *Listeria monocytogenes* is a rare cause of maternal meningitis during pregnancy and can cause miscarriage, stilbirth, preterm birth, and neonatal meningitis and sepsis. Maternal infection with rubella, Zika virus, toxoplasmosis, cytomegalovirus, herpes simplex virus, varicella zoster virus, and syphilis can result in fetal loss, or congenital anomalies.

When dystonia develops during pregnancy, it usually manifests acutely as a medication side effect, often related to an antiemetic. Chorea may develop during pregnancy, usually following streptococcal infection but occasionally spontaneously. Restless legs syndrome is experienced by 20% of pregnant patients, usually in the latter half of pregnancy; it subsides soon after delivery. Treatment of anemia and iron deficiency often improves symptoms.

Certain peripheral entrapment neuropathies are liable to develop in pregnancy and may lead to troublesome symptoms. Lumbar disk herniation causing radicular and low back pain must be distinguished from lumbosacral plexus compression in the pelvis. Familial brachial neuritis tends to relapse during pregnancy or the puerperium. Carpal tunnel syndrome and meralgia paresthetica occur during pregnancy, likely due to fluid retention and weight gain; the former is treated with wrist splints and tends to resolve after delivery. Obturator, femoral, sciatic, and common peroneal neuropathies may occur during

gynecologic surgery and in anesthetized patients in the lithotomy position. Electromyography, performed at least 3 weeks after onset of symptoms, may be helpful with localization of lesions and in determining prognosis for recovery. The incidence of idiopathic facial palsy (Bell palsy) is increased during pregnancy; corticosteroids increase the chance of a complete recovery when started within 5 days of symptom onset.

Peripheral neuropathy may develop due to nutritional deficiency in the setting of hyperemesis gravidarum. Guillain-Barré syndrome does not occur more commonly during gestation than at other times, and treatment and prognosis are identical to those for nonpregnant patients. Pregnancy may lead to an acute exacerbation of acute intermittent porphyria. During pregnancy, symptoms of myasthenia gravis may worsen in 19% to 50% of patients, and one-third experience an exacerbation after delivery. Vaginal delivery is possible. Regional anesthesia is preferred over general anesthesia, and neuromuscular blockade, especially with depolarizing agents, should be avoided in patients with myasthenia. Magnesium sulfate can precipitate myasthenic exacerbation and should be avoided. Infants born to myasthenic patients should be carefully watched during the first week after delivery for signs of neonatal myasthenia.

Patients with myotonic dystrophy have increased rates of spontaneous abortion. Weakness and myotonia may be aggravated by pregnancy, and labor may be abnormal due to failure of the uterus to contract normally. As in myasthenia, depolarizing neuromuscular blockade should be avoided.

QUESTIONS

1. A 23-year-old nulligravida presents to your clinic for a routine check-up. She has epilepsy and is followed by a neurologist, who prescribes her carbamazepine. She is sexually active but is not interested in becoming pregnant and asks about contraceptive choices. She is particularly interested in oral contraception because she has heard from some friends that this might also help with her menstrual cramps. Which of the following is the least appropriate response?
   a. Discuss an intrauterine device without a progestin because these are highly effective and do not interact with systemic medications.
   b. Offer oral contraceptives containing estrogen and progestin, since these can indeed be effective for dysmenorrhea.
   c. Discuss barrier methods.
   d. Offer oral contraceptives containing estrogen and progestin, but counsel her that carbamazepine may interfere with their effectiveness and an additional method of contraception is also recommended.

2. A 36-year-old nulligravida with epilepsy who is prescribed valproic acid and lamotrigine presents to your clinic for removal of her intrauterine device, since she is interested in becoming pregnant. Which of the following is not an appropriate part of counseling this patient?
   a. Suggest the patient speak with her neurologist to consider an anticonvulsant regimen that does not include valproic acid because of its association with major congenital malformations.
   b. Suggest the patient speak with her neurologist about the possibility of anticonvulsant monotherapy during her pregnancy to minimize the risk of fetal anomalies.
   c. Suggest the patient speak with her neurologist about stopping anticonvulsants during pregnancy, since the medications are a greater risk to the fetus than breakthrough seizures are to the patient.
   d. Emphasize the importance of continuing anticonvulsant medications during pregnancy due to the risk of seizures to the patient and fetus.
   e. Emphasize the importance of folic acid supplementation before conception and during pregnancy.

3. A 35-year-old primigravida at 15 weeks' gestation presents to the emergency department with a seizure. There was no head trauma associated with the seizure, and the semiology was typical. The patient has epilepsy and is prescribed lamotrigine. She states she has been adherent to her anticonvulsant prescription. The medical history is otherwise unremarkable, and no other medications are prescribed. The blood pressure is normal, as is the neurologic examination, and there is no proteinuria. Which of the following questions or diagnostic tests is least important?
   a. Lamotrigine level
   b. Was the patient's lamotrigine dose increased during the pregnancy?
   c. Was a lamotrigine level checked before conception?
   d. Noncontrast head computed tomography
   e. Has the patient been experiencing frequent vomiting and, if so, has she noticed her lamotrigine tablets in the emesis?

4. A 28-year-old G3P2 woman at 35 weeks' gestation presents to Obstetrics triage with a new headache. She has never had headaches before. There was no visual aura preceding this headache. She describes the pain as a sensation of severe bitemporal pressure, rates the pain at 7/10, and states it came on gradually but has been steadily worsening over the past 2 weeks. There is no fever and no stiff neck. The neurologic examination is normal. There is no papilledema. What is the most appropriate next step in this patient's management?
   a. Prescribe acetaminophen, metoclopramide, and intravenous fluids.
   b. Obtain a noncontrast head CT.
   c. Obtain a CT with and without contrast including a CT venogram.
   d. Obtain MRI of the brain.
   e. Obtain MRI of the brain and a magnetic resonance venogram.

5. A 33-year-old gravida 4, para 2 at 32 weeks' gestation presents to Obstetrics triage with sudden-onset difficulty speaking, right facial droop, and right arm weakness. She has no medical history and is only taking prenatal vitamins. She was asymptomatic 2 hours earlier. Which of the following is the most appropriate test to order?
   a. Noncontrast head CT
   b. Noncontrast head CT and CT angiogram of the head and neck
   c. MRI of the brain
   d. MRI of the brain, magnetic resonance angiography of the head and neck
   e. Lumbar puncture

6. In the treatment of acute ischemic stroke, up to what time after a patient was last seen at their neurologic baseline can intravenous thrombolysis be administered?
   a. 2 hours
   b. 3 hours
   c. 4.5 hours
   d. 5.5 hours
   e. 6 hours

7. A 25-year-old G1P0 at 12 weeks' gestation presents with abnormal movements. She states that for the past 3 weeks, she has noticed increasingly frequent uncontrollable movements of the right arm. It will often rise or abduct on its own, and the hand and elbow flex and extend uncontrollably as if the arm were "dancing to its own rhythm." Examination shows the described movements, as well as occasional shoulder movements and ipsilateral leg movements. Thyroid function tests, a complete blood count, calcium, and antistreptolysin O titers are normal, as are noncontrast MRI of the brain, echocardiography, antinuclear antibody, and antiphospholipid antibodies. Which one of the following statements is true?
   a. Treatment with antidopaminergic medications will likely be necessary to control the movements.
   b. The movements will likely resolve by the end of pregnancy or after delivery.
   c. The pregnancy should be terminated in order to eliminate the movements.
   d. The disorder may affect fetal growth and development.
   e. The disorder is probably psychogenic, and the woman should be referred for counseling.

8. A 29-year-old G1P1 woman complains of right leg weakness 2 days after vaginal delivery. She had epidural anesthesia, and for the first day after delivery did not get out of bed because of persistent bilateral leg weakness and numbness presumed to be due to lingering effect of the anesthetic. Her examination shows numbness over the anterior, medial, and lateral leg below the knee and the dorsum of the foot, as well as weakness of dorsiflexion, inversion, and eversion at the ankle. She denies back pain. The symptoms were not present before delivery. What is the most likely site of injury?
   a. L5 nerve root in the spinal canal due to an L5-S1 disk herniation
   b. Lumbosacral trunk due to compression from the fetal head against the pelvic brim
   c. Sciatic nerve due to improper positioning during labor
   d. Femoral nerve due to compression during labor
   e. Common peroneal nerve due to compression at the fibular head

9. A 37-year-old woman G3P2 woman at 14 weeks' gestation presents to Obstetrics triage with progressive numbness and weakness affecting her legs. The neurologic symptoms began approximately 2 weeks ago. The patient has had significant nausea and vomiting throughout her first trimester and has lost several pounds. She is concerned that the neurologic symptoms may be a sign of dehydration. On examination, she is mildly disoriented, has allodynia in the feet, and says touching her feet feels like "sandpaper." She has bilateral foot drop and walks with a wide-based, ataxic gait. If the appropriate intervention is not administered immediately, the patient is at risk for which of the following complications?
   a. Seizure
   b. Ischemic stroke
   c. Permanent short-term memory loss
   d. Hemorrhagic stroke
   e. Hearing loss

10. A 31-year-old woman with myasthenia gravis at 38 weeks' gestation presents to labor and delivery. Her pregnancy has been uncomplicated, and she has been planning for a vaginal delivery. She takes pyridostigmine and a low dose of prednisone, and her myasthenia is well controlled. Which of the following is not a consideration in the peripartum management of a patient with myasthenia?
    a. Avoidance of medications that can exacerbate weakness, including magnesium sulfate
    b. Avoidance of neuromuscular blocking agents, especially depolarizing agents such as succinylcholine
    c. Careful monitoring of the newborn infant for evidence of weakness during the first week after delivery
    d. Administration of a higher dose of corticosteroids immediately after delivery to prevent myasthenic crisis
    e. Regional anesthesia over general anesthesia if cesarean delivery is necessary

Management of Depression and Psychoses in Pregnancy and in the Puerperium

KIMBERLY A. YONKERS | ARIADNA FORRAY

(see *Creasy and Resnik's Maternal-Fetal Medicine, 9e: Ch 67*)

Summary

Mood disorders are common in pregnant and postpartum individuals, although prevalence rates vary among studies. The prevalence of a unipolar major depressive episode in pregnancy is 12.7%. Bipolar disorder occurs in about 1% to 2% of the population; its prevalence is similar in pregnant and nonpregnant individuals. The course of illness can vary: Some individuals become depressed in pregnancy and continue to be symptomatic into the postpartum period. Others improve shortly after delivery. About half of individuals who are depressed in the postpartum period had an onset of illness after the delivery. Individuals with schizophrenia and schizoaffective disorder have chronic conditions with symptoms that, ideally, are controlled by antipsychotic medication and mood-stabilizing drugs. Vulnerability to either schizophrenia or schizoaffective disorder is not affected by pregnancy or being in the postpartum period, although symptoms may be under slightly better control in pregnancy.

A diagnosis of major depressive disorder (MDD) is made when an individual has episodes of major depression but does not have episodes of mania or hypomania. Additional depressive symptoms include decreased interest in pleasurable activities, insomnia, change in appetite, decreased energy, excessive guilt or worthlessness, decreased concentration, psychomotor slowing or agitation, and suicidal ideation. Appropriate tools for assessment of depressive symptoms in pregnant individuals include the Edinburgh Postnatal Depression Scale, the Patient Health Questionnaire-9, the Inventory of Depressive Symptomatology, or the Primary Care Evaluation of Mental Disorders Patient Health Questionnaire. Depressive episodes are also experienced by individuals with bipolar disorder. However, for a diagnosis of bipolar disorder, an individual must have experienced an episode of mania or hypomania. Individuals who experience psychosis and are not in an episode of mania or depression may have a chronic psychotic condition such as schizophrenia or schizoaffective disorder. Schizoaffective disorder is differentiated from schizophrenia in that the former condition requires mood symptoms, including episodes of mania or major depression, that are prominent, although psychosis may also occur without mood symptoms.

Untreated depression among pregnant individuals is associated with preterm birth and low birth weight. Individuals with bipolar disorder are at higher risk of adverse birth outcomes, including preterm birth, microcephaly, gestational hypertension, and antepartum hemorrhage. Individuals with psychosis during pregnancy are at a heightened risk for cesarean delivery, antepartum hemorrhage, placental abruption, postpartum hemorrhage, premature delivery, stillbirth, premature rupture of membranes, and fetal abnormalities.

A treatment plan for a pregnant or postpartum individual with depression should begin with a determination of whether the patient has had recent or past symptoms of mania or psychosis because this can help determine the optimal treatment approach. In general, individuals with severe or recurrent unipolar MDD may need antidepressant treatment. Interpersonal psychotherapy and cognitive-behavioral therapy are empirically validated psychotherapies that may help individuals with a mild to moderate depressive episode in pregnancy remain stable. Because of the seriousness of bipolar disorder and the need for pharmacotherapy, pregnant individuals with bipolar disorder should be comanaged by a psychiatrist. Individuals who have a history of mania, whether they are in an episode of depression or not, should be treated with pharmacotherapy. Individuals who suffer from schizophrenia and schizoaffective disorder typically require pharmacologic treatment to control symptoms. Individuals with severe psychiatric illness are at high risk of relapse if medication is discontinued.

Antidepressant use has been widely studied in pregnancy. Selective serotonin reuptake inhibitors are the first-line treatment for major depression. With the exception of paroxetine, structural malformations are not a great risk. The greater concern relates to some of the perinatal risks such as persistent pulmonary hypertension of the newborn, although these events are uncommon. Lithium is the gold-standard treatment for bipolar disorder in nonpregnant populations, and while it may be considered the first-line mood stabilizer during pregnancy, there is inconsistency in the information and recommendations regarding its use in the perinatal period. Much of the conflicting evidence is due to the historical data, which overstated lithium's teratogenic effect. The risk of cardiac malformations is lower than previously thought, and potential adverse effects appear to be dose dependent. When maternal illness is included in statistical models that test for lithium exposure and risk of cardiac malformations, the risk is attenuated. Available data do not strongly associate fetal anomalies in general with antipsychotic medication use in pregnancy. Antipsychotic exposure has been associated with preterm birth. Mood stabilizers, such as sodium valproate and carbamazepine, should be avoided in pregnancy if possible.

QUESTIONS

1. Which of the following is NOT an appropriate tool for assessment of depressive symptoms in pregnant patients?
   a. Edinburgh Postnatal Depression Scale
   b. Patient Health Questionnaire-9
   c. Inventory of Depressive Symptomatology
   d. NIDA Quick Screen
   e. Primary Care Evaluation of Mental Disorders Patient Health Questionnaire

2. What is the most appropriate next step in the evaluation of a patient with anxiety, insomnia, difficulty making decisions, and loss of enjoyment of previously enjoyable activities?
   a. Start lorazepam 0.5 mg twice a day for her anxiety.
   b. Start trazodone 50 mg at bedtime for sleep.
   c. Reassure her that this is normal and will get better with time.
   d. Complete an Edinburgh Postnatal Depression Scale to screen for depression and start sertraline, if appropriate.

3. Which of the following is the most common pregnancy complication associated with antipsychotic use in pregnancy?
   a. Preterm birth
   b. Small for gestational age
   c. Gestational diabetes
   d. Ebstein anomaly

4. Which of the following is necessary to meet criteria for bipolar disorder?
   a. Anxiety
   b. Depression
   c. Insomnia
   d. Mania
   e. Suicidal ideation

5. Which of the following factors is most likely to increase the risk of decompensation of bipolar disorder during pregnancy?
   a. Dysregulation of sleep patterns
   b. Medication discontinuation
   c. Marital discord
   d. Substance use

6. Which of the following should be recommended at an initial prenatal visit in the first trimester for a patient taking lithium for bipolar disorder?
   a. Stop the lithium immediately due to potential teratogenic effects.
   b. Make no changes and continue to take the same dose of lithium throughout the pregnancy.
   c. Continue to take the lithium, and monitor lithium levels.
   d. Switch from lithium to quetiapine due to cardiac malformations associated with lithium.

7. At a 6-week postpartum visit a patient reports having difficulty sleeping, intrusive thoughts that something bad is going to happen to the baby, loss of appetite, and inability to sit still for more than a few minutes at a time. Which of the following is the most likely diagnosis?
   a. Postpartum psychosis
   b. Generalized anxiety disorder
   c. Major depressive episode
   d. Normal adjustment for a new parent

8. Which of the following is the most prevalent psychiatric disorder in women in their early 20s?
   a. Bipolar disorder
   b. Schizophrenia
   c. Schizoaffective disorder
   d. Major depressive disorder

9. Which of the following is the most appropriate next step in management in a patient with recurrent depression who previously responded to cognitive behavioral therapy?
   a. Reassurance that symptoms are mild and will improve on their own.
   b. Refer to prior psychotherapist and follow mood closely throughout the pregnancy.
   c. Start paroxetine.
   d. Start mirtazapine.

10. Which of the following is the only U.S. Food and Drug Administration–approved treatment specifically designed postpartum depression?
    a. Sertraline
    b. Escitalopram
    c. Brexanolone
    d. Fluoxetine

11. Which of the following is the most appropriate next step in a patient with postpartum depression started on sertraline 50 mg 2 weeks ago, who reports still feeling depressed and spends most of the day in bed, as well as daily suicidal thoughts including overdosing on Tylenol?
    a. Increase sertraline dose to 100 mg.
    b. Immediate evaluation by a mental health provider.
    c. Refer for psychotherapy.
    d. Reassure her that symptoms will improve in the next couple of weeks, and have the clinic social worker reach out in 1 week.

12. Which of the following perinatal complications has been associated with selective serotonin reuptake inhibitors exposure in pregnancy?
    a. Small for gestational age
    b. Noncardiac congenital malformations
    c. Low birth weight
    d. Persistent pulmonary hypertension of the newborn

Substance Use and Addiction in Pregnancy and the Postpartum Period

GREGORY JONES | SPENCER HANSEN

(see *Creasy and Resnik's Maternal-Fetal Medicine*, 9e: Ch 68)

Summary

Substance use disorders (SUDs) are characterized by impairment caused by the recurrent use of alcohol or other drugs (or both), including health problems, disability, and failure to meet major responsibilities at work, school, or home, and are diagnosed using criteria from Diagnostic and Statistical Manual of Mental Disorders—5. Past month substance use is less in pregnancy compared with nonpregnancy, and use decreases by trimester. Approximately 20% of people who stop using a substance in pregnancy continue abstinence postpartum. Continued use in pregnancy can be considered pathognomic for a substance use disorder. Substance use prevalence has been stable or decreasing in pregnancy for all substances except cannabis. Although pregnant individuals are considered a priority population for treatment, they are no more likely than nonpregnant women to receive treatment.

Universal screening for substance use disorder is recommended in pregnancy and the postpartum period. No one screening instrument appears superior in pregnant individuals. Biological drug testing using urine or other biological matrixes such as meconium or umbilical cord are not a substitute for screening for substance use, misuse, or addiction.

Pregnant people with SUD often experience discrimination from clinicians. Concern about untreated or undertreated pain is common for people with SUD, especially those with opioid use disorder (OUD). Medications for opioid use disorder (MOUD) do not provide analgesia, and people with addiction may need more pain medication during labor. MOUD should be continued at the same dose throughout the delivery hospitalization, and pain management should be multimodal, using nonopioid medications, regional anesthesia, and opioid agonists if needed. Preoperative and postoperative MOUD discontinuation is associated with overdose and should be avoided. Given the increase in both intentional and unintentional fentanyl use, pregnant and postpartum individuals and their support individuals should be counseled about naloxone use and the potential need to call emergency medical services, as multiple doses may be necessary to reverse an opioid overdose.

The American Academy of Pediatrics policy is that maternal substance use is "not a categorical contraindication to breastfeeding"; however, breastfeeding in the context of illicit substance use is not recommended due to a lack of data on neurodevelopmental outcomes among breastfed children in the setting of maternal illicit substance use. In addition, the vast majority of drug-related pregnancy-associated deaths occurred in the postpartum year.

In the United States, tobacco continues to be the most common substance used in pregnancy, with 9%—25% of pregnant individuals reporting smoking tobacco. While robust data support behavioral intervention among pregnant individuals who smoke, there is insufficient evidence for medications as few studies include this population. Alcohol affects all aspects of reproduction, including fertility, fetal anomalies, and lactation. There is no known lower safety limit for alcohol exposure in pregnancy to avoid the common and most severe associated outcomes: fetal alcohol spectrum disorder and stillbirth. Both screening and brief intervention are associated with a reduction in drinking in pregnancy, but abrupt cessation risks withdrawal. Although limited data on safety may be concerning to some, when contrasted with the known risks of alcohol, consideration of medication for the treatment of alcohol use disorder should be standard in clinical care.

The existing studies on cannabis use have mixed findings regarding the associated risks of fetal growth restriction, malformations, and stillbirth. Clinicians should be aware of the risk of cannabinoid hyperemesis syndrome. There is no specific screening tool for cannabis use in pregnancy. A combination of motivational enhancements, cognitive behavioral therapy, and contingency management produces the best abstinence outcomes for patients with cannabinoid use disorder.

QUESTIONS

1. As medical director of a maternal fetal medicine practice, you are discussing with care providers which screening instrument is best to identify substance use in pregnancy. According to published clinical trials, which screening instrument should you adopt in your clinic that has the greatest accuracy in identifying substance use in pregnancy?
   a. National Institute on Drug Abuse (NIDA) Quick Screen—ASSIST
   b. SURP-P (Substance Use Risk Profile—Pregnancy)
   c. CRAFFT
   d. WIDUS (Wayne Indirect Drug Use Screener)
   e. In the two trials comparing screening instruments among pregnant individuals, no instrument appears clearly superior.

2. A 28-year-old individual presents for a postpartum visit at 6 weeks after an uncomplicated term vaginal delivery. Medical history includes opioid use disorder, and the patient has been receiving methadone since the second trimester. The patient states, "I've been taking it like I should, but I'm thinking of getting off it. I'm doing really well and haven't had urges to use heroin since starting methadone. I mean, do you think it's really important I stay on it at this point?"
   According to best available evidence, if she were to stop taking methadone, what is the likelihood of return to opioid use within 1 year postpartum?
   a. 10%
   b. 30%
   c. 50%
   d. 80%
   e. 100%

3. A pregnant individual presents for an initial prenatal visit at 36 weeks' gestation. You ask what kinds of barriers to care occurred that prevented earlier initiation of care. The patient states, "I've been using methamphetamines this pregnancy but I was finally able to get off. I was worried I would lose custody of my baby." All of the following are true except
   a. State policies related to substance use in pregnancy are becoming less punitive in the United States.
   b. The assumption that addiction in pregnancy is associated with subsequent child abuse or neglect is not supported by clinical evidence.
   c. There is no evidence of benefit in terms of maternal health or child development from a child welfare report due to substance use in pregnancy.
   d. Implementing universal drug testing at time of delivery has shown to perpetuate racial inequities in child welfare reporting.

4. A 25-year-old individual presents for an initial prenatal visit. The patient is a gravida 2, para 1 at 16 weeks' gestation. The patient reports reducing cigarettes to 2 a day, down from 10 before pregnancy, and now wants to stop smoking completely but states, "For some reason I just blow up on my coworkers if I don't have that lunch or dinner cigarette. It's like the only thing that calms my anxiety when I get tired and stressed as the day goes on. What help can I get to stop completely?" Which of the following treatment recommendations shows the best evidence supporting tobacco smoking cessation during pregnancy?
   a. Cognitive behavioral therapy
   b. Contingency management
   c. Varenicline (Chantix)
   d. Nicotine patch, lozenge, or gum
   e. Both a and b

5. A 21-year-old presents to a prenatal visit requesting help to stop smoking. The patient is a gravida 1, para 0 at 22 weeks' gestation and reports smoking 7–10 cigarettes every day. Recently, the patient saw a commercial on television about varenicline and asks you to give her a prescription. Which of the following is true concerning the use of varenicline during pregnancy?
   a. Varenicline has been systematically studied among pregnant persons.
   b. Available safety data on varenicline in pregnancy, although limited, are reassuring.
   c. Varenicline administered to rats and rabbits at doses 36–50 times higher than human doses based on serum concentrations demonstrated increased risk of congenital anomalies.
   d. Four human cohort studies and one case report identified increased risk of maternal or fetal harm.

6. Which of the following is true concerning observed fetal growth restriction from cannabis exposure?
   a. Cannabis does not affect glucose and insulin regulation, and therefore there is no theoretical basis for fetal growth restriction.
   b. Most of the studies assessing association between cannabis exposure and fetal growth restriction are adequately controlled for concomitant tobacco exposure.
   c. Prospective studies show mixed data between prenatal cannabis exposure and fetal growth restriction.
   d. All of the above are true.

7. A 19-year-old presents for a first prenatal visit. The patient is a gravida 1 at 14 weeks' gestation. The patient has a history of heavy cannabis use, reporting, "I smoke weed all day long." The patient reports a significant reduction in cannabis use since pregnancy awareness but continues to smoke "a few hits in the evening because without it I just can't sleep." The patient asks you about a medication to help with cannabis use reduction. Which of the following would be the most appropriate medication for helping with cessation of cannabis use disorder?
   a. Gabapentin
   b. Olanzapine
   c. Naltrexone
   d. Currently, there is no effective pharmacotherapy available for cannabis use or cannabis use disorder.

8. The patient asks about nonpharmacologic options. You tell the patient that your clinic is holding a 12-week program for pregnant individuals who use cannabis. You explain that the program entails weekly group therapy sessions, monetary compensation for attendance and expected urine toxicology, and weekly individual therapy session. Which of the following is most effective?
   a. Contingency management
   b. Motivational enhancements
   c. Cognitive behavioral therapy
   d. A combination of all three
   e. None of the above

9. A 32-year-old patient has an uncomplicated vaginal delivery at 39 weeks' gestation. Medical history is complicated by stimulant use disorder with last use of cocaine at 34 weeks' gestation after entering a residential treatment program. As you head out of the room into the hallway, you are pulled aside by the patient's nurse. The nurse asks you, "We know the patient used cocaine during pregnancy. Can you help me understand if prenatal cocaine exposure will affect the child's intelligence?" What is the most appropriate response to the nurse?
   a. "Most likely the child is going to have a lower IQ and will require a lot of extra help and tutoring."
   b. "The home environment is more predictive of child intelligence quotient (IQ) than prenatal cocaine exposure."
   c. "Because of the prenatal cocaine exposure, cognitive development and function are likely to be impaired."
   d. "Since the patient used cocaine during pregnancy, the infant will have the best chance for achievement in another family."

10. An 18-year-old pregnant individual arrives to the emergency department with a severe headache of 2 hours' duration, nausea, and feeling generally unwell. The patient is a gravida 3, para 2 at 32 weeks' gestation. Blood pressure on arrival is 180/120. The patient reports using cocaine 2 hours before arrival. Which of the following medications is contraindicated to treat severe-range blood pressure?
   a. Labetalol
   b. Hydralazine
   c. Nifedipine
   d. Methyldopa

11. A 22-year-old pregnant individual comes to your office for a first prenatal visit. The patient is a gravida 4, para 2 at 16 weeks' gestation. After completing her NIDA Quick Screen—ASSIST, the patient is positive for use of heroin. After furthering evaluation, the patient endorses several symptoms over the past year. Which of the following symptoms are most consistent with opioid use disorder?
   a. "I've tried to stop using, but I just can't."
   b. "I've been dreaming about using."
   c. "I've gone to some sketchy place to meet my dealer. It's really scary and I've had to do things I didn't want to do just to get my fix."
   d. "I shared needles a few times because I just need the withdrawal to stop."
   e. All of the above are symptoms of opioid use disorder.

12. A 32-year-old gravida 3, para 2 at 39 weeks' gestation undergoes an uncomplicated elective repeat low transverse cesarean delivery. The medical history is significant for opioid use disorder and has been well controlled on methadone 80 mg daily. Eight hours after low transverse cesarean section, the patient reports significant pain. Vital signs are 37°C (98.6°F), pulse is 70/min, respirations are 12/min, and blood pressure is 124/74 mm Hg. On evaluation, the patient is alert, oriented, and not sedated. Which of the following is FALSE regarding pharmacologic management in this patient?
   a. The patient's methadone should be discontinued.
   b. Pain management should be multimodal.
   c. Opioid agonist medications can be used for analgesia.
   d. Nonopioid medications can be used for analgesics.
   e. The patient is at risk of undertreated pain.

13. A 21-year-old presented for a 6-week postpartum visit. The patient is a gravida 1, para 1 after an uncomplicated vaginal delivery. The patient has alcohol use disorder that was in remission during pregnancy and reports returning to heavy alcohol use (more than four drinks/day) in the postpartum period. The patient desires to continue breastfeeding for the infant's health benefits of breast milk. After discussion of treatment options for alcohol use disorder, which of the following is most accurate?
   a. Breastfeeding is an absolute contraindication.
   b. Use shared decision making to determine risks/benefits of continued breastfeeding.
   c. Breastfeeding is always preferred regardless of alcohol use.
   d. Alcohol is not transferred via breastmilk.
   e. There are no means of limiting alcohol concentration in breast milk.

14. A 25-year-old individual presents to the office for a 2-week postpartum visit after a repeat low transverse cesarean section. The patient is a gravida 3, para 3 with opioid use disorder and reports that while hospitalized, buprenorphine/naloxone was discontinued. The patient reports remission of opioid use disorder for the previous 1 year while taking buprenorphine/naloxone. The patient notes that withdrawal symptoms prompted a return to heroin use after discharge. Which of the following can be considered the most significant risk factor for respiratory depression, overdose, and death in this patient?
    a. Recent pregnancy
    b. Recent discontinuation of buprenorphine/naloxone
    c. Previous buprenorphine/naloxone use
    d. Opioid withdrawal symptoms
    e. Cesarean delivery

15. A 28-year-old patient presents for a prenatal visit. The patient is gravida 1, para 1 and 3 months postpartum with medical history significant for alcohol use disorder. The patient was recently admitted to inpatient medicine unit for monitoring alcohol withdrawal and detoxification. The patient reports no alcohol use since discharge but is concerned about alcohol cravings. Which of the following medications is a U.S. Food and Drug Administration–approved pharmacotherapy for maintenance of alcohol use disorder at this time?
    a. Naltrexone
    b. Sertraline
    c. Bupropion
    d. Gabapentin
    e. Lorazepam

16. A 22-year-old presents to the emergency department with a chief complaint of migraine headache. The patient is a gravida 1, para 0 at 8 weeks' gestation. The patient reports using the substance kratom at a local store to aid her chronic migraine symptoms. Which of the following substances is kratom most similar to pharmacologically?
    a. Amphetamine
    b. Opioid
    c. Benzodiazepine
    d. Cannabis
    e. Cocaine

17. A 32-year-old pregnant individual comes to the office. The patient is a gravida 3, para 2 at 16 weeks' gestation with daily heroin use. The patient meets criteria for opioid use disorder and is interested in initiating medication for treatment with buprenorphine/naloxone. In addition to counseling on buprenorphine/naloxone initiation, which of the following should be prescribed to the patient?
    a. Ondansetron
    b. Clonidine
    c. Trazodone
    d. Methadone
    e. Naloxone

18. A 27-year-old presents for a prenatal visit. The patient is a gravida 2, para 1 at 21 weeks' gestation and using alprazolam 1 mg three times daily that was prescribed by the primary care physician. The patient states that the alprazolam helps with anxiety symptoms and is interested in starting psychotherapy. The patient reports a history of taking alprazolam more often than prescribed, leading to the need for early prescriptions, and denies legal consequences, withdrawal, or attempts to cutback in the past. Which of the following is the most likely diagnosis?
    a. Benzodiazepine use disorder
    b. Generalized anxiety disorder
    c. Panic disorder
    d. Benzodiazepine misuse
    e. Sedative misuse

69

The Skin and Pregnancy

VIVIANA DE ASSIS

(see Creasy and Resnik's Maternal-Fetal Medicine, 9e: Ch 69)

Summary

Common skin changes induced by pregnancy include hyperpigmentation, which occurs with at least 90% of pregnant women. It is thought to result from increased levels of melanocyte-stimulating hormone, beta endorphin, estrogen, and progesterone. Pigmentation is most accentuated in the areolar and genital skin. All pigmentary changes typically regress after delivery. Hydroquinone 4%, tretinoin, and hydrocortisone can be useful if hyperpigmentation persists beyond pregnancy. Pregnancy can produce new melanocytic nevi or enlarged preexisting nevi; however, the incidence of changes in nevi and formation of melanoma seem to be no greater than for nonpregnant women. Most melanomas exhibit asymmetry, an irregular border, variegated colors (i.e., red or white in addition to black or blue), and a diameter greater than 6 mm. Suspicious lesions should be excised immediately.

Vascular changes in pregnancy include proliferation and dilation of blood vessels. Telangiectasias, spider angiomas, palmar erythema, and pyogenic granulomas are all common vascular changes in pregnancy. Pyogenic granuloma refers to a red, nodular, often pedunculated, exuberant proliferation of blood vessels and inflammatory cells. The surface is often ulcerated, with yellowish purulence. They are more commonly found on the scalp, upper trunk, fingers, and toes. They are especially common on the gums, often resulting from gingivitis or trauma, and have been called *epulis gravidarum*. The terms *lobular capillary hemangioma*, *pregnancy tumor*, and *granuloma gravidarum* are other synonyms for pyogenic granuloma. Connective tissue changes include striae, which can be red or purple, atrophic bands over the abdomen, breasts, thighs, buttocks, groin, and axillae. They represent linear tears in dermal connective tissue. Striae occur in 50% to 80% of pregnancies, and they are severe in about 10%, especially in teenagers. Women with striae have an increased incidence of subsequent pelvic organ prolapse.

The hair cycle is divided into three phases of different duration. The growing phase (anagen) persists about 3–4 years, the transitional phase (catagen) lasts 2 weeks, and the resting phase (telogen) lasts several weeks. Newly forming hair causes shedding of older hair in the telogen phase. During the last portion of pregnancy there is an increased number of hairs in anagen and fewer hairs in telogen. After hormone withdrawal postpartum, the number of hairs in telogen can increase to 35% and in some severe cases 40%–50%. This diffuse hair loss is known as telogen effluvium. Regrowth is likely to occur by 9 months post delivery without intervention.

Medications to be used in pregnancy for dermatoses vary. Options include emollients, calamine lotion, cold compresses or baths, and topical corticosteroids. Clobetasol is a high-potency topical corticosteroid that has potential for significant absorption if used on large body surface areas. Antihistamines such as fexofenadine and desloratadine have insufficient data but are still used in pregnancy. Hydroxyzine is not recommended in the first trimester because it is associated with increased rate of congenital malformations (5.8%). Cetirizine, chlorpheniramine, cyproheptadine, diphenhydramine, and loratadine are more regularly used for patients with bothersome pruritus and are considered category B. Systemic corticosteroids appear to be relatively safe for use in severe disease. A modest increase in birth defects with corticosteroids was reported. Fluorinated corticosteroids should be avoided, since they lead to higher concentrations of active drug reaching the fetus. Infants of mothers treated with systemic corticosteroids in high doses and for long durations should be monitored for adrenal insufficiency.

Pruritic urticarial papules and plaques of pregnancy are characterized by erythematous papules, plaques, and urticarial lesions that begin in the third trimester. Approximately 80% of patients experience itching. Lesions begin in the abdomen and spare the umbilicus. The rash usually resolves before or within weeks after delivery. There is no increased risk of fetal morbidity or mortality, and the rash does not tend to recur in subsequent pregnancies. Topical corticosteroids are adequate for management of patients.

Atopic eruption of pregnancy is also known as *prurigo gestationis* and *folliculitis of pregnancy*. This condition is an intensely pruritic skin eruption in which excoriation predominates, suggesting a prominent emotional component. Patients may have a genetic predisposition for atopic dermatitis. The lesions consist of excoriated papules or nodules that occur mostly over the extremities, usually beginning in the middle of pregnancy. Elevation of liver enzymes is sometimes associated with this condition. The eruption clears by 3 months post delivery.

Pemphigoid gestation (previously termed herpes gestationis) is a rare, autoimmune, blistering dermatosis of pregnancy and immediate postpartum period. It is not associated with herpes simplex virus (HSV). Onset usually occurs during the second or third trimester; however, cases have been reported with onset in the first trimester or postpartum period. High frequency of human leukocyte antigen haplotype B8 and DR3/DR4 has been reported. Lesions begin around the umbilicus and involve the trunk, buttocks, and extremities. Face and mucosal membranes are usually not affected. Vesicles and bullae are present. Mortality rate for infants is as high as 30%. Systemic corticosteroid treatment for severe cases reduces the fetal risk. Postpartum flares are present in 50%–75% of patients. Exacerbation typically begins within 24–48 hours after delivery and can last from weeks to months. A portion of women will continue to experience recurrences of skin lesions with subsequent use of oral contraceptives. Placental antibody deposition may result in placental insufficiency. Topical corticosteroids can be used for mild disease. If severe disease is present, then systemic corticosteroids like prednisone can be used and titrated to the minimum dose that will prevent further blister formation. In postpartum periods, higher doses of systemic corticosteroids can be employed.

Impetigo herpetiformis is a severe, generalized, pustular dermatosis associated with pregnancy. It is unrelated to the bacterial or viral infection as its name implies. It's likely to represent pustular psoriasis in pregnancy. Onset is usually in the third trimester, but cases have been documented in the first trimester. The disease subsides between pregnancies but can recur with subsequent ones. It may be accompanied by hypoparathyroidism, hypocalcemia, hypophosphatemia, decreased vitamin D levels, elevated erythrocyte sedimentation rate, and leukocytosis. It is clinically recognized by hundreds of translucent, white, sterile pustules that arise on irregular erythematous basses or plaques. Common areas include the axillae, inframammary areas, umbilicus, groin, and gluteal

crease. It can be accompanied by fever, chills, nausea, vomiting, and diarrhea with severe dehydration. Systemic corticosteroids therapy is the treatment of choice. Systemic antibiotics may be necessary for secondary infections. Intravenous fluids and electrolyte replacement are also important.

Autoimmune progesterone dermatitis is a rare and poorly defined, urticarial, popular, vesicular, eczematous, or pustular eruption thought to be caused by hypersensitivity to progesterone in ovulating women. It may be associated with spontaneous abortion. Patients with a severe eruption may benefit from systemic corticosteroids.

Pregnancy has various effects on acne. Tetracycline should be avoided because of the risks of fatty liver of pregnancy to mother and damage of fetal dentition. Atopic dermatitis can worsen in more than half of pregnancies. Overall, most skin rashes in pregnancy are itchy and tend to resolve after pregnancy.

QUESTIONS

1. Hyperpigmentation occurs in approximately ____% of pregnant women.
   a. 2
   b. 10
   c. 50
   d. 90

2. Which of the following characteristics are concerning for melanoma?
   a. Regular border
   b. Symmetrical edge
   c. Diameter < 6 mm
   d. Variegated colors

3. A 25-year-old G2P1 at 33 weeks' gestation presents for evaluation of a gum lesion that appeared 2 days after a dental cleaning. On examination the lesion appears red, nodular, and pedunculated. The top surface of the lesion appears ulcerated, and some yellow purulence is noted. The most likely diagnosis is:
   a. Herpetic gingivostomatitis
   b. Pyogenic granuloma
   c. Oral candidiasis
   d. Aphthous ulcer

4. Linear tears in the dermal connective tissue represent:
   a. Pyogenic granuloma
   b. Striae
   c. Hyperpigmentation
   d. Chloasma

5. Women with striae have an increased incidence of the following:
   a. Deep venous thrombosis
   b. Pelvic organ prolapse
   c. Diverticulitis
   d. Melanoma

6. A 38-year-old G1P1 at 6 weeks postpartum presents for her postpartum visit. On review of systems, she reports significant hair loss causing her distress. Which is the best treatment option for this patient?
   a. Observation and reassurance
   b. Referral to dermatology for further evaluation
   c. Scalp biopsy
   d. Minoxidil 5% for daily use

7. Which medications should be avoided due to higher concentrations of the active drug reaching the fetus?
   a. Fluorinated corticosteroids
   b. Nonfluorinated corticosteroids
   c. Oral antihistamines
   d. Topical corticosteroids

8–11. Match the following description to the best answer choice.
   a. Pruritic urticarial papules and plaques of pregnancy
   b. Pemphigoid gestationis
   c. Atopic eruption of pregnancy
   d. Impetigo herpetiformis

8. Rare, autoimmune, blistering dermatosis of pregnancy and immediate postpartum period. Onset usually occurs during the second or third trimester. A high frequency of human leukocyte antigen haplotype B8 and DR3/DR4 has been reported. Vesicles and bullae are present. The mortality rate for infants is as high as 30%.

9. Characterized by erythematous papules, plaques, and urticarial lesions that begin in the third trimester. Lesions begin in the abdomen and spare the umbilicus. There is no increased risk of fetal morbidity or mortality, and the rash does not tend to recur in subsequent pregnancies.

10. Severe generalized pustular dermatosis associated with pregnancy. Unrelated to bacterial or viral infection. Onset is usually in the third trimester, but cases have been documented in the first trimester. May be accompanied by hypoparathyroidism, hypocalcemia, hypophosphatemia, decreased vitamin D levels, elevated erythrocyte sedimentation rate, and leukocytosis. Clinically recognized by hundreds of translucent, white, sterile pustules that arise on irregular erythematous bases or plaques.

11. Intensely pruritic skin eruption in which excoriation predominates, suggesting a prominent emotional component. The lesions consist of excoriated papules or nodules that occur mostly over the extremities, usually beginning in the middle of pregnancy. Elevation of liver enzymes is sometimes associated with this condition. The eruption clears by 3 months post delivery.

Anesthetic Considerations for Complicated Pregnancies

JOY L. HAWKINS

(see *Creasy and Resnik's Maternal-Fetal Medicine, 9e: Ch 70*)

Summary

When caring for the complicated patient who is pregnant, anesthesiologists contribute their experience in the labor and delivery (L & D) unit, a strong background in critical care, and their expertise caring for a wide variety of patients and conditions in the operating room and procedural areas. These conditions may require acute management of complications during the peripartum period.

Amniotic fluid embolism in its most severe form requires early intubation and ventilation with 100% oxygen and positive end-expiratory pressure to correct hypoxia. High-quality cardiopulmonary resuscitation is needed at some point in many cases. Resuscitation with pressors and inotropes should be guided by invasive monitoring and transesophageal echocardiography if possible. Consider extracorporeal membrane oxygenation if ventricular dysfunction is unresponsive to medical management. Coagulopathy is diagnosed by traditional labs and point-of-care testing such as thromboelastography (TEG) and treated with a 1:1:1 ratio of packed red blood cells, fresh-frozen plasma, and platelets with other products.

Maternal cardiac arrest is managed similarly to nonpregnant patients with the following adaptations: (1) Include the neonatal team when activating the maternal cardiac arrest team, (2) Place the patient supine on a backboard and provide manual left uterine displacement rather than tilt, (3) Place the hands slightly higher on the sternum but deliver the usual rate and depth of chest compressions, (4) Defibrillate per Advanced Cardiac Life Support guidelines but remove the fetal scalp electrode if present, (5) Secure the airway with an endotracheal tube to improve ventilation and reduce aspiration, (6) Obtain intravenous or intraosseous access for medications *above* the diaphragm, (7) Consider diagnoses unique to pregnancy (e.g., amniotic fluid embolism) or to L & D (e.g., local anesthetic toxicity), and (8) actively begin preparing for delivery as soon as cardiac arrest is confirmed to achieve delivery within 5 minutes of starting CPR.

Cardiac disease is the leading cause of maternal mortality in the United States. Using the New York Heart Association classification at delivery will help determine level of care required. Classes III and IV require antepartum optimization with the cardiology team, invasive monitoring during labor and delivery, and postpartum care in a cardiac intensive care unit (ICU). The highest-risk lesions in pregnancy are stenotic valvular lesions, severe pulmonary hypertension from any cause, right-to-left intracardiac shunting, Marfan syndrome with a dilated aortic root, and peripartum myocardial infarction. Antepartum planning with the patient's cardiologist must consider site of delivery (ICU, main operating room, or L & D), mode of delivery (e.g., induction of labor vs. cesarean), need for invasive monitoring, type of anesthetic, obstetric medications with adverse side effects to be avoided, and site of postpartum care. Cardiac procedures required during pregnancy can be performed with good outcomes for mother and fetus.

Hemorrhage >1000 mL that is ongoing should be managed with a massive transfusion protocol that includes administration of tranexamic acid, use of cell salvage (especially if a patient refuses blood products), embolization by Interventional Radiology, and placement of the Resuscitative Endovascular Balloon Occlusion of the Aorta (REBOA) device if available.

Preeclampsia/Eclampsia can lead to stroke. If vasodilator infusions (e.g., nicardipine) are needed to reduce blood pressure lower than 160/110 mm Hg, an arterial line should be provided. All fluids should be limited. Neuraxial anesthesia may be contraindicated if the platelet count falls below 70K or there are other forms of coagulopathy. Eclamptic seizures markedly increase maternal morbidity. They are managed with magnesium sulfate, high-flow oxygen while in the lateral position, and airway management if aspiration occurs, but eclampsia alone is not an indication for emergent operative delivery.

Respiratory diseases seen commonly during pregnancy include asthma, pulmonary thromboembolism, and, beginning in 2020, coronavirus disease 2019 (COVID-19). Patients with asthma should be medically optimized before their delivery and then maintained on their inhalers and medications intrapartum. If thromboembolism requires anticoagulation, use of neuraxial anesthesia will be determined by national guidelines for managing anticoagulants. If intubation is required in any of these situations, the most experienced provider should prepare induction medications, use a video laryngoscope, have a supraglottic airway as backup, and call for experienced assistance in case a difficult airway is encountered.

Sepsis must be treated rapidly and aggressively using antibiotics after cultures are obtained, fluids, pressors, and source control. Invasive monitors will help direct care. Respiratory support including intubation may be required. Initial management may occur in L & D before transfer to the ICU. Using an ICU bundle to direct care has been shown to improve outcomes.

Substance abuse in pregnancy often involves methamphetamines or opioids; each requires different acute management. Controlling sympathetic stimulation and hemodynamics is key after acute amphetamine or cocaine use, while managing tolerance, withdrawal, and analgesia are primary concerns for opioid users. Women with opioid use disorder may be on methadone or buprenorphine for medication-assisted treatment, which will alter pain management during labor and after cesarean delivery, but these medications should be continued throughout the peripartum period.

Trauma management begins with obtaining all needed imaging and providing any treatment that benefits the mother while monitoring the fetus as appropriate for gestational age. Rarely is emergency cesarean delivery required. Obstetricians and anesthesiologists from L & D should provide advice on alterations of physiology in pregnancy (e.g., need for left uterine displacement), avoidance of medications with potential teratogenic effects, steroids and magnesium sulfate administration for select premature fetuses, and delivery for fetal indications or if the gravid uterus is interfering with intraabdominal repairs. Postoperative care may involve fetal monitoring and observation for preterm labor.

In summary, multidisciplinary collaboration among anesthesiologists, obstetricians, consultant specialists, and nursing staff is the key to best management of complicated pregnancies.

QUESTIONS

1. What is the most common cause of maternal mortality after live birth in the United States?
   a. Hemorrhage
   b. Thrombotic pulmonary embolism
   c. Infection or sepsis
   d. Cardiovascular conditions
   e. Hypertensive disorders of pregnancy

2. What is a normal physiologic change during pregnancy?
   a. Increased alveolar ventilation leading to reduced arterial pO_2
   b. Expanded plasma volume leading to anemia
   c. Elevated lower esophageal sphincter tone causing reflux or heartburn
   d. Reduced minute ventilation leading to hypercarbia
   e. Reduced albumin levels that reduce the risk of pulmonary edema

3. You are caring for a G1 at term with severe primary pulmonary hypertension who presents for cesarean delivery for breech presentation. Which medication could worsen her pulmonary hypertension and should be avoided during her peripartum course?
   a. Prostaglandin $F_{2\alpha}$ (carboprost tromethamine)
   b. Nifedipine
   c. β-agonist tocolytic agents (terbutaline)
   d. Oxytocin in high concentrations
   e. Magnesium sulfate

4. You are called to the emergency department to evaluate a G2P1 at 28 weeks' gestation with known asthma who is having an exacerbation. She has received an albuterol treatment in the ED in addition to her usual medications at home. The results of her arterial blood gas have just come back: pH 7.3, pO_2 80 on 2L nasal cannula, and pCO_2 42. What is an appropriate level of care for her at this time?
   a. Home with precautions
   b. Further observation in the emergency department
   c. L & D to monitor the fetus
   d. ICU for higher level of care

5. Which of the following is recommended management of cardiac arrest in a pregnant woman?
   a. Place a wedge under the backboard to achieve left uterine displacement.
   b. Obtain femoral intravenous access for medications.
   c. Avoid defibrillation until the fetus is delivered.
   d. Call the neonatal team if she has not had return of spontaneous circulation in 10 minutes.
   e. Administer resuscitation drugs in usual doses per current American Heart Association guidelines.

6. When cardiac arrest occurs in a pregnant patient in L & D, transport immediately to the operating room to perform expedited cesarean delivery under sterile conditions.
   a. True
   b. False

7. An actively laboring parturient on L & D becomes acutely unresponsive with unobtainable blood pressure and appears cyanotic. Brisk vaginal bleeding ensues. A presumed diagnosis of amniotic fluid embolism (AFE) is made. In addition to intubation, ventilation, and CPR, what other management strategies should be initiated?
   a. Transeophageal echocardiography to guide pulmonary vasodilators and inotropes
   b. 1.5 mL/kg bolus of intralipid
   c. Recombinant Factor VIIa as an early therapy for coagulopathy
   d. Avoidance of thromboelastography (TEG), which may give erroneous results in this setting
   e. Avoidance of initiating extracorporeal membrane oxygenation to minimize bleeding

8. A G1 at 28 weeks with known severe rheumatic mitral stenosis presents with congestive heart failure. After a difficult course in the ICU achieving initial medical stabilization by the cardiology team, a catheter balloon commissurotomy is suggested. How would you counsel the patient about having this procedure performed while she is pregnant?
   a. The fetus cannot be shielded from radiation in the cardiac catheterization laboratory.
   b. Third trimester is too late in pregnancy to perform surgery or other procedures.
   c. There is a high chance the fetus will not survive the procedure.
   d. Because medical management of her mitral stenosis has been difficult, this procedure may be her best option to prevent morbidity for her and her baby.
   e. The anesthetic drugs she will require are teratogenic for the fetus.

9. A G1 at 30 weeks' gestation is being induced for pre-eclampsia with severe features because of worsening laboratory values. She is on a magnesium sulfate infusion but has not required additional antihypertensive agents. You are called emergently to her labor room, where a grand mal seizure is in progress. What steps should be taken?
   a. Turn off her magnesium infusion to prevent toxicity.
   b. Place her supine in Trendelenburg position.
   c. Perform endotracheal intubation immediately to prevent aspiration.
   d. Administer high-flow oxygen by mask to compensate for the patient's high metabolic demands.
   e. Proceed emergently to the operating room for cesarean delivery.

10. A patient who delivered by cesarean and was found to have an undiagnosed placenta percreta is in the operating room with uncontrolled massive hemorrhage. She is increasingly unstable despite ongoing resuscitation. Which of the following statements about the resuscitative endovascular balloon occlusion of the aorta (REBOA) device is true?
    a. The balloon catheter acts as an internal aortic occlusion device to be used until hemorrhage is controlled.
    b. The REBOA can only be placed in the Interventional Radiology suite.
    c. It should be advanced to Zone I above the renal arteries for obstetric hemorrhage.
    d. The balloon must be deflated every 2 hours to prevent lower limb and organ ischemia.
    e. It is inserted via the femoral vein on either side.

11. Neuraxial anesthesia (spinal or epidural) is contraindicated in parturients infected with COVID-19 because of the risk of infecting the cerebrospinal fluid with virus and causing meningitis or encephalitis.
    a. True
    b. False

12. You are meeting a patient for the first time who is transferring care because of her new diagnosis of severe fetal growth restriction. She tells you that she is on prescribed Suboxone (buprenorphine and naloxone) and asks if she should stop taking it before her delivery date. How should you respond?
    a. Her usual daily doses should be taken during labor and her postpartum stay to prevent withdrawal.
    b. Her daily dose should be doubled for the week before her delivery.
    c. She will be transitioned to methadone to improve her baby's outcome and lessen neonatal withdrawal symptoms.
    d. She should discontinue her Suboxone the day before her delivery, since we will use neuraxial anesthesia for pain control during labor or cesarean delivery.
    e. Because Suboxone includes naloxone in its formulation, nonsteroidal anti-inflammatory drugs will not be helpful for her postpartum analgesia.

13. A patient with known asthma at 30 weeks' gestation has been admitted from the emergency department to the ICU. She now requires intubation for worsening arterial blood gases and unresponsiveness to medical management. After induction of anesthesia, the anesthesiologist has made two unsuccessful attempts at intubation with a video laryngoscope, was unable to mask ventilate between attempts, and is now attempting unsuccessfully to place a laryngeal mask airway. Another anesthesiologist from the operating room is there to assist. The patient's oxygen saturations have decreased to the 80s. What is the next step in the difficult airway algorithm?
    a. Attempt laryngoscopy with a different type of videolaryngoscope.
    b. Call for the fiberoptic bronchoscope from the main operating room.
    c. Halt attempts while additional bronchodilators are administered.
    d. Prepare to obtain a surgical airway by cricothyroidotomy or operative tracheotomy.
    e. Deliver the fetus to improve perfusion and oxygenation.

14. During postpartum hemorrhage >1000 mL following cesarean delivery for placenta previa, a dose of tranexamic acid (TXA) 1 g has been administered. The hemorrhage continues despite ongoing resuscitation and other usual care. Which of the following is true?
    a. The first dose of TXA should have been given before delivery because the patient was at risk for PPH and TXA doesn't cross the placenta.
    b. There is increased risk of thrombotic complications after administration of more than 2 g in a 24-hour period.
    c. TXA is extremely expensive, so others medications should be tried first.
    d. Unless the TEG or rotational thromboelastometry shows fibrinolysis, there is no reason to administer TXA.
    e. TXA will act as a uterotonic and improve uterine atony.

15. An otherwise healthy parturient has Raynaud disease and is receiving medical therapy from her PCP for increasingly severe symptoms. She is at risk of uterine atony after delivery of twins. Which uterotonic should be avoided if postpartum hemorrhage occurs?
    a. Oxytocin
    b. Methylergonovine
    c. Prostaglandin E2
    d. Misoprostol
    e. Calcium

16. An asymptomatic COVID+ mother requires an emergency cesarean delivery for cord prolapse under general anesthesia. The operating room is not a negative pressure room. What precautions should be taken to extubate her safely?
    a. A member from the nursing team and obstetrics team should be present to assist in case she needs rapid reintubation.
    b. Before extubation, she should be moved to a negative-pressure room in L & D, and nonanesthesia personnel should wait outside the door for 15 minutes.
    c. She should be moved to the main operating room postanesthesia care unit for extubation so that extra nursing assistance is close by.
    d. After extubation, she should be placed on high-flow nasal cannula.
    e. Medications to prevent postoperative nausea and vomiting should not be given in this scenario.

17. A parturient on methadone medically assisted treatment for opioid addiction had a cesarean delivery and received neuraxial morphine for postoperative pain control. She is complaining of severe itching and requests treatment. What is the best option for her?
    a. Nalbuphine 5 mg IV
    b. Diphenhydramine 25 mg IV
    c. Butorphanol 0.5 mg IV
    d. Naloxone 40 µg IV, repeated as needed
    e. Switch her treatment from methadone to buprenorphine

18. A G1 parturient is scheduled for induction of labor at term. Her antepartum course was complicated by deep vein thrombosis and pulmonary embolism requiring full anticoagulation. She is currently receiving unfractionated heparin 10,000 U three times daily. She would like to have the option of an epidural for labor analgesia. What would you say about how her heparin dosing will be managed?
    a. She will be changed to a heparin infusion on arrival to L & D, which will allow an epidural to be placed.
    b. She should hold her heparin dose the previous evening and the morning of her induction, and a PTT will be drawn on arrival.

c. She will be changed to enoxaparin 2 weeks before delivery to allow for ease of testing her coagulation status.
d. A dose of protamine will be given 1 hour before epidural placement to reverse the heparin anticoagulation.
e. Neuraxial analgesia is not possible for her. She will be given patient-controlled analgesia for labor and general anesthesia if cesarean delivery is required.

19. A patient is admitted to L & D acutely intoxicated with cocaine. She appears to be in active labor with concern for abruption. Her vital signs include blood pressure 195/120, heart rate 133, and temperature 36.5°C. What medication(s) should not be used acutely in this setting to control her hemodynamics?
    a. Hydralazine
    b. Labetalol
    c. Nicardipine + metoprolol
    d. Esmolol + nitroprusside

20. You will be caring for a patient with placenta percreta and extensive pelvic involvement. She is refusing blood products due to her Jehovah's Witness faith despite extensive counseling. What options could be discussed in her multidisciplinary antepartum care conference to try to improve her outcome?
    a. Administration of erythropoietin with iron therapy to improve her antepartum hematocrit
    b. Delivery in a hybrid operating room so that embolization catheters could be placed by Interventional Radiology
    c. Use of closed-circuit cell salvage setup by the perfusionist team to meet Jehovah's Witness requirements
    d. A surgical plan to leave the placenta in situ with hysterectomy scheduled in several weeks
    e. All of the above

Intensive Care Considerations in Obstetrics

LAUREN A. PLANTE | STEPHEN LAPINSKY

(see *Creasy and Resnik's Maternal-Fetal Medicine, 9e: Ch 71*)

Summary

Between 1 and 10 women per 1000 maternities are admitted to an intensive care unit (ICU); many more require high-acuity care outside of a traditional ICU. Although the maternal-fetal medicine specialists will have experience dealing with common obstetric critical care conditions (e.g., hemorrhage, hypertensive emergencies), others, such as sepsis and acute respiratory distress syndrome (ARDS), are less common.

Most obstetric patients who need a higher level of care require additional nursing interventions or more intensive monitoring rather than actual life support technologies and could be cared for in a stepdown, high-dependency, or intermediate-care unit rather than a level 3 ICU. These are generally patients at risk of, but not yet in, organ failure. Nevertheless, there are some critically ill obstetric patients who require support for organ failure, which can only be provided in an ICU, such as mechanical ventilation, extracorporeal circulatory support, and intraaortic balloon counterpulsation.

In busy maternity units, a high-dependency unit can often be colocated on a labor ward so as to manage patients who need intravenous antihypertensives or post-hemorrhage care. This may be a defined area within the labor and delivery floor or may be achieved by assigning a single nurse, with adequate training, to carry out required monitoring and interventions without moving the patient out of the labor or postanesthesia care unit.

The majority of obstetric admissions to an ICU (generally >80%) are postpartum rather than antenatal. Most women admitted to an ICU antepartum have nonobstetric causes for admission, most commonly pneumonia, severe asthma exacerbation, pyelonephritis, diabetic ketoacidosis, status epilepticus, pulmonary embolus, appendicitis, and pancreatitis. Women admitted postpartum usually have an obstetric reason for admission: hemorrhage, post-cesarean surgical complications, preeclampsia/eclampsia, anesthetic complications, and obstetric infection. ICU length of stay is short for most women (1–2 days), and mortality is much lower than for other patients admitted to an ICU.

Other chapters in this textbook address many of the conditions relevant to an ICU. This chapter focuses on two paradigmatic critical care syndromes: sepsis and ARDS.

SEPSIS

Infection alone is not the critical feature in sepsis. Instead, sepsis is now defined as "life-threatening organ dysfunction caused by a dysregulated host response to infection." This is a paradigm shift.

Clinical criteria found to correlate best with sepsis—in an infected patient not already in the ICU—are any two of the following criteria:

1. Systolic blood pressure ≤100 mm Hg
2. Respiratory rate ≥22/min
3. Altered mental status

This brief bedside assessment constitutes the quick Sequential Organ Failure Assessment (qSOFA) score. qSOFA is not diagnostic for sepsis, but a score of 2 predicts a heightened risk for prolonged ICU stay or mortality and should prompt the physician to look for organ dysfunction, step up therapy, and increase monitoring or transfer outright to higher levels of care. For patients already in the ICU, however, the full Sequential Organ Failure Assessment score is used to assess organ dysfunction: an increase of 2 or more points suggests sepsis be considered. Note that fever is neither necessary nor sufficient in determining whether sepsis is present.

Septic shock has been redefined as "a subset of sepsis in which underlying circulatory and cellular metabolism abnormalities are profound enough to substantially increase mortality." Operationally, this equals hypotension (mean arterial pressure [MAP] ≤65 mm Hg) requiring vasopressors, plus serum lactate level above 2 mmol/L, despite adequate volume resuscitation.

Normal physiology of pregnancy has not yet been incorporated into a modification of Sepsis-3 or qSOFA score. The World Health Organization (WHO) has, however, proposed a new definition of maternal sepsis, as follows: "A life-threatening condition, defined as organ dysfunction resulting from infection during pregnancy, childbirth, post-abortion, or the postpartum period."

New organ dysfunction in a previously healthy woman should raise the suspicion of sepsis. Fever is not required but may be present.

The crucial points are to have a high index of suspicion and low threshold to initiate antibiotic therapy promptly, within the first hour of suspicion of sepsis. Initial empiric therapy should be broad enough to cover all possible microbial pathogens, with the plan to narrow the spectrum of the antimicrobial agent when the causative microorganism/s are identified. Because these patients are identified by instability, frequency of monitoring and reevaluation must be increased: they cannot simply be left to usual clinical care. When sepsis is suspected, after antibiotics are begun and cultures obtained, a search should begin for a focus of infection amenable to source control. Imaging is often required. If a specific focus is identified, steps should be taken, such as curettage for retained products of conception or drainage of an abscess. Source control has been demonstrated to reduce mortality in sepsis and, although it has not been specifically studied in obstetric sepsis, is expected to be beneficial. Many cases of sepsis in obstetrics localize to the uterus and are easily accessible to source control. Source control should be attained within the first 6 to 12 hours, or "as soon as possible following successful initial resuscitation," because there appears to be a decrement in survival when control is delayed beyond this period.

If hypotension or hypoperfusion is present, then fluid resuscitation should immediately follow initiation of antimicrobials. Fever, venodilation, and capillary leakage all leave the septic patient inadequately preloaded. Not all septic patients can be resuscitated with fluids alone. The purpose of vasopressors is to constrict the pathologically dilated systemic circulation characteristic of sepsis and thereby maintain adequate perfusion. The clinician should not hesitate to administer norepinephrine to a septic pregnant patient when it is indicated for blood pressure support.

ACUTE RESPIRATORY DISTRESS SYDROME

Respiratory failure occurs when normal alveolar gas exchange is not maintained. It may be type 1, which manifests as hypoxemia, or type 2, in which hypercapnia is present. Type 2 hypercapnic respiratory failure is also referred to as *ventilatory failure*. Pure ventilatory failure need not be pulmonary in origin: anything that impairs neuromuscular function or central control of ventilation can cause hypercapnea or ventilatory failure.

ARDS is a relatively common cause for respiratory failure. The rate of ARDS in pregnancy appears to have risen. Figures from the United States show 37.5 cases per 100,000 live births in 2006, rising to 59.6 in 2012. These estimates are, however, an order of magnitude higher than in Canada, where the rate of ARDS in obstetric patients was calculated as 5.5 per 100,000 delivery hospitalizations.

ARDS is a nonspecific response of the lung to a variety of inciting events, defined as "a syndrome of inflammation and increased permeability that is associated with a constellation of clinical, radiological, and physiologic abnormalities that cannot be explained by, but may coexist with, left atrial or pulmonary capillary hypertension." The lungs are stiff and resist expansion. The cornerstone of treatment is effective positive-pressure mechanical ventilation, to improve hypoxemia, help mobilize edema fluid, and decrease the work of breathing. However, positive-pressure ventilation, the mainstay of treatment, itself may cause further damage to the lung. It is now well established that lower tidal volume in mechanical ventilation is associated with lower mortality and more ventilator-free days (in nonpregnant adults). This strategy allows hypercapnia and respiratory acidosis to occur but minimizes inflation pressures and stretch-induced lung injury. There are no data on outcomes of a lung-protective or lower-tidal-volume ventilation strategy for pregnant women with ARDS. In fact, there are no randomized controlled trials of ventilator strategies in an obstetric population. Maternal acidemia does affect fetal acid-base status, which suggests that continuous fetal monitoring could be useful, specifically in determining the lower acceptable limits of maternal pH. Delivery does not improve maternal survival in ARDS.

Administration of humidified high-flow oxygen via specialized nasal cannula may stave off intubation and has been used with success in pregnancy.

When planning to intubate a pregnant woman, remember that this is considered a more difficult airway and that the reduced functional residual capacity makes the progression to profound hypoxemia more likely. Because of pregnancy-related airway edema, a smaller endotracheal tube should be used (e.g., 7.0 mm rather than 8.0 mm).

In contemporary practice, the usual approach to management of ARDS is a volume-controlled ventilation strategy. The MFM physician will seldom be the physician setting the ventilator, but the following is a suggested strategy to start. Set the starting tidal volume to 6 to 8 mL/kg, based not on actual body weight but rather ideal body weight: the equation for ideal body weight in kilograms is $45.5 + 0.91$ (height in cm—152.4). The pressure generated for this tidal volume will depend on lung compliance, but the plateau pressure should not exceed 30 to 35 cm H_2O. (Pregnancy does increase intraabdominal pressure and decreases lung compliance.) If airway pressure is above this level, decrease tidal volume. Set initial PEEP at 5 cm H_2O. Starting Fio_2 should be 1.0 and starting frequency between 10 and 15/min. Check arterial blood gas and patient status within 30−60 minutes. Adjust the ventilator settings. In most cases, further ventilator adjustments will be made by the intensivist, in conjunction with the respiratory therapist, rather than by the obstetrician-gynecologist or maternal-fetal medicine physician.

Extracorporeal life support (ECLS) has been used during pregnancy, most notably during the influenza A H1N1 epidemic of 2009 to 2010 and the COVID-19 epidemic of 2019-2021. Complications include bleeding (related to the need for anticoagulation), thromboembolic events, and cannulation-related injuries. A systematic review of ECLS in pregnancy identified 358 cases of ECMO, including VV-ECMO for ARDS and VA-ECMO for amniotic fluid embolism and peripartum cardiomyopathy, among other causes. Aggregated maternal survival was 75%, and fetal survival was 65%, with complications including bleeding and intracranial neurologic events. The risk for bleeding complications is high, however, and the role extracorporeal life support should play in severe respiratory failure during pregnancy remains unclear.

Whenever a pregnant or postpartum patient is admitted to the ICU, she is entitled to equity in both maternity care and critical care. The team of professionals caring for her must be multidisciplinary, flexible, and able to communicate with both one another and the patient and her family. Goals for care and recovery should be incorporated into treatment.

Ongoing weakness, myopathy, and neuropathy are common among ICU survivors in general, as is psychologic distress (e.g., depression and posttraumatic stress disorder [PTSD]). Planning for hospital discharge should take into account that ICU survivors may have additional physical, rehabilitation, cognitive, or emotional needs. Almost nothing is known about recovery from critical illness during pregnancy, though a recent qualitative study points to weakness, frustration, isolation, anxiety, panic attacks, depression, and PTSD after the critical-illness hospitalization.

QUESTIONS

1. Which of the following statements are true regarding hemodynamic monitoring with the pulmonary artery catheter (PAC)?
   a. The PAC is an invasive intervention, contraindicated during pregnancy.
   b. PAC measurements can be used to accurately diagnose sepsis during pregnancy.
   c. The PAC is a useful intervention for long-term hemodynamic monitoring in the unstable pregnant patient.
   d. Studies have demonstrated that PAC use is associated with an increased mortality.
   e. An advantage of PACs is the ability to provide a continuous readout of cardiac output.

2. Which of the following statements regarding sepsis during pregnancy is INCORRECT?
   a. The incidence of sepsis correlates with income level and socioeconomic status.
   b. The diagnosis requires isolation of a causative organism.
   c. A significant risk factor is cesarean delivery.
   d. Initial treatment with broad-spectrum antimicrobials is appropriate.
   e. Inotrope therapy (e.g., norepinephrine) may be essential for management of the pregnant woman with septic shock.

3. A 26-year-old G1P0 is diagnosed with pyelonephritis-related sepsis. Management of sepsis requires which of the following to reduce mortality?
   a. Early broad-spectrum antibiotic administration
   b. Early administration of boluses of crystalloid for fluid resuscitation
   c. Early administration of boluses of colloid (albumin) for fluid resuscitation
   d. Antibiotics to be initiated after culture and sensitivity results
   e. Placement of a pulmonary artery catheter to direct hemodynamic management

4. A 22-year-old G2P1001 with preeclampsia develops acute respiratory distress syndrome (ARDS) in pregnancy. Which of the following is true regarding ARDS?
   a. It is less common than in the general population due to young age and lack of comorbidity.
   b. It is difficult to diagnose as normal pregnancy is associated with an increased respiratory rate and decreased partial pressure of carbon dioxide ($PaCO_2$).
   c. It may occur related to pregnancy complications.
   d. If mechanical ventilation is required, prompt delivery should be undertaken.
   e. When ventilated, it requires minimization of tidal volume at 6 mL/kg actual weight.

5. Which of these does not require vascular cannulation?
   a. Measurement of central venous pressure
   b. Calculation of systemic vascular resistance
   c. Measurement of inferior vena cava diameter
   d. Pulse contour analysis

6. A 30-year-old G6P5015 undergoing cesarean delivery has a successful resuscitation for an intraoperative cardiac arrest. Which of the following is the best unit for her recovery?
   a. Intensive care unit
   b. Intermediate care unit
   c. Post–acute care area of the surgical suite
   d. Labor and delivery ward

7. A 38-year-old G3P2002 at 18 weeks' gestation is admitted to the neurointensive care unit with acute hemorrhagic stroke. Which of these statements is correct regrding her management?
   a. Teratogenesis remains a concern for the next few weeks.
   b. Neuroimaging should be performed as indicated.
   c. The risk of miscarriage is above 50%.
   d. The pregnancy should be terminated.

8. A 30-year-old patient comes to the obstetrical triage unit at 31 weeks complaining of increasing dyspnea. Her S_pO_2 is 92% on room air and 95% on 40% Venturi mask (F_IO_2 0.4). Her respiratory rate is 28/min, heart rate 120/min, blood pressure 90/62, temperature 38°C (100.4°F), and the fetal heart rate is 160 bpm. She is uncomfortable but can answer your questions. Which of the following best reflects her qSOFA score?
   a. 0
   b. 1
   c. 2
   d. 3

9. Six hours after admission to the hospital, a patient with respiratory illness has a respiratory rate of 32/min and her SpO_2 has decreased to 91% on a 40% Venturi mask. All of the following are appropriate interventions to consider EXCEPT:
   a. Change to 100% F_IO_2 via nonrebreather.
   b. Change to high-flow nasal cannula at 50 L/min and 100% oxygen (F_IO_2 1.0).
   c. Intubate and begin mechanical ventilation at F_IO_2 1.0 with PEEP 5 cm H_2O, respiratory rate 14, assist-control mode, tidal volume 6–8 mL/kg.
   d. Undertake cesarean delivery under general anesthesia.

10. Among ICU survivors, quality of life can be affected for a long time. What is known about long-term outcomes after maternal critical care?
    a. Rates of psychologic distress and neuromuscular dysfunction are more common among ICU survivors who were pregnant during their ICU admission, compared with women who were not pregnant during ICU admission.
    b. Rates of psychologic distress and neuromuscular dysfunction are less common among ICU survivors who were pregnant during their ICU admission, compared with women who were not pregnant during ICU admission.
    c. Women who survived an ICU admission during pregnancy are grateful.
    d. Women who survived an ICU admission during pregnancy have additional needs and concerns.

Pregnancy as a Window to Future Health

JANET CATOV | C. NOEL BAIREY MERZ

(see Creasy and Reskink's Maternal-Fetal-Medicine, Ch 72)

Summary

Cardiovascular disease (CVD) is the leading cause of mortality among women in the United States and developed countries. Women on average experience CVD mortality about 10 years later than men. However, women experience a higher fatality rate following a first myocardial infarction, and despite an overall decline in the CVD death rate in the United States, the rate of decline has been slower for women compared with men. In addition, the death rate is 70% higher in African-American women compared with White women. Two-thirds of coronary heart disease sudden deaths occur in women with no previous symptoms, compared with one-half of sudden deaths in men. It is now evident that this excess mortality is due in part to an increased death rate among premenopausal women, although little is known regarding coronary artery disease among this group. From 1995 to 2014, myocardial infarction (MI) hospitalizations increased in young women but not in men; relative to men, young women with MI had a higher comorbidity index and a lesser likelihood of being managed with guideline-based medications. Although the risk for CVD increases after menopause, this is indistinguishable from aging; further, risk factors that are elevated before menopause increase proportionally post menopause. Thus detection of elevated risk during reproductive years may provide a critical opportunity to delay or prevent onset of CVD in women.

Healthy pregnancy requires profound maternal vascular, immune, and metabolic adaptations to support placentation and fetal growth. It is now well established that an impaired ability to mount these adaptations contributes to adverse pregnancy outcomes (APOs) such as hypertensive disorders of pregnancy, preterm birth, fetal growth restriction, stillbirth, and gestational diabetes mellitus (GDM). Indeed, pregnancy now can be viewed as a "stress test" of these systems, with adverse pregnancy outcomes being a harbinger of excess cardiometabolic risk and CVD morbidity and mortality. Leveraging this possibility may help mitigate this high-risk trajectory and delay or prevent CVD in women, and guidelines now identify women with adverse pregnancy outcomes as a high-risk group for CVD.

Despite advancements in management, however, CVD remains a significant cause of morbidity and mortality. This is particularly true in women who often present with atypical symptoms and are frequently misdiagnosed and undertreated. Women are more likely to have nonobstructive CAD, yet their mortality remains significantly elevated. This has been attributed in part to the increased recognition of coronary microvascular dysfunction and other coronary-related and non–coronary-related disorders that contribute to ischemia and related adverse cardiovascular outcomes in these patients. Along these same lines, as diagnosis remains challenging in this population, so does risk stratification. Risk stratification has traditionally been insensitive in women, as existing risk scores tend to categorize most women as low risk. This has led to a move toward more sex-specific risk stratification with inclusion of alternative markers such as high-sensitivity C-reactive protein (hsCRP) in the Reynolds risk score or inclusion of stroke in the ACC/AHA atherosclerotic cardiovascular disease (ASCVD) risk score. However, another area that has remained underappreciated is the potential predictive value of a history of adverse pregnancy outcomes. These conditions often occur in young, otherwise healthy women who under the "stress test" of pregnancy demonstrate future tendencies toward metabolic and cardiovascular conditions such as hypertension and diabetes.

There has been some progress. GDM and hypertensive disorders of pregnancy are now included in CVD risk stratification guidelines for women, and other adverse pregnancy conditions are becoming more widely recognized. However, cardiovascular (CV) risk calculators such as the Framingham risk score, Reynolds risk score, and 2013 ASCVD calculator do not incorporate these adverse pregnancy conditions, leading to potential underestimation of lifetime CV risk in women. A major reason for the lack of sufficient evidence to incorporate these adverse pregnancy conditions into risk calculators is that the large population registries able to link pregnancy history to CV events lack data on traditional risk factors, such as cholesterol levels, required as input for the risk calculators. Furthermore, most large cohorts that follow women to collect data on these CV risk factors have failed to collect information regarding their history of pregnancy complications. In part, this is caused by questions about the accuracy of maternal recall of pregnancy complications. For example, an initial review evaluating maternal recall of hypertensive disorders in pregnancy demonstrated relatively poor accuracy. However, women recall GDM, infant birth weight, and length of gestation much more accurately (92% sensitivity, and correlations ranging from 0.95 to 0.85). Thus maternal recall of these common pregnancy complications may prove useful to screen for CVD risk. Indeed, a recent large, multiethnic cohort of women who are more densely phenotyped, with longer-term follow-up and APO adjudication from the Women's Health Initiative, convincingly show that hypertensive disorders of pregnancy and low birth weight are independently associated with future CVD in women after adjustment for established risk factors and other APOs, suggesting that this risk enhancement should be incorporated into a new ASCVD risk score for women. Accordingly, research is needed to determine whether incorporation of reliably reported pregnancy history data will improve

CV risk scoring systems for women. Early evidence using older-age cohorts has yielded null prediction benefit, but more work is needed. Further, should these ASCVD scores be useful for detection and treatment, it will behoove us to mandate coding of APOs in the electronic health record (EHR), which currently is not done. Specifically, medical and surgical history are mandatory elements in the EHR, while pregnancy history is not. Policy action is needed to (1) add pregnancy or APO history to required EHR fields in medical and surgical history, (2) identify and enter APOs into the EHR at the time of delivery, (3) increase access to APO EHR history by clinicians and continuity of care systems over women's life courses, and (4) calculate ASCVD risk scores adding APO history to improve CVD in women.

QUESTIONS

1. What adverse pregnancy outcomes are associated with excess cardiovascular disease? Check all that apply:
   a. Hypertensive disorders of pregnancy
   b. Preterm delivery
   c. Gestational diabetes
   d. Small for gestational age
   e. Stillbirth
   f. All
   g. None

2. What cardiovascular risk factors are the largest contributors to cardiovascular disease events in women? (check two most important)
   a. Hypertension
   b. Dyslipidemia
   c. Obesity
   d. Psychosocial Stress
   e. Poor sleep
   f. Smoking
   g. Physical inactivity

3. Are APOs linked to cardiovascular disease events via classic risk factors or novel factors?
   a. Traditional
   b. Novel
   c. Both

4. Is high parity associated with excess CVD events?
   a. Yes, due to biologic mechanisms
   b. Yes, due to shared lifestyle and environmental factors
   c. No, no biologic, lifestyle, or environmental factors link high parity with CVD

5. What proportion of women are affected by hypertensive disorders of pregnancy in the United States?
   a. 2%–3%
   b. 5%–7%
   c. 15%
   d. 20%

6. Is the risk of CVD among women with gestational diabetes due to progression to type 2 diabetes?
   a. Yes, exclusively
   b. No, GDM is not associated with CVD
   c. Combination, some of the risk is due to progression to T2DM and some appears to be a direct association without progression to T2DM

7. Preterm birth is a heterogenous condition, and are subtypes of preterm birth according to clinical presentation (spontaneous and indicated; early and late preterm birth) each associated with CVD in mothers?
   a. Risk of CVD is eightfold higher in women with preterm births.
   b. CVD risk is highest for indicated preterm birth but still detectable for spontaneous preterm birth.
   c. There is no risk of CVD following spontaneous PTB.

8. What is the pathophysiology linking small-for–gestational age births to maternal CVD?
   a. Poor placentation
   b. No association between SGA delivery and maternal CVD
   c. Unknown

9. Sex-specific risk CVD stratification with inclusion of alternative markers can include what?
   a. High-sensitivity C-reactive protein (hsCRP) in the Reynolds risk score
   b. Inclusion of stroke in the ACC/AHA ASCVD risk score
   c. A history of adverse pregnancy outcomes can be used to improve sex-specific risk stratification in women
   d. All of the above

10. Maternal recall of hypertensive disorders in pregnancy has relatively poor accuracy—are there useful components with better recall?
    a. Women recall GDM, infant birth weight, and length of gestation much more accurately.
    b. Women do not recall GDM, infant birth weight, and length of gestation much more accurately.

11. Women with a history of adverse pregnancy conditions may benefit from additional or more frequent CV risk stratification including annual screening of blood pressure, lipids, and fasting glucose. What are current guidelines?
    a. Women with preeclampsia or gestational hypertension should follow up with a physician for a blood pressure check within 1 week of delivery.
    b. Women with GDM should have repeat glucose testing at 6 weeks postpartum.
    c. All of the above.

12. Accurate measurement of blood pressure is essential to categorize blood pressure, stratify cardiovascular risk, and guide management, and a target blood pressure of less than 130/80 mm Hg is recommended for adults with confirmed hypertension and cardiovascular disease or a 10-year atherosclerotic cardiovascular disease risk of 10% or more. What is the role of nonpharmacologic therapeutic lifestyle change?
    a. Adults with elevated blood pressure or stage 1 hypertension whose estimated 10-year risk of atherosclerotic cardiovascular disease is less than 10% should be treated with nonpharmacologic interventions.
    b. Adults with elevated blood pressure or stage 1 hypertension whose estimated 10-year risk of atherosclerotic cardiovascular disease is less than 10% should not be treated with nonpharmacologic interventions.

13. The American College of Obstetricians and Gynecologists Task Force recommends that women with a history of preeclampsia and preterm birth or recurrent preeclampsia should have what screening?
    a. An annual assessment of their lipid profile, blood pressure, body mass index, and fasting blood glucose
    b. A one-time assessment of their lipid profile, blood pressure, body mass index, and fasting blood glucose

14. The ASCVD risk assessment guideline provides a lifetime risk estimator that is crucial for women to understand their long-term risk and to motivate lifestyle changes to improve ASCVD risk. It often demonstrates short-term risk is low—why is this useful?
    a. Because 10-year risk is often lower in women
    b. Because lifetime risk is higher for most of those 20 to 59 years of age
    c. Because risk assessment can be useful to enhance the discussion for improvement in risk factors through lifestyle optimization at younger ages
    d. All of the above

15. Why is pregnancy considered a "stress test"?
    a. Pregnancy is a time of significant hemodynamic, vascular, and metabolic adaptations.
    b. Pregnancy occurs in young women when life is stressful.

16. Are physicians at an increased risk of adverse pregnancy outcomes compared with nonphysicians?
    a. Female physicians may be at slightly higher risk of severe maternal morbidity.
    b. This association appeared to be mediated by their tendency to delay childbearing compared with nonphysicians.
    c. All of the above.

17. Are newborns of physicians at an increased risk of morbidity compared with newborns of nonphysicians?
    a. Newborns of physicians appear to experience less morbidity.
    b. Newborns of physicians appear not to experience less morbidity.

18. Are non-White women at an increased risk for APOs that are associated with increased maternal CVD risk?
    a. True
    b. False

The Neonate

Neonatal Morbidities of Prenatal and Perinatal Origin

JAMES M. GREENBERG

(see *Creasy and Resnik's Maternal-Fetal Medicine, 9e: Ch 73*)

Summary

The best care for neonates requires close collaboration with the obstetric provider and aligned communication with the mother and her supporters. Many complications of pregnancy have implications for neonatal outcomes. Careful planning will optimize care by allowing appropriate preparation for potential neonatal morbidities. Maternal conditions of note include insulin resistance, chorioamnionitis, hypertensive disorders, autoimmune disorders, hemorrhagic conditions, nutritional disorders such as anorexia, substance abuse disorders, and multifetal gestation. Congenital malformations are often detected many weeks before delivery and should prompt proactive planning around site of delivery and provisions for appropriate deployment of skilled delivery room personnel. Prenatal discussions with the mother and her supporters should include plans for resuscitation and neonatal transfer if appropriate.

Prematurity: Infants born before term may experience a wide variety of comorbid conditions including feeding difficulties, respiratory distress syndrome, intraventricular hemorrhage, retinopathy of prematurity, necrotizing enterocolitis, and bronchopulmonary dysplasia. The risk of experiencing a complication of prematurity is inversely related to gestational age at birth. Although late preterm births (32–38 weeks' gestation and/or 1500-2500 gm) are unlikely to experience severe complications of prematurity, problems such as hypoglycemia, apnea, and feeding difficulties require extended inpatient nursery stays compared with full-term counterparts. Avoiding elective delivery before 38 weeks is preferable. Extreme prematurity (<28 weeks' gestation) carries a high risk of morbidity and mortality. The threshold of viability for preterm infants has declined over the past 30 years. Survival at 22 weeks has been described, and most specialty perinatal centers now offer the option of delivery room resuscitation once the pregnancy has reached 22–24 weeks. There is some variation in this threshold among centers across the United States. Local data and the specific circumstances of each delivery must be considered. Discussions among families, delivery room personnel, obstetric providers, and neonatal providers regarding resuscitation and postdelivery neonatal intensive care unit care should be a high priority if delivery during the periviable period is anticipated. Ethical consultation can be a valuable resource.

Respiratory Problems: Newborns, especially those born preterm, are prone to respiratory difficulties. Some, such as transient tachypnea of the newborn, are self-limiting and almost always respond to supportive care. Respiratory distress syndrome is a consequence of functional pulmonary surfactant deficiency. This is most common before 34 weeks' gestation with severity increasing as gestational age at delivery decreases. Early provision of pulmonary surfactant and/or continuous positive airway pressure are effective treatments. However, some will progress to develop neonatal chronic lung disease as bronchopulmonary dysplasia. This disorder is characterized by heterogeneous distribution of pulmonary atelectasis, fibrosis, and parenchymal cysts. Severely affected infants may require treatment with systemic steroids, chronic positive pressure ventilation, and supplemental oxygen. Some may also develop pulmonary vascular hypertension. Pulmonary hypoplasia is typically a consequence of diminished or absent amniotic fluid exposure during pregnancy due to preterm, prelabor, and prolonged rupture of membranes. Pneumothorax is an early complication along with pulmonary hypertension. Pulmonary hypoplasia with pulmonary hypertension is also a common sequela of severe congenital diaphragmatic hernia. Treatment with pulmonary vasodilators is useful, although severe cases are refractory. With the decline in postdate deliveries, meconium aspiration syndrome is now a less common cause of pulmonary hypertension. Most cases respond well to pulmonary vasodilator therapy.

Gastrointestinal Problems: Hyperbilirubinemia is by far the most common gastrointestinal problem affecting newborns. The vast majority require only observation or noninvasive treatment with phototherapy. Severe cases may require double volume exchange transfusion, especially those due to pathologic hemolysis. The goal for all neonates is prevention of kernicterus, a devastating complication of severe hyperbilirubinemia that results in irreversible brain injury and death. Feeding difficulties associated with prematurity are a common gastrointestinal problem. The typical preterm has limited endurance for enteral feedings with poorly coordinated suck and swallow. These issues resolve with time in the neurologically intact neonate and require only supportive care such as gavage feedings to optimize growth and development. The most devastating gastrointestinal complication of prematurity is necrotizing enterocolitis. This condition occurs most often in preterm infants born before 32 weeks and is characterized by inflammation and necrosis of the intestine. The etiology is not well understood. Treatment is supportive and prevention is best achieved through prevention of extreme preterm delivery.

Neurologic Problems: Hypoxic-ischemic encephalopathy is a consequence of impaired cerebral blood flow during the antepartum and/or peripartum period. Detection before delivery is difficult due to the limited specificity and sensitivity of fetal heart rate monitoring. Postnatal neuroimaging may assist with diagnosis and timing of injury. Brain cooling through head or systemic cooling are excellent neuroprotective strategies for those with moderate or severe insults. Among preterm infants born before 32 weeks, intraventricular hemorrhage represents an important cause of brain injury. Hemorrhage that extends into the surrounding brain parenchyma carries the highest potential for long-term neurologic deficits. Posthemorrhagic obstructive hydrocephalus may occur, and in severe cases this requires surgical shunting. Perinatal stroke and periventricular white matter injury may occur as complications of ischemic injury or on an idiopathic basis. Mechanisms are still unknown, and the best strategy for mitigation remains prevention of preterm birth. Similarly, cerebral palsy is attributed to brain injury during prenatal, perinatal, or postnatal life and can be associated with genetic abnormalities, hypoxic-ischemic events, head injury, or central nervous system infection. Premature birth and low birth weight are the most important identifiable risk factors associated with cerebral palsy. Perinatal infection and placental dysfunction are also implicated in the pathophysiology of cerebral palsy.

Neonatal Infection: Throughout the world, neonatal infection remains an important cause of morbidity and mortality. The neonatal immune system, especially the preterm immune system, is less mature, especially when considering acquired immune function. Signs and symptoms of neonatal infection are often nonspecific. Lethargy, poor feeding, low tone, new-onset apnea, and altered cutaneous perfusion may be seen, although by the time these are recognized, the infection may be at an advanced stage. Among bacterial causes, group B streptococcus and gram-negative rods are most common. *Staphylococcus* including methicillin-resistant strains are also concerning. Careful screening of contacts for carrier status and survey cultures of environmental surfaces may assist mitigation of outbreaks in nursery settings. While COVID-19 disease is a significant maternal concern during pregnancy, the virus has not proven to be a major contributor to neonatal infectious disease morbidity or mortality.

QUESTIONS

1. Neonatal conditions associated with preeclampsia include all of the following except:
   a. Thrombocytopenia
   b. Hypocalcemia
   c. Hypernatremia
   d. Polycythemia

2. During the early neonatal period, the infant of a diabetic mother should be closely monitored for:
   a. Hypoglycemia
   b. Anemia
   c. Hearing loss
   d. Overeating

3. Neonates exposed to opioids in utero must be evaluated for neonatal opioid withdrawal syndrome (NOWS). True statements about NOWS include:
   a. All opioid-exposed neonates develop NOWS.
   b. Symptoms of NOWS include excessive irritability, loose stools, and feeding difficulty.
   c. Nonpharmacologic treatment for NOWS can be effective.
   d. a, b, and c
   e. b and c

4. Late preterm infants:
   a. Are small for gestational age
   b. Are more likely to have temperature instability
   c. Should be managed like term infants
   d. Are at risk of having hyperglycemia and polycythemia
   e. a and b

5. Transient tachypnea of the newborn
   a. Is a mild, self-limiting respiratory disorder
   b. Is less common following a cesarean delivery
   c. Only occurs in term infants
   d. Improves with surfactant treatment
   e. All of the above

6. Antenatal corticosteroid treatment
   a. Reduces pulmonary morbidity from meconium aspiration
   b. Accelerates lung maturation
   c. May promote long-term behavioral-emotional problems
   d. b and c only
   e. a, b, and c

7. Which of the following statements about bronchopulmonary dysplasia (BPD) are true?
   a. BPD is a complication of respiratory distress syndrome.
   b. BPD is a common respiratory complication of late preterm birth.
   c. Most infants with BPD require mechanical ventilation beyond the age of 1 year.
   d. The diagnostic chest x-ray criteria of BPD must include cystic changes, focal shifting atelectasis, and hyperinflation.

8. Neonatal findings exhibiting the highest risk for hypoxic-ischemic encephalopathy include which of the following?
   a. Five-minute Apgar score <3
   b. Severe metabolic acidosis in arterial blood sampled from the umbilical artery or a peripheral artery
   c. Abnormal tone on initial neurologic exam
   d. Abnormal electroencephalogram or early-onset clinical seizure activity
   e. All of the above

9. Complications of necrotizing enterocolitis include all the following except:
   a. Long-term feeding problems
   b. Intestinal atresia
   c. Growth failure
   d. Cerebral palsy and developmental delay

10. Which one of the following statements about neonatal hyperbilirubinemia is false?
    a. Most cases of neonatal jaundice have no long-term effects and may have physiologic benefit.
    b. Unrecognized hemolysis is an important risk factor.
    c. Exclusively breast-fed neonates are more likely to require treatment for severe jaundice.
    d. Preterm infants are protected from hyperbilirubinemia by lower rates of polycythemia.

11. Intraventricular hemorrhage:
    a. Is most common among preterm infants younger than 32 weeks' gestation
    b. Originates in the subarachnoid space
    c. Is a common complication of vacuum-assisted delivery
    d. Is caused by neonatal hydrocephalus

12. The most common identifiable risk factor for cerebral palsy is
    a. A 1-minute Apgar score of <3
    b. A 5-minute Apgar score of <3
    c. Preterm birth
    d. Middle cerebral artery infarction

13. Which of the following statements about meconium-stained amniotic fluid and meconium aspiration syndrome are true?
    a. Routine tracheal suctioning is a best practice for delivery room management of neonates born through meconium-stained amniotic fluid.
    b. Amnioinfusion will prevent meconium aspiration syndrome.
    c. Meconium aspiration syndrome is uncommon (<5%) in the setting of meconium-stained amniotic fluid.
    d. The incidence of meconium aspiration syndrome has increased over the past decade.

14. Bronchopulmonary dysplasia is a multifactorial pulmonary disorder. Which of the following does NOT contribute to the known pathogenic pathways of BPD?
    a. Preterm birth
    b. Oxygen exposure
    c. Mechanical ventilation
    d. In utero opioid exposure
    e. Chorioamnionitis

15. Which maternal condition(s) is/are NOT considered safe to breastfeed?
    a. HIV
    b. Hepatitis B and Hepatitis C
    c. HIV and COVID
    d. Hepatitis B, Hepatitis C, HIV, and COVID

16. Which one of the below statements about HSV is TRUE?
    a. Neonatal HSV most commonly presents with symptoms within 48 hours of birth.
    b. Recurrent maternal HSV infection has a higher incidence of neonatal HSV than a primary maternal infection.
    c. All infants born to a mother with an active genital HSV lesion need to be evaluated for HSV, regardless of mode of delivery.
    d. Oral acyclovir is the initial treatment of choice for neonatal HSV infection.

17. What maternal condition(s) does/do NOT have a therapy available to infants at birth to try to prevent transmission?
    a. Hepatitis B
    b. Hepatitis C
    c. Hepatitis B and C
    d. HIV

ANSWERS

Chapter 1

1. c
2. b
3. c
4. d
5. b
6. c
7. a
8. c
9. b
10. b
11. c
12. d
13. c
14. a
15. c
16. b
17. a
18. b
19. c
20. d

Chapter 2

1. b
2. c
3. d
4. b
5. b
6. c
7. d
8. c
9. c
10. b
11. d
12. d
13. c
14. a
15. a
16. c
17. a
18. b
19. c
20. d

Chapter 3

1. d
2. c
3. b
4. e
5. a
6. e
7. d
8. e

9. a
10. d
11. e
12. d
13. a
14. e
15. b
16. c
17. a
18. a
19. c
20. e

Chapter 4

1. c
2. d
3. b
4. b
5. c
6. b
7. b
8. d

Chapter 5

1. a
2. a
3. b
4. c
5. d
6. d
7. a
8. c
9. c
10. d

Chapter 6

1. c. In contrast to nonpregnant, where blood flow is equally distributed between the endometrium and myometrium, in mid to late pregnancy roughly 80%–90% of blood flow is directed to the placenta.
2. b. Genetic defects in synthesis and assembly of the extracellular matrix components collagen and elastic fibers contribute to cervical insufficiency.
3. a. In contrast to most other species, progesterone synthesis does not decline during pregnancy. As the human placenta makes progesterone, circulating P4 levels do not decline until after delivery of the placenta.

4. d. The peptide hormone relaxin is reported to inhibit uterine contractility.
5. a. A reduction in collagen crosslink density contributes to reduced mechanical strength of the cervix during the softening phase.
6. c. Cervical softening spans most of the pregnancy and is achieved in the progesterone-dominant phase of pregnancy.
7. b. Onset of labor is associated with an increase in estrogen function, which in part regulates uterine activation and potentially aspects of cervical ripening/dilation.
8. b. The fetal adrenal produces DHEAS, an androgen precursor required for estrogen synthesis in the placenta.
9. c. PGDH is responsible for the degradation of PGE2 and PGF2a and is regulated by cytokines and steroid hormones.
10. a. Matrix metalloproteases are enzymes that degrade proteins. They are not considered DAMP molecules.

Chapter 7

1. d
2. a
3. d
4. b
5. b
6. a
7. b
8. d
9. d
10. d
11. d
12. c
13. a
14. d
15. d
16. b
17. c
18. d
19. a
20. c

Chapter 8

1. a
2. b
3. b
4. b
5. c

Chapter 9

1. a
2. c
3. a
4. b
5. d
6. b
7. b
8. a
9. b
10. a
11. d
12. b
13. d

Chapter 10

1. d. Implantation occurs approximately 8 to 10 days after ovulation in most successful pregnancies. Previously it was thought to take place between 6 and 7 days. Implantation requires a series of complex steps from the apposition of the blastocyst to the endometrium to the remodeling of the capillary bed and formation of the trophoblastic lacunae. This process is thought be complete by day 10 in which the blastocyst is completely encased in uterine stromal tissue.

2. c. hCG can be detected as soon as 1 week before the next menses and is one of the earliest hormones produced of the embryo even before implantation. In in vitro fertilization studies, hCG was detected as early as the eight-cell stage. Therefore it is one of the earliest biochemical markers of pregnancy.

3. a. In a female with virilization and elevated 17-hydroxyprogesterone level, the most likely cause is 21-hydroxylase deficiency, which leads to the accumulation of substrate 17-hydroxyprogesterone in the steroid pathway. This leads to shunting of the pathway to produce adrenal androgens and causing adrenal hyperplasia.

4. a. A significantly elevated testosterone-to-dihydrotestosterone ratio suggests a deficiency in the conversion of testosterone to dihydrotestosterone. Dihydrotestosterone is important in the virilization and maturation of male external genitalia. In a karyotypically male infant with ambiguous genitalia, the low levels of dihydrotestosterone suggest that the phenotype of the infant will be hypovirilized external male genital structures.

5. e. 5-Alpha reductase converts local testosterone to dihydrotestosterone and is important to the final maturation of external male genital structures. In a male infant with ambiguous genitalia and hypovirilization with an elevated testosterone-to-dihydrotestosterone ratio, it is suspected that there is a deficiency in the steroid conversation by 5-alpha reductase.

6. c. hCG is one of the earliest hormones produced by the embryo before implantation and can be detected in the serum as early as 7−8 days before expected menses. The drop in hCG levels likely signify a biochemical pregnancy loss.

7. e. The corpus luteum produces progesterone that is essential for maintenance of early pregnancy. Later in pregnancy, the placenta produces sufficient progesterone to maintain pregnancy. Therefore removal of the corpus luteum before the seventh week usually results in abortion. Removal of the corpus luteum after the ninth week does not appear to influence the pregnancy. Progesterone supplementation is required if corpus luteum function is compromised before 9 to 10 weeks' gestation.

8. b. Vascular endothelial growth factor (VEGF) regulates placenta angiogenesis and cytotrophoblast invasion, and aberrancies in these processes are observed in preeclampsia. Serum VEGF is significantly lower in women with severe preeclampsia.

9. a. High levels of inhibin A are associated with trisomy 21 and high levels of beta hCG. Trisomy 21 is associated with low AFP and low estriol. These serum markers are used in screening tests for fetal chromosomal abnormalities.

10. e. It is recommended that a pregnant patient is screened for gestational diabetes even though her pregestational screen was negative. Insulin resistance increases during the pregnancy state, and therefore a diabetes screen outside of pregnancy is out reflective of the metabolic changes that occur in pregnancy.

11. d. Metabolic changes seen in pregnancy include increased insulin resistance with hyperinsulinemia, as well as relative fasting hypoglycemia and increased circulating lipids. Prolonged fasting in pregnancy is accompanied by exaggerated hypoglycemia without the increase of gluconeogenesis. There is no significant difference in glucagon levels in nongravid and late pregnancy values.

12. b. Ulipristal acetate is a selective progesterone receptor modulator, or antiprogestin, that is a U.S. Food and Drug Administration−approved emergency contraceptive to prevent pregnancy within 5 days of intercourse. It is not an abortifacient. Progesterone plays a role in the maintenance of early pregnancy through its production by the corpus luteum. However, before implantation, which is complete 8−10 days after ovulation, the use of ulipristal acetate is to inhibit follicular rupture to prevent pregnancy.

13. a. Overall, progesterone levels do not change with the onset of labor in humans. However, progesterone regulates uterine contractions on the basis of the ratio of its two receptor subtypes: PR-A and PR-B. The expression of PR-B exceeds that of PR-A during uterine quiescence and relaxation, and the expression of PR-A exceeds PR-B at the time of labor.

14. d. When the fetus and the placenta lack sulfatase, pregnancies have dysfunctional onsets of labor leading to posterm gestations. This disorder is localized on a gene on the short arm of the X chromosome affecting the male infant. In the first few months of life, the male infant is noted to have ichthyosis, or a skin-scaling condition.

15. c. Oxytocin receptors and oxytocin increase shortly before the onset of labor. Oxytocin rises during labor, especially in the second stage of labor, and can stimulate the production of prostaglandins. Corticotropin-releasing hormone is associated with labor and myometrial contractility and is found to be higher throughout pregnancy in women with preterm labor. Progesterone regulates uterine contractions but does not change at the onset of labor.

Chapter 11

1. d
2. c
3. b
4. d
5. e
6. d
7. a
8. d
9. e
10. e
11. e
12. e
13. a

14. e
15. c
16. d

Chapter 12

1. b
2. a
3. c
4. b
5. d
6. c

Chapter 13

1. e
2. b
3. e
4. e
5. b
6. c
7. d
8. a
9. c
10. b

Chapter 14

1. a and b
2. c
3. b
4. a
5. a
6. c and e
7. a and b
8. c
9. b
10. b
11. d
12. b
13. c
14. c
15. a
16. a
17. b
18. b
19. b
20. b

Chapter 15

1. d. Case-control studies are generally less time consuming and less expensive than cohort studies.
2. a. Randomized controlled trials, if well done, should have little concern about confounding. The process of randomization should balance potential confounders equally between the groups.
3. b. Good practice suggests that subgroup analyses of randomized controlled trials be planned a priori on the basis of a biologically plausible rationale for anticipated differences.
4. d. Case-control studies are most appropriate for the study of rare outcomes, such as hydranencephaly.
5. d. Recall bias is a concern in many studies of teratogen exposure, which there may be differential recall of an exposure based on whether a disease develops.
6. a. Only an odds ratio can be calculated for data from a case-control study. Relative risks and risk differences can be assessed in cohort studies and randomized clinical trials.
7. c. Both stratified analysis and multivariable modeling are reasonable approaches to assess and control for confounding factors in an observational study.
8. d. Odds ratios are generally not a measure of effect in a randomized controlled trial and, therefore, are not used in a sample size estimate. Answers a−c are all essential components of a sample size calculation for a randomized controlled trial (in addition to minimal detectable relative risk).
9. c. The sentence describes the positive predictive value, which is something that we can use to counsel patients after a test result has returned.
10. c. A receiver operating characteristic curve is an appropriate graphical representation for this relationship. Funnel plots are used to assess for publication bias in a meta-analysis.

Chapter 16

1. c
2. b
3. c
4. a
5. d

Chapter 17

1. c
2. b
3. a
4. c
5. a
6. b
7. a
8. b
9. a
10. b

Chapter 18

1. a
2. b

3. a
4. c
5. a
6. a
7. c
8. c
9. b
10. b
11. c
12. a
13. b
14. b
15. c
16. a
17. a
18. d

Chapter 19

1. a
2. b
3. d
4. b
5. c
6. d
7. a
8. c
9. a
10. c

Chapter 20

1. c
2. a
3. d
4. b
5. e
6. c
7. e
8. b
9. a
10. b
11. a
12. c
13. d
14. e
15. a
16. b

Chapter 21

1. d
2. c
3. a
4. a
5. a
6. d
7. e
8. c
9. e
10. a
11. d

12. b
13. e
14. d
15. b
16. e
17. d
18. b
19. e
20. e
21. e
22. d
23. d

Chapter 22

1. d
2. c
3. a
4. a
5. c
6. b
7. a
8. d
9. a
10. d
11. d
12. d
13. b
14. b
15. e

Chapter 23

1. b. Increased first-trimester nuchal translucency thickness is a risk factor for congenital heart disease in the fetus. A family history of congenital heart disease in a first-degree relative would also increase this risk.

2. d. If the left side of the fetal heart appears larger than the right side of the fetal heart, further cardiac evaluation is warranted. Normally, the right side of the fetal heart is larger than the left.

3. a. The "twig sign" represents an abnormal pulmonary venous confluence behind the left atrium. This finding suggests total anomalous pulmonary venous return and is not seen in the other listed congenital heart defects.

4. a. Supraventricular tachycardia, particularly when sustained or associated with congenital heart disease, can cause fetal congestive heart failure and hydrops. Conditions with severely regurgitant valves (such as Ebstein anomaly with severe tricuspid regurgitation) and cardiomyopathies are also potential causes. The circulation in HLHS, transposition of the great arteries, and tetralogy of

Fallot with pulmonary atresia, in the absence of confounding factors, is generally well tolerated by the fetus.

5. c. Persistent left-sided superior vena cava, which usually drains to the coronary sinus, can be associated with obstructive left-sided cardiac lesions. This may possibly be a result of a dilated coronary sinus causing reduced inflow through the mitral valve and, subsequently, other left-sided cardiac structures. Coarctation of the aorta is a type of left-sided obstructive lesion.

6. d. In complete atrioventricular canal defect, typical fetal echocardiographic findings include a primum atrial septal defect, inlet ventricular septal defect, and a lack of normal offsetting of the atrioventricular valves, all of which are seen on 4CV. Small membranous ventricular septal defects can readily be missed on 4CV, and evaluation for these defects warrants dedicated imaging with the ultrasound beam perpendicular to the septum.

7. a. Tricuspid valve regurgitation is a typical finding in Ebstein anomaly. Associated findings in more severe cases can include pulmonary hypoplasia, supraventricular tachycardia, and hydrops. Tricuspid valve regurgitation cannot be present in tricuspid atresia, which is characterized by the absence of a patent tricuspid valve orifice.

8. c. HLHS is one of the most severe forms of critical congenital heart disease, requiring prostaglandin infusion for systemic circulation postnatally until the initial surgical intervention (typically performed within the first several days of life). Due to the necessity of early postnatal intervention, as well as a relatively high likelihood of acute circulatory problems, delivery must be planned at a tertiary care center with pediatric cardiology and cardiac surgical expertise. The circulation is generally well tolerated in utero, and emergent delivery by caesarean section for this diagnosis alone is not warranted. Premature delivery appears to confer an increased risk of morbidity and mortality in these patients.

9. a. Valvar aortic stenosis in the fetus has the potential to evolve to HLHS. Fetuses with aortic stenosis require close follow-up by fetal echocardiography for this reason.

10. b. Tetralogy of Fallot with absent pulmonary valve is associated with dilated or aneurysmal branch pulmonary

arteries. The ductus arteriosus is usually absent in this lesion.

11. c. Newborns with D-TGA should be started on prostaglandin postnatally, at least until its necessity can be evaluated with a complete postnatal cardiac evaluation in a highly monitored setting. In cases with a restrictive or intact atrial septum, severe hypoxemia and acidosis can develop rapidly, and emergent balloon atrial septostomy may be required as a rescue measure before the arterial switch operation. While the atrial septum should be evaluated in all fetuses with D-TGA, fetal echocardiography in the current era cannot reliably predict which patients will ultimately require balloon atrial septostomy postnatally. The potential need for this intervention is therefore appropriate to convey during prenatal counseling.

12. b. Truncus arteriosus is highly associated with DiGeorge syndrome (22q11 microdeletion). While a broad range of congenital heart defects can be seen with trisomy 21, the most common are ventricular septal defect and atrioventricular canal defect. Noonan syndrome is associated with pulmonary stenosis and hypertrophic cardiomyopathy. Turner syndrome is associated with coarctation of the aorta and bicuspid aortic valve.

13. a. The description of multiple echogenic, homogeneous, well-circumscribed masses in the ventricles is consistent with cardiac rhabdomyomas. These are seen in tuberous sclerosis.

14. d. Premature atrial contractions represent the most commonly detected type of fetal cardiac arrhythmia and are generally well tolerated. They are usually not associated with other cardiac problems and do not require treatment, even when present in a pattern of bigeminy. There is a low risk of development of associated supraventricular tachycardia, but surveillance/follow-up is prudent.

15. b. Dexamethasone may represent an important approach to prevent progression to complete heart block in fetuses with maternal anti-SSA antibodies and a prolonged mechanical PR interval.

16. c. Ventricular inversion with transposition of the great arteries, also referred to as "congenitally corrected transposition," is commonly associated with abnormalities of the tricuspid valve, a ventricular septal defect, pulmonary stenosis, and/or heart block.

17. b. Flow through the ductus arteriosus is normally right to left in the fetus with normal cardiac anatomy and a normal circulatory pattern. In the presence of severe left-sided obstructive disease, flow through the ductus arteriosus typically remains right to left, with increased flow. In the presence of severe right-sided obstructive disease, the flow through the ductus arteriosus is typically left to right.

18. b. An atrial septal defect in fetal life rarely leads to dilation of the right heart and/or elevation of the ductus arteriosus pulsatility index. Left-sided obstructive lesions such as mitral atresia, however, do result in dilation of the right heart, increased flow through the ductus arteriosus, and an elevated ductus arteriosus pulsatility index.

19. c. Tetralogy of Fallot with absent pulmonary valve commonly presents with cardiomegaly related to severe pulmonary regurgitation. In many cases, the degree of tricuspid regurgitation is sufficient to lead to hydrops. The other defects noted do not typically lead to heart failure or hydrops in the fetus. Atrial bigeminy is well tolerated in the fetus.

20. d. Turner syndrome commonly presents with aortic stenosis and/or coarctation of the aorta, frequently in association with a pleural effusion. The pulsatility index in the ductus arteriosus is elevated because of increased right-sided output in the context of left-sided obstructive lesions. Many affected fetuses with Turner syndrome develop hydrops and suffer fetal demise.

Chapter 24

1. a. Chylous ascites carries the best prognosis for survival. Hydrops and metabolic storage disease are often fatal; urinary ascites can be associated with bladder outlet obstruction, which can lead to bilateral obstructive renal dysplasia and renal failure.

2. b. Duodenal atresia produces the characteristic "double bubble" sign, representing the dilated stomach and fluid-filled proximal duodenum. Esophageal atresia will produce a small or absent stomach bubble; jejunal atresia is suspected with multiple dilated loops of bowel; and an imperforate anus may produce a dilated rectum but is often not detected prenatally.

3. d. With gastroschisis, the abdominal wall defect is typically located to the right of the abdominal cord insertion; left-sided defects are much less common. If the cord passes through the fetal extracorporeal intestinal mass, this is more likely a ruptured omphalocele. If there is bowel located exiting superior to the umbilicus, one should suspect limb body–stalk anomaly.

4. a. The sonographic finding of omphalocele imparts a 40% risk of aneuploidy, with half being trisomy 18. If the omphalocele sac contains only bowel, but *without* liver, this increases the risk of aneuploidy compared with cases where the fetal liver is also extruded into the sac. Giant omphalocele carries a lower risk of aneuploidy; fluid in the omphalocele sac is common and does not change the aneuploidy risk.

5. c. Ovarian cysts can be seen in up to 30% of female neonates, representing normal follicular cyst(s), stimulated by elevated maternal HCG levels. Other cystic abdominal lesions are significantly less common.

6. c. Harmonic imaging enhances sonographic imaging by improving image quality but can overexaggerate the finding of echogenic bowel, with increased edge artifacts. Lower gain and low-frequency transducers decrease image quality and make the sonographic picture darker and perhaps less detailed. While through transmission will improve acoustic quality, it is not expected to produce greater echogenicity of the visualized bowel.

7. b. Polyhydramnios is common in esophageal atresia, with or without TE fistula, because the fetus is unable to efficiently swallow to regulate the amniotic fluid volume. Central nervous system abnormalities (e.g., anencephaly, fetal akinesia conditions) and duodenal atresia can also produce polyhydramnios.

8. c. Bladder outlet obstruction (e.g., posterior urethral valves) can lead to rupture of an overdistended bladder and/or proximal urinary system, leaking urine into the fetal abdomen and producing isolated ascites. Fetal gastroschisis, esophageal atresia, and diaphragmatic hernia are not typically associated with ascites.

9. b. Omphalocele carries a 40% risk of aneuploidy, half of which is due to trisomy 18. Duodenal atresia and esophageal atresia each carry a 30% risk of aneuploidy; the risk of aneuploidy with gastroschisis is low.

10. d. Ectopia cordis (extracorporeal fetal heart) is associated with Pentalogy of Cantrell: omphalocele, diaphragmatic hernia, absent diaphragmatic pericardium, congenital heart anomalies, and inferior sternal defects. The sternal defects can be large enough to produce ectopia cordis.

11. d. The omphalocele diameter-to-abdominal circumference ratio is used to predict the ability to achieve primary closure of the omphalocele. If the omphalocele diameter-to-abdominal circumference ratio is ≥ 0.24, this imparts a seven-fold higher risk that the omphalocele will not be able to be closed primarily.

12. a. The most predictive factor for perinatal mortality with an umbilical vein varix is concomitant abnormalities (including sonographic findings suggestive of aneuploidy). Although turbulent flow within the umbilical vein varix can suggest the need for increased surveillance, and perhaps preterm delivery, these do not have as high a predictive value for perinatal mortality. The finding of an umbilical vein varix should prompt careful fetal sonographic evaluation for other fetal abnormalities.

Chapter 25

1. d. Per the 2014 Multidisciplinary Consensus Statement, renal dilation >4 mm is considered abnormal up to 28 weeks' gestation; after 28 weeks, renal dilation >7 mm is abnormal.

2. a. Only autosomal dominant polycystic kidney disease will produce increased corticomedullary differentiation. Autosomal recessive polycystic kidney disease, obstructed cystic dysplasia, and Meckel-Gruber syndrome produce echogenic kidneys with decreased corticomedullary differentiation.

3. d. Only obstructive cystic dysplasia will produce *smaller* kidney(s), with involution of the damaged nephron units. PKD and Meckel-Gruber syndrome will result in larger kidneys. With autosomal recessive PKD and Meckel-Gruber syndrome, the kidneys are typically *massively* enlarged, filling the fetal abdomen.

4. a. Multicystic dysplastic kidney(s) will produce irregular noncommunicating

cysts within the kidney(s), which appear echolucent. The kidneys are typically enlarged, and the renal parenchyma will have increased echogenicity due to compression by the cysts causing renal dysplasia. If there is advanced bilateral disease, oligohydramnios may be present.

5. a. While both PUVs and MMIHS will produce an enlarged fetal bladder, in contradistinction to posterior urethral valves, polyhydramnios is a prominent feature of MMIHS. The bowel often appears unremarkable (i.e., not echogenic in either condition, and microcolon may not be sonographically evident).

6. b. Ureteroceles are most often associated with renal duplication. While a finding of PUVs is associated with megacystis and bilateral ureteroceles can occasionally cause lower uterine tract obstruction with resultant megacystis, these conditions and pelvic kidney(s) are not typically associated with ureteroceles.

7. c. Bladder exstrophy should be suspected if there is a persistently absent bladder on sonographic imaging, an isoechoic mass inferior to the abdominal cord insertion, and possibly ambiguous genitalia. However, VUR is not associated with bladder exstrophy, as the bladder contents are drained directly into the abdominal cavity, with no back pressure to cause reflux.

8. b. The most common cause of 46,XX ambiguous genitalia is congenital adrenal hyperplasia, which causes virilization of the female genitalia. Approximately 90% of these cases are due to 21-hydroxylase deficiency.

9. b. If MRI detects a uterus, the baby will likely be assigned as a female. "Ovaries" could be undescended testes (cryptorchidism), and a small phallus/clitoris is nondiagnostic. The pubic ramus angle is not helpful in determining gender assignment.

10. c. In general, the upper pole moiety is obstructed and the lower pole moiety is associated with reflux. Obstruction of the ureter from the upper pole moiety entering the bladder results in an ureterocele, and the ureter and upper pole renal pelvis become dilated. Resultant pressure on the renal parenchyma produces cystic renal dysplasia of the upper pole moiety.

11. d. Absent renal arteries on color Doppler imaging is pathognomonic for bilateral renal agenesis. Nonvisualization

of the fetal bladder can be due to bladder exstrophy; empty renal fossae can be due to horseshoe or pelvic kidney(s); and anhydramnios can have multiple other etiologies (e.g., prelabor rupture of membranes, placental insufficiency).

12. c. Fetal ureters are not usually sonographically apparent, unless they are dilated, as with ureterovesical junction obstruction or congenital megaureter. While color Doppler imaging can distinguish a dilated ureter from vascular structures, they cannot identify the ureters per se; fetal urination does not significantly alter the appearance of the fetal ureters.

Chapter 26

1. d. The most common *lethal* skeletal dysplasia is thanatophoric dysplasia (35%), followed by osteogenesis imperfecta type II (25%) and achondrogenesis (7%); collectively, these account for nearly half of all diagnosed skeletal dysplasias.

2. d. Heterozygous achondroplasia accounts for 10% of all skeletal dysplasia and is nonlethal. Rhizomelic dysplasia is also nonlethal but less common. Homozygous achondroplasia appears similar to thanatophoric dysplasia and is lethal, while heterozygous achondrogenesis carriers are typically asymptomatic.

3. a. Rhizomelia affects the proximal bones (femur, humerus); mesomelia alters the intermediate bones (radius, ulna, tibia, fibula); and acromelia involves the distal limbs (hands, feet). Micromelia suggests the entire limb is shortened.

4. b. Approximately 85% of polydactyly is postaxial with an extra digit on the ulnar or fibular side of the distal extremity. Preaxial (13%) and mesoaxial (2%) polydactyly are significantly less common.

5. a. The Ponseti method is the most common initial treatment for clubfoot, with serial casting and abduction bracing. The French physiotherapy method includes initial daily stretching and taping, followed by splinting. Approximately 40% will require subsequent tendon release surgery, regardless of initial treatment. Ambulating on clubfeet, with or without crutches/walker, often perpetuates the clubfoot and worsens long-term prognosis for normal ambulation.

6. d. Only type IV sacrococcygeal teratoma will be entirely contained internally without any external components. Type I–III sacrococcygeal teratomas all have external tumors, with the mass extending internally to the presacral area (type I) or intrapelvic extension (type II) or extending to within the fetal abdomen/pelvis (type III).

7. a. While maternal teratogenic exposures (e.g., medications, pelvic radiation) can produce congenital birth defects, sacral agenesis is more often due to maternal hyperglycemia interrupting growth of pluripotential somatic stem cells at the caudal eminence. Maternal seizure disorder is also associated with an increased risk of congenital birth defects but unlikely to cause sacral agenesis.

8. c. Myeloschisis is the term for an open neural tube defect without any overlying sac. It is generally thought to result from a ruptured myelomeningocele or meningocele sac overlying the open neural tube defect. Myelodysplasia is a form of bone marrow cancer.

9. b. Nonvisualization of the brainstem, fourth ventricle, or cisterna magna on first-trimester imaging is suggestive of a Chiari malformation and would be suspicious for a fetal open neural tube defect (e.g., spina bifida). The brainstem-to–brainstem-to-occipital bone ratio is abnormal if it is *greater* than 1, suggesting the area of the cisterna magna is small or obliterated due to a Chiari malformation. The sonographic findings of lemon sign and cerebral ventriculomegaly seen with open neural tube defects are often not sonographically apparent until later in pregnancy.

10. c. A strawberry-shaped fetal calvarium (flattened occiput and pointed frontal bones) is most often associated with trisomy 18. While brachycephaly can be associated with trisomy 13 and trisomy 21, this finding is relatively nonspecific.

11. d. Sacrococcygeal teratoma is considered to be a "closed" neural tube defect and is unlikely to cause abnormal curvature of the spine. However, disruptions of the fetal spine (open neural tube defect) or fetal torso (body stalk abnormality or amniotic band sequence) can be associated with scoliosis and other abnormal appearance of the fetal spine.

12. b. The umbilical cord is involved with amniotic bands in approximately 30% of cases but accounts for a high risk of perinatal loss (67%) compared with cases without umbilical cord involvement (19%).

Chapter 27

1. b
2. b
3. a
4. c
5. d
6. c
7. b
8. a
9. b
10. d
11. c
12. a

Chapter 28

1. b
2. e
3. e
4. d
5. a
6. e
7. a
8. b
9. c
10. d

Chapter 29

1. b
2. d
3. d
4. c
5. b
6. a
7. b
8. b
9. d
10. c
11. a
12. d
13. d
14. a
15. d
16. c
17. c
18. b
19. d
20. d

Chapter 30

1. b
2. c

3. d
4. c
5. a
6. d
7. b
8. a
9. c
10. e
11. b
12. d
13. a
14. d
15. e
16. b
17. b
18. e
19. d
20. c

Chapter 31

1. b
2. c
3. e
4. c
5. c
6. d
7. d
8. b
9. d
10. c
11. a
12. d
13. c
14. d
15. d
16. e
17. e
18. c
19. d
20. a
21. a
22. e
23. d

Chapter 32

1. c
2. d
3. c
4. a
5. c
6. e
7. a
8. e
9. e
10. c

Chapter 33

1. b. The fetal heart, like the adult heart, has intrinsic pacemaker activity via the

sinoatrial node, atrioventricular node, and His-Purkinje system. A fetus with complete heart block will have a fetal heart rate of 60–80 beats/min.
2. c. The vagus nerve is responsible for transmission of impulses causing beat-to-beat variability. Tonic influence of the vagus nerve would cause a decrease, not an increase, in the FHR. Oscillatory influence of the vagus nerve results in variability. A persistent blockade of this influence eliminates variability but does not cause decelerations.
3. c. The mean arterial pressure of the mother is 100 mm Hg. The spiral arteries reduce this pressure to 70 mm Hg. The fetal mean arterial pressure is approximately 55 mm Hg. The intervillous space has a mean arterial pressure of approximately 10 mm Hg, gently bathing the chorionic villi with maternal blood.
4. a. The fetal scalp electrode measures the R wave directly on the fetal electrocardiogram, giving the most accurate FHR tracing and the true beat-to-beat variability.
5. a. Hypoxemia or acidemia of a previously healthy fetus, leads to redistribution of blood flow favoring vital organs (brain, heart, adrenal glands). This response allows fetus to survive up to 30 minutes with a limited oxygen supply without compromise or decompensation.
6. a. Cord compression, as in cord prolapse, decreases the umbilical cord perfusion. This leads to increase fetal levels of carbon dioxide and decreased levels of oxygen, leading to respiratory acidosis.
7. a. A low pH is a more prognostic factor for adverse neonatal outcomes. Even more than base deficit in depressed neonates at birth. Low arterial cord pH correlated to neonatal mortality and composite morbidity, as well as long-term outcomes such as cerebral palsy as studied by Yeh P et al.
8. e. Therapeutic hypothermia is generally initiated in near-term infants (>36 weeks' gestation) for management of neonatal encephalopathy resulting from acidemia if they are within 6 hours of delivery and meet 1 of the following criteria: umbilical cord pH of <7.0, base excess >16 mMol/L, or moderate to severe encephalopathy on clinical examination.
9. e. The ACOG, Royal College of Obstetricians and Gynecologists, and Royal College of Midwives recommend

routine cord blood measurements for all cesarean deliveries and instrumented deliveries for "fetal distress." In addition, the ACOG recommends cord blood measurements for low 5-minute Apgar score, severe fetal growth restriction, abnormal fetal heart tracing, maternal thyroid disease, multifetal gestation, and intrapartum fever.

10. c. Fetal hypoxia is associated with decreased or absent fetal heart rate variability. In addition, nonhypoxic causes of decreased or absent FHR variability include anencephaly, narcotized or drugged higher cerebral centers, and a vagal blockade defective cardiac conduction system.

Chapter 34

1. c. Diagnosis of TTTS is based on amniotic fluid level volume and bladder size discrepancies among between monochorionic twins. According to Quintero staging, this patient would be considered stage 3 given polyhydramnios in the recipient and oligohydramnios in the donor twin, absence of a bladder in donor twin, and abnormal Doppler values.
2. b. During open fetal surgery procedures, hysterotomies are performed to expose the fetus. This precludes patients from a trial of labor given increased risks of uterine rupture, and delivery should take place at 37 weeks unless indications arise earlier.
3. c. After congenital diaphragmatic hernia is diagnosed, the first goal is to exclude additional abnormalities including via genetic analyses and detailed imaging of the fetal structures which can occur are present in 30% to 40% of cases.
4. c. In a recent meta-analysis review of conservative management versus interventions for twin reversed arterial perfusion sequence, the authors found that intervention using either cord occlusion or ablation conferred a better survival rate compared with conservative management.
5. d. Conservative management seems justified as there is no progressive deterioration, and Doppler studies are normal when taking the contralateral side as a reference.
6. a. The most important limiting factor for survival of neonates born with congenital diaphragmatic hernia is the inability to ventilate patients with severe lung hypoplasia.

7. a. Tumor hemorrhage and arteriovenous shunting leading to circulatory failure remain the largest contributors to mortality. In one study, hemorrhagic mortality represented 70% of the overall mortality in the neonatal period.
8. a. This statement is accurate. Overall, the survival rate for both twins after laser photocoagulation for TTTS is approximately 67%.
9. c. On the basis of ultrasonographic findings, this pregnancy does not meet criteria for TTTS (twin A's fluid is normal), even though oligohydramnios and abnormal umbilical artery Dopplers are present. These findings are also commonly encountered as the result of severe fetal growth restriction.
10. c. This statement is accurate. None of the studies done in animals and humans have shown teratogenic effects when given at usual clinical doses. In multiple animal models, neonatal exposure to anesthetics is associated with persistent learning deficits. Yet it remains to be seen whether similar effects are experienced by human fetuses and later children.

Chapter 35

1. c
2. a
3. c
4. b
5. a
6. c
7. a
8. c
9. b
10. b
11. d
12. d
13. c
14. c
15. b
16. a
17. b

Chapter 36

1. a
2. b
3. d
4. d
5. b
6. d
7. b
8. d
9. d

10. b
11. c
12. d
13. d
14. d
15. c
16. d

Chapter 37

1. b
2. a
3. d
4. a
5. a
6. e
7. a
8. c
9. d
10. e
11. c
12. b
13. a
14. c
15. c

Chapter 38

1. b
2. a
3. b
4. c
5. c
6. c
7. d
8. a
9. a
10. a

Chapter 39

1. b
2. d
3. a
4. c
5. b
6. c
7. d
8. d
9. a

Chapter 40

1. b. Labor progression in the 21st century is different than that described by Friedman et al. More conservative definitions for active labor help counsel patients and reduce the rate of cesarean deliveries. Active labor begins when the rate of cervical dilation begins to change more rapidly, but it may not be abrupt especially in

nulliparous women. In multiparous patients, the inflection point is at 5–5.5 cm, with the 5th percentile for rate of dilation as <1 cm/hr. The average length of the active phase, as described by Zhang's group, was 5.5 hours compared to 2.5 hours in Friedman's labor curves.

2. d. This patient is experiencing a prolonged latent phase, which is defined as >12 hours for nulliparous patients. Due to the patient's discomfort in the setting of a reported history of regular contractions, it is not reasonable to discharge to home without offering an intervention. Similarly, reassessing in 2 hours without an intervention prolongs the patient's discomfort. Since this patient's gestational age is less than 39 weeks and she does not have a medical indication for induction of labor, it would not be reasonable to induce her labor, and offering an epidural for labor analgesia without another initial intervention could lead to iatrogenic intervention. Either augmentation of labor with oxytocin or therapeutic narcosis can result in the resumption of normal cervical dilation. One regimen for therapeutic narcosis is morphine sulfate 15-20 mg, with an additional 10-15 mg if the patient does not become somnolent.

3. a. The 95th percentile for expected time to dilate from 6 to 7 cm is 1.8 hours for nulliparas and 1.2 hours for multiparas. Therefore, since cervical dilation has remained unchanged for more than 2 hours in this patient, intervention is recommended to address this protraction disorder. In the presence of oxytocin augmentation, the patient would meet criteria for arrest of descent if there has been no cervical change for more than 4 hours with a sustained contraction pattern of greater than 200 Montevideo units, or for more than 6 hours if a contraction pattern of greater than 200 Montevideo units cannot be sustained. Placement of an intrauterine pressure catheter would not be indicated without first titrating pitocin. However, on the subsequent cervical check, if no further cervical change, placement of an intrauterine pressure catheter would be warranted to measure Montevideo units.

4. d. Risk factors for shoulder dystocia include prolonged second stage of labor, as well as fetal macrosomia, diabetes, and a history of shoulder dystocia in a previous birth. Prolonged second stage has also been associated with perinatal mortality in deliveries without an epidural, as well as admission to the neonatal intensive care unit (NICU) and composite serious neonatal morbidity. However, none of the other choices are independently associated with a prolonged second stage. Maternal risks include chorioamnionitis, severe perineal lacerations, uterine atony, and blood transfusion.

5. b. A shoulder dystocia is considered an obstetric emergency. Use of any maneuvers is most successfully employed only after making an overt announcement of the diagnosis and implementing a coordinated team approach to management. McRobert's maneuver is conventionally the first maneuver, following which all other maneuvers are employed. Suprapubic pressure oriented over the posterior aspect of the anterior fetal shoulder can be used in conjunction with McRobert's, after which Rubin, Woods, or delivery of the posterior arm can be attempted. Although not done routinely, if perineal soft tissues limit the feasibility of these maneuvers, an episiotomy can be considered.

6. c. Risk factors for retained placenta include maternal age >30 years, preterm delivery between 24 weeks 0 days and 26 weeks 6 days compared with delivery after 34 weeks 0 days, and stillbirth. Placenta accreta is a rare cause of retained placenta and can be a cause of postpartum hemorrhage, but this patient does not have risk factors for placenta accreta, the manual removal does not appear to have been technically difficult, and the placenta appears intact.

7. b. The accepted definition for failed induction of labor requires an attempt at both oxytocin administration and artificial or spontaneous rupture of membranes prior to diagnosis. Cervical ripening alone is insufficient to meet this diagnosis, and cesarean delivery following induction of labor should be classified by the most precise terminology, including but not limited to failed induction of labor, arrest of dilation, arrest of descent, or nonreassuring fetal status. There is some data to show that the presence of fetal fibronectin (fFN) in cervical and vaginal secretions is a means for predicting the success of induction of labor, but it is not widely practiced and the absence of fFN does not predict nor diagnose failure. Conservatively diagnosis failed induction is central to a strategy to decrease the nulliparous, term, singleton, vertex (NTSV) cesarean birth rate.

8. e. If induction of labor occurs prior to term or prior to when delivery would be medically indicated, it increases the chance of neonatal surfactant deficiency. Additionally, normal parturition is associated with a decrease in fetal lung fluid. If induction is pursued instead, "wet lung syndrome" can exacerbate respiratory morbidity and, if severe, can be associated with persistence of fetal circulation and need for mechanical ventilation in the neonate. Gestational age is most accurate when based on objective data and data obtained before 20 weeks'.

9. b. This patient has fetal malpresentation as well as oligohydramnios, defined by maximum vertical pocket <2 cm. If persistent, this is a contraindication to external cephalic version for breech presentation. There are no randomized trials for route of delivery in preterm patients with breech presentation; therefore, offering induction of labor at this gestational age would not be evidence-based and, moreover, induction with oxytocin has been associated with increased perinatal death among planned breech vaginal deliveries. Additionally, oligohydramnios is a medical indication for preterm delivery between 36 weeks 0 days gestation and 37 weeks 6 days gestation, so cesarean delivery within this range of gestational ages would be the best recommendation.

10. e. All of the choices aside from choice (e) are criteria for allowing a trial of labor in a breech presentation. An extended fetal head is a contraindication to vaginal delivery.

11. b. While suspected fetal macrosomia has been associated with decreased success of external cephalic version, it is not a contraindication. Of note, obvious cephalopelvic disproportion is a contraindication to this procedure. Other factors associated with reduced success include primiparity, maternal obesity, advanced gestation, and anterior implantation of the placenta. The overall success rate of external version is 65%, and the risk

of cesarean delivery is reduced by 50% among patients undergoing external version for breech presentation at 36 weeks.

12. e. Intravenous analgesia may be associated with sedation and/or overdose. If excessive sedation with respiratory depression is noted in either patient or neonate, naloxone may be administered as an opioid antagonist. Options include fentanyl, remifentanil, meperidine, butorphanol, and nalbuphine. Shorter acting narcotics are preferred to decrease neonatal sedation. Epidural anesthesia is also more likely to provide effective analgesia than parenteral agents.

13. b. Vacuum extraction should not be performed prior to 34 weeks of gestation because of the risk of fetal intraventricular hemorrhage. All of the other answers are contraindications to both forceps deliveries and vacuum extractions.

14. e. Cesarean delivery has been associated with increased respiratory morbidity at all gestational ages, and risk is higher in prelabor cesarean compared with patient who are delivered by cesarean during labor. In nulliparous women, forceps-assisted vaginal delivery was associated with decreased postpartum hemorrhage; vacuum extraction was associated with decreased endometritis; and both routes had lower wound complications compared to cesarean delivery. However, both forceps and vacuum were associated with increased cervical/sulcal lacerations. Multiparous patients had a decreased overall composite morbidity and blood transfusion compared to cesarean delivery. For nullipara neonatal outcomes, forceps-assisted vaginal delivery had a decreased overall composite, lower sepsis, and respiratory morbidity; both forceps and vacuum deliveries had less neonatal ICU admissions. In multiparous forceps-assisted vaginal deliveries only, neonatal birth trauma was less than cesarean deliveries.

15. d. In a large meta-analysis of patients undergoing trial of labor after cesarean, the intended route of delivery, the presence of an unknown type of scar, and the use of oxytocin made no difference in the rate of uterine wound dehiscence. The study also showed that maternal febrile morbidity was lower after a trial of labor than after an elective repeat cesarean, and

the odds of perinatal death was higher in patients with a trial of labor compared to elective repeat cesarean (OR 2.1, CI 1.3-3.4).

Chapter 41

1. c
2. b
3. a
4. c
5. b
6. d
7. d
8. a
9. c
10. a

Chapter 42

1. e
2. c
3. d
4. a
5. b
6. b
7. d
8. e
9. c
10. e

Chapter 43

1. d. In 80% of bleeding occurring in the second half of pregnancy, early labor, or local lesion of the lower tract or no source identified.

2. b. Transabdominal ultrasound has been shown to be inferior to transvaginal ultrasound for definitive placental localization.

3. b. Placenta accreta is suspected on ultrasound when there is loss of normal hypoechoic boundary between bladder wall and uterus, increased vascularity in the placenta-uterus interface, sonolucencies, or lacuna in the placenta. A normal placenta is homogeneous in appearance.

4. a. Placenta accreta is suspected on ultrasound when there is loss of normal hypoechoic boundary between bladder wall and uterus, increased vascularity in the placenta-uterus interface, sonolucencies, or lacuna in the placenta. The timing of elective delivery via cesarean hysterectomy is usually between 34 and 36 weeks.

5. c. Vaginal bleeding followed by fetal distress is common in vasa previa. A risk factor for vasa previa is velamentous cord insertion. Because all the

fetal cardiac output passes through the cord, it can take less than 10 minutes for fetal exsanguination.

6. d. The Society of Maternal Fetal Medicine recommends delivery of patients with vasa previa between 34 and 35 weeks.

7. d. In large retrospective studies and meta-analysis, subchorionic hemorrhage is associated with spontaneous abortion, abruption, and preterm delivery.

8. e. Known risk factors for placental abruption include prior history, which increases the risk 20-fold. Hypertension and preeclampsia are also risk factors, while smoking is one modifiable risk factor. Multiple retrospective and prospective studies have shown no increased risk of abruption with factor V Leiden mutation.

9. b. Risk factors for placental abruption including smoking and hypertension. Abruption is commonly accompanied by uterine contractions. A Kleihauer-Betke test is of no diagnostic value in abruption.

10. d. Coagulopathy develops in 10% of placenta abruptions and is related to severity of event, massive hemorrhage, and fetal demise.

Chapter 44

1. c
2. b
3. d
4. c
5. e
6. c
7. c
8. b
9. e
10. b
11. d
12. d
13. b
14. d
15. e
16. a
17. c
18. e
19. d
20. a

Chapter 45

1. a
2. c
3. b
4. d
5. a
6. c

7. d
8. b
9. a
10. b
11. c
12. b
13. a
14. d

Chapter 46

1. b
2. a
3. c
4. b
5. b
6. d
7. a
8. a
9. d
10. c
11. c
12. d
13. a
14. b
15. b

Chapter 47

1. d
2. c
3. a
4. a
5. c
6. c
7. b
8. c
9. a
10. b

Chapter 48

1. e
2. b
3. a
4. a
5. c
6. d
7. d
8. b
9. c
10. e
11. d
12. b
13. a
14. c
15. c
16. b
17. a
18. b
19. d
20. b

Chapter 49

1. d. Chikungunya. Symptomatic illness occurs in 72%−97% of infected individuals, whereas in the other infections asymptomatic infections are more commonly observed than symptomatic disease.

2. e. Parvovirus B19 disease. When the classic lacy, reticular rash appears in Parvovirus B19 disease, the infection has already resolved and there is no further risk of transmission. The rash in all other conditions is present when individuals are infectious.

3. d. <1%. Women with an undetectable serum HIV virus load on established antiretroviral therapy have a vertical transmission risk of <1%. Although the risk is minimal, it is not considered to be zero. In 1994, an 8% transmission risk was reported in the PACTG 076 trial in the arm that received Zidovudine during pregnancy as an infusion during labor to the mother and with postexposure prophylaxis to the infant versus 25% risk of transmission observed in the placebo arm of that early study. Forty percent risk of transmission is an estimate of the risk of an infant acquiring HIV infection from an untreated mother combining risks accruing in utero, intrapartum, and 12 months of breastfeeding with no maternal treatment.

4. d. Ganciclovir IV. The infant has clinical findings consistent with symptomatic congenital CMV infection. Given the severe manifestations of disease, treatment should be initiated intravenously with ganciclovir.

5. b. Rubella. Vertical transmission of rubella virus causing congenital rubella syndrome is unlikely beyond 20 weeks of gestation. Varicella, HSV-2, Chikungunya, and HIV can be transmitted late in pregnancy at the time of labor and delivery.

6. c. HSV-2. Vertical transmission of both HSV-1 and HSV-2 to the infant can cause disseminated disease in the infant, which is clinically indistinguishable from bacterial sepsis. Infants with perinatally acquired HIV or Hepatitis C are asymptomatic at birth. Congenital rubella syndrome has clinical features that are distinct from neonatal sepsis. Neonates of mothers with Parvovirus B19 do not present with a sepsis-like picture at birth.

7. d. Rubella. Infants with congenital rubella syndrome often present with congenital heart defects.

8. a. CMV. Congenital cytomegalovirus is the most common infectious cause of sensorineural hearing loss in infants and young children. Rubella can also cause sensorineural hearing loss; however, it is no longer common due to global immunization efforts. The other infections are not associated with sensorineural hearing loss.

9. b. Chikungunya. CMV and West Nile virus have both been associated with neonatal microcephaly cases in the United States. Zika virus can cause microcephaly in a woman who never went to an endemic area through infection of her spouse and sexual transmission to a pregnant mother with transmission of the virus to the infant. Chikungunya is not likely to cause microcephaly, not a virus that circulates in the United States, and not sexually transmissible.

10. d. Varicella. Infants with congenital varicella virus no longer shed the virus at birth, as the infection is resolved by the time they are delivered. All other viruses can be identified early in neonatal life in congenitally infected infants.

11. d. The influenza vaccine is safe during any trimester. The safety of the influenza vaccine is well established and safe at any time during pregnancy.

12. d. Nasopharyngeal RT-PCR. Nasal midturbinate or anterior nasal swab PCR is also acceptable. The sensitivity of the antigen test is lower than both rapid and laboratory-based nucleic acid amplification tests, so a negative result should be interpreted with caution. Serologic testing (IgM and IgG) can be used to identify past infections.

13. d. 90%. While Ebola has a reputation for being highly contagious, the basic reproductive number is estimated to be as low as 2, and the household attack rate is approximately 15%. The risk of maternal mortality is estimated to be as high as 90% without treatment, although 28-day mortality dropped to 35% in a randomized clinical trial with Ebanga, which included pregnant women. The risk of perinatal mortality is approximately 100%.

14. a. 6 and 11. LR-HPV genotypes 6 and 11 are largely responsible for respiratory papillomatosis (laryngeal papilloma). HR-HPV genotypes 16 and 18 cause the majority of cervical cancer cases in the United States.

15. a. Spontaneous abortion. Increased rates of atrial septal defects, neural tube defects, and fetal growth restriction have not been reported with mumps infection in the first trimester.

Chapter 50

1. b
2. d
3. c
4. b
5. b
6. b
7. c
8. e
9. c
10. c
11. a
12. e
13. b
14. c
15. d
16. d

Chapter 51

1. a. Rubella immunity is lifelong. Second infections are not associated with congenital infection or evidence of clinical disease. This is the reason that vaccination campaigns have greatly reduced or eliminated congenital infection. GBS is associated with clinical disease no matter which infection or colonization has occurred. Both *T. gondii* and CMV have been demonstrated to have disease with reinfection. *T. pallidum* reinfection is associated with maternal and congenital infection.

2. e. The data on antibody avidity and likelihood of primary versus recurrent infection have only been demonstrated to be useful in the setting of IgG and IgM positive serologies. IgM can be positive with both primary and recurrent infection or reactivation.

3. a. Early treatment (<3 weeks from seroconversion) of *T. gondii* has been demonstrated to be marginally protective against fetal transmission. In areas where serologic screening occurs routinely or in patients with a known exposure (e.g., veterinarians), treatment should begin early to prevent congenital infection.

4. a. One of the primary medications for *T. gondii* is pyrimethamine, which is teratogenic. Thus spiramycin is preferred earlier in pregnancy, and

the treatment medication regimen is dependent on gestational age.

5. b. The best studies estimate 2%–7% risk of Congenital Zika syndrome with maternal ZIKV infection. This did not include miscarriages and terminations, so it is likely an underestimate; thus, 5%–10% is the best answer. The incidence of microcephaly is 3%.

6. c. All herpesviruses including varicella zoster virus, herpes simplex viruses, and cytomegalovirus have an acute infection followed by latency. These viruses can all reactivate (recurrent herpes outbreaks, zoster or shingles, and CMV reactivation).

7. b. Of the answers, IgM positive, IgG positive and IgG low avidity is the best answer. IgG positivity with IgM negativity represents a history of infection, and avidity testing is not indicated (answers a, e, and g). Although serum PCR is the gold standard for diagnosis of CMV infection, it can be positive with reactivation or recurrent infection (c). A positive amniocentesis (d) is suggestive of congenital infection but not maternal primary infection and can occur with reactivation.

8. d. The measles, mumps, and rubella vaccine is not recommended in pregnancy because the vaccine contains live attenuated rubella virus and there are concerns for potential teratogenicity. Influenza, TdaP, and severe acute respiratory syndrome–coronavirus 2 vaccination are recommended in pregnancy. Although the Yellow fever vaccine is live, there has been no adverse risk demonstrated with administration. If a patient is traveling to an endemic area, vaccination should be considered. The hepatitis B vaccine is recommended in some circumstances in pregnancy.

9. c. Parvovirus B-19, *T. gondii* and varicella are not shed in the lower reproductive tract and are vertically acquired only with transplacental transmission.

10. a. The P antigen or globoside protein is on the surface of the syncytiotrophoblast, as well as erythrocyte precursors, and is the primary mechanism of parvovirus B19 binding for viral entry.

11. a. Parvovirus B-19 causes anemia and cardiogenic hydrops from severe anemia by destroying the erythrocyte precursors on fetal bone marrow. GBS and *E. coli* are associated with prematurity, stillbirth, and early- and

late-onset neonatal sepsis but not hydrops. Listeria infection is associated with pregnancy loss (miscarriage, stillbirth) and preterm delivery. Varicella is more classically associated with congenital varicella syndrome. Other pathogens associated with hydrops include CMV and *T. pallidum*.

12. c.

13. e. Thrombocytopenia in a PUBS sampling at the time of IUT has been correlated to severity of bone marrow suppression and disease. Fetuses with severe thrombocytopenia have been demonstrated to have a worse prognosis. MCA Dopplers, not umbilical cord or umbilical artery Dopplers, can estimate fetal anemia and need for PUBS/IUT. The level of viremia or avidity has not been demonstrated to have prognostic value.

14. d. With the implementation of intrapartum GBS prophylaxis, *E. coli* has surpassed GBS as the major cause of EOS.

15. c. *L. monocytogenes* can be acquired vertically through transplacental transmission but is not considered teratogenic. The other pathogens including Zika virus, cytomegalovirus, *T. gondii* and *T. pallidum* are considered teratogenic.

16. c. Transplanted organs and their recipients are routinely typed for CMV and *T. gondii*. Both can cause disease in immunosuppressed individuals, and mismatching is important to recognize. With pregnancy in a transplant patient, knowing this typing is important for understanding perinatal risk of acquisition and exposure to these pathogens.

17. d. Placental listeriosis is characterized by abscess development. Both microabscesses and macroabscesses have been described. The other pathologic findings are not consistent with *L. monocytogenes* infection.

18. d. This patient is either susceptible for infection or has an acute infection. Repeat serologies can be considered if the IgM comes back negative in 1 week, but 8 weeks is too long. Amniocentesis or cordocentesis can be considered for congenital infection but is invasive and MCA Doppler is a noninvasive way to evaluate for fetal risk from infection.

19. b. Both *L. monocytogenes* and *T. gondii* can be transmitted through contaminated food. Classically, *L. monocytogenes* is transmitted through unpasteurized

cheeses or with epidemic outbreaks. *T. gondii* is present in undercooked meat and can be present in high amounts in some game meats.

20. b. GBS culture should be sent in women who present at 36 weeks with a beta-lactam allergy. Antibiotic sensitivities cannot be performed by PCR. Routine intrapartum prophylaxis with vancomycin is not recommended. If the isolate is clindamycin sensitive, then clindamycin is preferred over vancomycin for intrapartum prophylaxis. The question does not indicate if this is a high- or low-risk allergy and would need additional information to determine if she is a candidate for allergy testing or if cefazolin should be used. There are no data that antepartum antibiotic use decreases the incidence of EOS.

21. d. Women with a travel exposure without ongoing exposure and no symptoms are not recommended to have routine testing and can have consideration of testing after discussion with a provider. The likelihood of a positive result is low in this scenario. An ultrasound and amniocentesis are not indicated.

22. a. Women with ongoing, recurrent exposure to endemic areas should have testing three times during pregnancy including at presentation to care. Testing subtypes are evolving, but either subtype is a reasonable approach for testing. After the initial pandemic, ongoing circulating ZIKV has declined, making it unnecessary to perform an amniocentesis or ultrasound. A detailed discussion might be helpful for the patient but is not required for testing in this scenario.

23. c. CMV is the most common congenitally acquired infection. It can cause these ultrasound findings and is thus the most likely infectious cause of the options listed.

Chapter 52

1. d. This is a common finding in pregnancy, as the heart is moved somewhat leftward as the uterine size increases. PACs are relatively common during pregnancy.

2. b. Elective cesarean section is not generally recommended for women with history of obstructive hypertrophic cardiomyopathy during labor.

3. c. There is no evidence of Eisenmenger physiology. The PDA must be closed in the future, but this is not urgent.

4. a. ASD: excessive *flow* into the right heart is present with ASD, but excessive *pressure* and flow into the right ventricle (VSD) and pulmonary arteries (PDA) are not generally present. The risk of developing irreversible pulmonary hypertension with ASD is low in childbearing age.

5. b. Genetic testing for Marfan is reasonable (though will likely be negative). Assessment of the aortic valve area and ascending aortic diameter can be measured with echocardiography, which would eliminate the radiograph and contrast exposure with a chest CT scan.

6. e. All of these factors can contribute to neonatal events.

7. c. Novel oral anticoagulants (NOACs) are currently contraindicated during pregnancy with a mechanical valve, as is the combination of aspirin and clopidogrel. Enoxaparin can be used later in pregnancy, but at this point in her pregnancy, warfarin remains the medication of choice.

8. b. Hydrochlorothiazide is usually well tolerated; the other medications should be avoided during pregnancy.

9. a. Moderate to severe mitral stenosis can lead to significant pulmonary hypertension as pregnancy proceeds and cardiac output increases.

10. d. The patient is at moderate risk for coronary disease given her familial hypercholesterolemia and chest pain (though it is not classic for angina). Coronary CT scan and coronary angiography would expose the patient to intravenous contrast, which could worsen renal dysfunction. Exercise echo or nuclear scans are more accurate than exercise ECG tests and do not worsen renal function.

11. c. The patient most likely has SCAD. Coronary angiography can worsen the dissection, so it may not be the best diagnostic test (especially when the patient is responding to medical treatment). Nuclear perfusion and echocardiography can assess for ischemia but do not adequately image the coronary arteries.

12. a. Younger women are less likely to develop PPCM than older women (especially older women with multifetal pregnancies).

13. d. Moderate to severe aortic regurgitation, unless acute, is generally tolerated well.

Chapter 53

1. c. All three components of the triad, including hypercoagulability, venous stasis, and tissue injury increase during pregnancy, contributing to an increased VTE risk.

2. c

3. c. Higher levels of factors VII, VIII, and X, fibrinogen, and von Willebrand factor.

4. d. Reduced activity of protein S and increased resistance to activated protein C.

5. b. Any of: positive test for lupus anticoagulant, moderate-high positive levels of IgG or IgM anticardiolipin antibodies, or moderate-high positive levels of anti-beta-2-glycoprotein-I antibodies on two occasions 12 weeks apart.

6. a. There is no evidence that any treatment improves outcome in such individuals. APS requires both specific clinical features and confirmatory laboratory testing. Clinical features include three or more unexplained early pregnancy losses. Treatment in this case is not supported by evidence and would be considered experimental.

7. d. The appropriate treatment would be full anticoagulant doses of LMWH and low-dose aspirin through pregnancy and 6 weeks postpartum. This individual may qualify for life-long anticoagulation. Hydroxychloroquine may prove to be useful as well.

8. a

9. c

10. a. LMWH has not been shown to improve pregnancy outcomes in individuals with any thrombophilia. Anticoagulation may be appropriate to decrease risk of VTE but should not be used to improve pregnancy outcomes.

11. c. Incidental thrombocytopenia of pregnancy is common, occurs in up to 5% of pregnant people, and accounts for more than 70% of maternal thrombocytopenia. It is mild (>70,000 platelets/μL), asymptomatic, and often first observed by the clinician after a complete blood cell count (CBC) is obtained as part of a routine automated prenatal screening test.

12. d. The main treatments are corticosteroids and IVIG. Platelet transfusion is reserved for bleeding, surgery, and neuraxial anesthesia. Rarely, splenectomy, immunosuppressive drugs, and biologics may be used in refractory cases.

13. c. It is difficult to distinguish TTP from other conditions associated with thrombocytopenia such as aHUS and HELLP syndrome. TTP involves thrombocytopenia and hemolytic anemia, as do the other conditions. The most reliable test is decreased levels of ADAMTS13 activity (<20%). However, this test may take several days to obtain results. Platelets are very low and may be associated with purpura. LDH is elevated, there are usually neurologic symptoms, and there is not typically proteinuria.

14. c. Plasmapheresis is the gold standard treatment for TTP and has dramatically improved survival. Corticosteroids or other immunosuppressive therapy may be useful, and cytotoxic immunosuppressive agents are considered in refractory cases. Platelet transfusion should be AVOIDED because they may precipitate the disease. Delivery should be considered in refractory cases, if HELLP is possible, and at later gestational ages.

Chapter 54

1. d
2. a
3. c
4. b
5. c
6. e
7. a
8. c
9. a
10. d

Chapter 55

1. a
2. c
3. d
4. b
5. b
6. b
7. e
8. d
9. e
10. a
11. c
12. d
13. a
14. b
15. a
16. a
17. e
18. d
19. a
20. a

Chapter 56

1. b. IR-guided biopsy of an adnexal mass is not recommended. This may result in pathologic upstaging, and the sample may not be representative of the entire mass. Additional imaging and tumor markers may help to better define this mass and provide a baseline for tumor markers if malignancy is diagnosed. Surgical intervention is ideally timed for early second trimester.

2. a. Germ cell tumors are the most common ovarian cancers diagnosed in pregnancy. The incidence of sex cord stromal tumors and epithelial ovarian cancer in pregnancy is low.

3. d. Cervical biopsy is safe and accurate in pregnancy. A visible lesion warrants a diagnostic test to rule out malignancy. Cervical biopsy is safer and less invasive than conization. A Pap test is a screening test. Magnetic resonance imaging would be appropriate for further characterization if malignancy is diagnosed.

4. f. If the patient were not pregnant or this were not a desired pregnancy, immediate definitive therapy would be recommended with radical surgery or definitive chemoradiation. Though data are limited, delays in definitive therapy between 3 and 32 weeks to allow for pregnancy continuation did not result in significantly worse outcomes than expected. Thus, if this is a desired pregnancy, a detailed anatomy scan and aneuploidy screening, as well as consultation with maternal fetal medicine, would be recommended. Given the size of the tumor, we would recommend neoadjuvant chemotherapy with definitive therapy either at the time of delivery or shortly thereafter (~6 weeks). Vaginal delivery would not be recommended in a patient with cervical cancer due to potential for bleeding and/or seeding of vaginal/perineal lacerations.

5. b. The most commonly associated complications of cytotoxic chemotherapy in pregnancy include intrauterine growth restriction, low birth weight, and preterm delivery (often iatrogenic). Oligohydramnios is less common with cytotoxic chemotherapy, though it has been associated with use of trastuzumab in pregnancy. Cardiac anomalies/neurocognitive delay/limb defects

are not thought to be significantly associated with chemotherapy in the second and third trimesters.

6. c. Tocolytics in the second trimester have not been shown to decrease the risk of pregnancy complications after abdominal surgery.

7. a. Evaluation of a suspicious breast mass should not be delayed due to pregnancy. Imaging with mammogram or ultrasound would be an appropriate first step in the evaluation.

8. d. Delivery before 37 weeks has been associated with worsened neonatal outcomes and has not been shown to improve maternal outcomes in most settings. Chemotherapy in the second and third trimesters is associated with intrauterine growth restriction/low birth weight, and thus monitoring growth with serial ultrasounds is recommended. Chemotherapy should be held 3−4 weeks before planned delivery to avoid significant myelosuppression in the mother/neonate, which may increase risk of infection/bleeding. Patients should be counseled NOT to breastfeed while receiving chemotherapy.

9. a. Melanoma is the most common malignancy to metastasize to the placenta. The placenta should be sent to pathology for evaluation for any patient with a history of melanoma.

10. c. This patient's history is concerning for colon cancer. Colon cancer in pregnancy is associated with a poor prognosis, in part owing to delayed diagnosis. Though pregnancy is generally a relative contraindication to colonoscopy, a history like this warrants immediate investigation.

11. c. Delays in treatment portend a worse prognosis. For patients with apparently localized disease before gestational viability, surgical resection would be recommended.

12. b. A firm and immobile mass is concerning for malignancy. Fine-needle aspiration is less accurate than excisional or core biopsy, so this would be the next best step. Additional imaging would be based on the results of the excisional/core biopsy. Delaying workup until completion of pregnancy would not be recommended. Antibiotic therapy is not indicated in this setting.

13. c. Chemotherapy in the first trimester is associated with congenital anomalies and pregnancy loss. In the absence of respiratory compromise or

severe B symptoms, chemotherapy may be deferred until after the first trimester to minimize the risk for teratogenicity.

14. a. Rituximab is an anti-CD20 monoclonal antibody that targets malignant and normal B cells bearing CD20. This agent can deplete normal B cells in treated patients for 3−6 months, and this effect may persist in infants after birth for up to 4 months.

15. c. Nilotinib is an oral tyrosine kinase inhibitor. These agents are teratogenic, and while data are sparse, severe fetal malformations have been reported. Thus, in this setting, observation off therapy for CML is appropriate.

Chapter 57

1. a. Ovarian hyperstimulation syndrome (OHSS) is most likely to result in acute renal failure in pregnancy; this condition typically occurs in the early aspect of pregnancy after stimulation by exogenous hormones given for fertility purposes. The acute renal failure is typically secondary to a prerenal etiology from vascular permeability (third spacing).

2. d. The majority of patients who become pregnant after autologous donation of a kidney have normal renal function and an unremarkable pregnancy outcome. Some studies show an increased risk of preeclampsia compared with the baseline population; however, the majority of patients do not develop gestational hypertension or preeclampsia.

3. d. Mycophenolate mofetil is teratogenic; the benefits of the medication do not outweigh the known association of fetal birth defects including oral cleft, congenital heart defect, tracheoesophageal malformations, dysmorphic facial features, conductive deafness, and microtia/anotia. The other medications may be used in pregnancy for patients who need immunosuppression for their kidney transplant; these medications do not have the known association of teratogenicity that mycophenolate mofetil has.

4. a. A multidisciplinary team ideally aims for a patient with a renal transplant to conceive 12 months after the transplant when the patient is well established on an immunosuppression treatment without significant teratogenic risk and without rejection episodes in the past 12 months, a creatinine under 1.5 mg/dL, and absence or minimal presence of proteinuria.

5. b. The majority of patients with ESRD do not become pregnant spontaneously; however, if patients do become pregnant while on dialysis, the most likely etiology is a preterm delivery as up to 80% of pregnant patients will develop spontaneous labor or an iatrogenic indication for preterm delivery including fetal growth restriction, preeclampsia, or placental abruption.

6. d. The majority of patients with nephrolithiasis in pregnancy will have spontaneous passage of the stone without surgical management using intravenous hydration and pain management alone. If there is concern for impaction or infection, a cystoscopy with stent placement or nephrostomy tube placement may be necessary.

7. e. In the third trimester, the most likely inherited condition that will result in bilateral enlarged echogenic kidneys in the third trimester in the fetus is autosomal dominant polycystic kidney disease; 50% of parents with the condition will pass this condition to their offspring; however, the condition may not be recognized in the fetus on ultrasound.

8. b. Patients with preexisting diabetes are at increased risk of preeclampsia; patients with diabetic nephropathy have an even stronger association of developing preeclampsia.

9. c. Patients who develop the rare condition of thrombotic thrombocytopenic purpura need urgent treatment with plasmapheresis. If a clinician has a high clinical suspicion for TTP on the basis of clinical presentation, blood smear, and other laboratory values, plasmapheresis should be instituted even before the ADAMTS13 result returns typically days later.

10. b. Patients with an increased risk of preeclampsia including renal disease, chronic hypertension, multiple gestation, preexisting diabetes, a history of preeclampsia, and other moderate risk factors are recommended to initiate low-dose aspirin daily beginning in the late first trimester to reduce the risk of preeclampsia.

11. a. Delivery is advised for patients who develop acute renal insufficiency in the setting of preeclampsia. Typically, serum creatinine is lower in pregnancy compared with the nonpregnant individual. A creatinine of 1.3 mg/dL demonstrates a significant reduction in kidney function in pregnancy most commonly secondary to prerenal etiology. Delivery is warranted as renal insufficiency secondary to preeclampsia is known as a "severe feature" and expectant management is not recommended. Attempts at hydration will typically result in ongoing third spacing from endothelial dysfunction of preeclampsia and may result in pulmonary edema.

12. b. The majority of patients with chronic renal disease have stable or transient worsening of their kidney function during pregnancy, although pregnancy-related conditions such as preeclampsia may occasionally induce permanent worsening of kidney function.

Chapter 58

1. d
2. a
3. b
4. d
5. d
6. b
7. c
8. a
9. d
10. d
11. a
12. c
13. b
14. b
15. d
16. b
17. c
18. a
19. c
20. c

Chapter 59

1. a
2. c
3. b
4. d
5. d
6. a
7. c
8. e
9. c
10. a
11. c
12. a

Chapter 60

1. d
2. d
3. b
4. c
5. b
6. d
7. a
8. c
9. d
10. c
11. d
12. c
13. b
14. b
15. a
16. b
17. c
18. a
19. b
20. c
21. d

Chapter 61

1. c. Although it is preferred that labs determine gestational TSH ranges, the normal range in pregnancy for many assays can be generally estimated to be ~0.1–4.0 mIU/L (or subtract 0.5 from the upper end and subtract 0.4 mIU/L from the lower range of the institutional nonpregnant range to account for the effect of hCG). Since >99% of T4 and T3 are bound to TBG, which increases rapidly in early pregnancy due to the stimulatory effect of estrogen on TBG, indirect analog immunoassays, most commonly used to measure free T4 (FT4), are not more accurate than using the TT4 and adding the appropriate percent increase for the gestational age. Because there is less circulating T3 than T4, indirect analog immunoassays are even less accurate in measuring FT3; therefore, T3 is best assessed using the TT3 assay. The TT4 and TT3 increases in normal pregnancy can be estimated by multiplying 5% for each week starting at 7 weeks' gestation (i.e., at 12 weeks, multiply the reference range by 30% and at and after 16 weeks onward, multiple by 50%). Because most commercially available free T4 assays are not more accurate and both her TSH and TT4 are within the normal range for her gestation, there is no need to order any further labs or treat her. Palpitations and fatigue are nonspecific in pregnancy, and nausea is more likely to be related to hCG than thyroid hormone levels.

2. e. More than 90% of hypothyroidism diagnosed in pregnancy is subclinical. In pregnancy, the prevalence of SCH is 2%–5% (higher risk in patients with autoimmunity) and ~2% for isolated hypothyroxinemia. Most societal guidelines consider an isolated TSH ≥10 mIU/L with a normal free T4 (FT4) overt hypothyroidism rather than SCH due to the expected lower TSH in pregnancy. The TSH has a log linear relationship to the FT4 and will rise long before the free T4 decreases outside the normal range. Therefore, a TSH <10 is extremely unlikely to result in a low FT4 and her diagnosis, even without a FT4, is overwhelmingly likely to be SCH. SCH is defined by an elevated TSH (<10 mIU/L) with a normal FT4. Many patients will not demonstrate a low FT4 until TSH levels rise >20 or even 40 mIU/L. By far the most common etiology for her elevated TSH is due to Hashimoto thyroiditis, accompanied by TPO antibodies. With Hashimoto thyroiditis, the TSH first increases and later, if there is continued autoimmune destruction of the gland, the FT4 may fall (overt hypothyroidism). The T3 is spared until late and is last to fall, so there is no reason to check it in this case. Sometimes it can be helpful to check TPO antibodies in patients with a borderline TSH of 4–6 to confirm that the patient has Hashimoto thyroiditis and is at risk for further increases in her TSH with the increasing demand of thyroid hormone production in pregnancy. However, her TSH of 8 is clearly elevated for pregnancy and there is no consensus about the definite need for TPO antibodies.

3. b. Giver her TSH is modestly elevated, especially for the first trimester of pregnancy, and she has a normal FT4 for pregnancy, she has SCH, which is commonly due to Hashimoto thyroiditis. There remains controversy about the definite need to obtain TPO antibodies in SCH, as well as its treatment. Although the presence of TPO antibodies would be further supportive of Hashimoto thyroiditis, 10% of patients with SCH do not have Hashimoto antibodies. It can be helpful to check TPO antibodies in patients, especially with a borderline TSH of 4–6, given its diurnal variation and to rule out lab error to confirm the diagnosis of Hashimoto thyroiditis. Although TSH has a diurnal variation and can vary slightly due to assay reproducibility, a TSH of 8.0 in the first trimester would be considered much higher than expected by either process or even if both were operating together. Individuals with elevated TPO antibodies, even with a normal TSH, have up to a 20% chance of developing SCH in pregnancy, and some patients with SCH will go on to develop overt hypothyroidism with the increasing thyroid hormone demands of pregnancy. Those with high TPO antibodies are also at a much higher risk (up to 50%) for postpartum thyroiditis. Although it has not been clearly demonstrated with SCH (defined by a TSH <10 mIU/L with a normal T4) that treatment with low doses of LT4 improves pregnancy outcomes or offspring IQ, most studies included women with lower levels of TSH elevation (5–6 mIU/L) and treatment trials did not start until 15 weeks. Treatment for SCH is usually started at 50 mcg of LT4, which is much lower than a full replacement dose (~2 mcg/kg in pregnancy) and will not result in hyperthyroidism. Given the degree of her TSH elevation, treating with a low dose of LT4, especially if she was found to have TPO antibodies, is highly unlikely to do any harm and may have benefit this early in pregnancy. Giving her a full replacement dose (2 mcg/kg or 150 mcg in her case) is also unlikely to result in hyperthyroidism after the first week of therapy (due to the T4 half-life of 1 week) since her own T4 production will be suppressed by exogenous LT4. However, a full replacement dose is usually reserved for patients with overt hyperthyroidism. Retrospective data treating subclinical hypothyroidism during early pregnancy before the fetus is capable of synthesizing any thyroid hormone (14 weeks) demonstrate potential neurologic benefit. In this case, the TSH elevation is clearly higher than would be expected from laboratory error, it is higher than the median TSH in most randomized treatment trials, the individual is early in pregnancy, and treatment is extremely unlikely to do any harm and may be of some benefit. However, due to the lack of consensus and her strong

preference to not start therapy, repeating the TSH in 4 weeks to see if it has increased and obtaining TPO antibodies, which further supports the diagnosis of Hashimoto thyroiditis, is also an option. If treatment is still not elected, the TSH should be followed during pregnancy given that the patient may not be able to meet the increasing demands of thyroid hormone production as pregnancy continues and developing overt hypothyroidism as defined by a TSH >10 mIU/L is a risk and should definitely be treated.

4. b. Graves disease, gestational thyrotoxicosis, toxic nodule, and toxic multinodular goiter are considered in the differential diagnosis for this patient. Graves is usually associated with a diffusely enlarged thyroid and symptoms predating the pregnancy. It may be associated with exophthalmos and, when severe, pretibial myxedema. Typically, nausea and vomiting are not associated with Graves disease outside of pregnancy but rather due to high hCG levels, which also stimulates the thyroid gland due to its ability to bind to the TSH receptor. Generalized symptoms and signs of mild hyperthyroidism (tachycardia, heat intolerance, palpitations, diaphoresis, and hyperreflexia) are not specific and can be seen in both gestational thyrotoxicosis and Graves disease. This patient's presentation is most consistent with hCG-induced hyperthyroidism (i.e., hyperemesis gravidarum [nausea, vomiting, plus 5-lb weight loss] with mild hyperthyroidism signs and symptoms). Unlike Graves, gestational thyrotoxicosis is not associated with a thyroid goiter or exophthalmos. In Graves disease, the T3 is typically proportionally higher than the T4 due to increased peripheral conversion of T4 to T3. However, in this case, the TT3 is what would be expected for this stage of pregnancy (TT3 demonstrates a 5% increase per week starting at 7 weeks up to a 50% increase at ≥16 weeks). At 14 weeks, her TT3 would be estimated to be 40% increased or ~260 ng/dL, so it is normal for this gestational age. Toxic multinodular goiters or a toxic nodule can typically be distinguished from Graves on examination or a thyroid ultrasound. Her tachycardia will likely to respond to intravenous fluids, and a low-dose beta blocker may be considered if she remains tachycardic until her TRAB or TSI returns. Gestational thyrotoxicosis should not be treated with antithyroid drugs given it typically resolves by 16–18 weeks when hCG levels fall and treatment could have unintended consequences such as causing fetal hypothyroidism or maternal liver toxicity.

5. b. Overt hypothyroidism can result in all of the maternal risks as outside of pregnancy (e.g., heart failure, anemia, neurologic symptoms) and places the fetus at risk for neurodevelopmental delay, especially before 18 weeks when the fetus is entirely dependent on maternal T4 for normal neurologic development. Armour thyroid is porcine thyroid extract, which contains much more T3 than the human thyroid makes. Because T3 does not cross the placenta well and the fetal brain primarily has T4 receptors, T3 supplements should NOT be used in pregnancy. Even at physiological human doses (T4:T3 at 12-14:1), T3 is used selectively outside of pregnancy. In the case of a TSH ≥10 or overt hypothyroidism (low FT4), typically a full replacement dose of LT4 is started in pregnancy (~2 mcg/kg) compared with 1.6 mcg/kg outside of pregnancy. Since this patient is athyreotic from her thyroidectomy, she is likely to need at least a 25% increase in LT4 dose early in pregnancy. This patient's total replacement dose is likely to be approximately 225 ug/day (~2 mcg/kg) or 1600 mcg/week, which can be achieved by taking 2 extra tablets of the 175 mcg LT4 each week. Given that the half-life of thyroid hormone is ~1 week, this can be easily achieved by adding 2 tablets a week of a patient's thyroid dose taken before pregnancy. The TSH should be rechecked in 4 weeks to determine if further increases are needed.

6. a. This degree of overt hyperthyroidism can result in high cardiac output heart failure if allowed to persist, which occurs more commonly during pregnancy than thyroid storm. Even if the patient does not have high Graves antibodies, this degree of hyperthyroidism in a mother can result in growth restriction and fetal tachycardia. Since the patient is TRAB and TSI negative, the fetus should not develop a goiter (which occurs with high TRAB or TSI or severe maternal hypothyroidism from overtreatment with antithyroid drugs or from iodine deficiency) and the newborn is at highest risk for neonatal central hypothyroidism from suppression of fetal pituitary thyrotropes from undertreatment of high levels of T4 that cross the placenta.

7. d. It is not uncommon for a patient with this degree of overt thyrotoxicosis to have modestly elevated liver function tests (<3× normal), just from hyperthyroidism alone. Therefore, at this time, there is no need to consider plasmapheresis or preparation for surgery to treat her hyperthyroidism. It is important to avoid overtreating with antithyroid drugs and to titrate the antithyroid medication doses every 2–4 weeks to keep the FT4 (or TT4 corrected for gestation) at the upper limit of the normal range. An equivalent dose of PTU to MMI is about 20:1; 5 mg twice daily of MMI is neither an equivalent dose to her previous dose of PTU nor sufficient for this degree of hyperthyroidism. Given that the patient is not likely to have hepatotoxicity from PTU (i.e., she hasn't taken it in a long while) and her TT3 is relatively more elevated than her FT4 (TT3 is >3× elevated and FT4 is <2.5× elevated), it would be reasonable to start her back on 150 mg every 8 hours of PTU. This is considered a medium dose and might be slightly better than MMI at decreasing peripheral conversion of T4 to T3 and decreasing her TT3. However, MMI may have less hepatotoxicity and is likely to be effective at equivalent doses of PTU; starting her at 12.5 every 12 hours of MMI is an acceptable alternative. Judicious use of short-acting beta blockers such as propranolol or metoprolol is recommended until the PTU or MMI takes effect as long as the patient does not have evidence of heart failure.

8. a. At least 20% of patients have both Graves (TRAB or TSI) or Hashimoto (TPO or TG) antibodies, and it is not uncommon for these concurrent autoimmune diseases to present as a relapsing Graves or Graves that over time goes into remission (due to partial destruction of the gland from Hashimoto). The hyperthyroid phase of postpartum thyroiditis due to Hashimoto antibodies tends to recur earlier (1–3 months postpartum) compared with an exacerbation from Graves antibodies, which typically

occurs 4−8 months postpartum. The cause of the hyperthyroid phase from postpartum thyroiditis is due to partial destruction of the thyroid by Hashimoto antibodies, releasing stored thyroid hormone, and is not due to increased synthesis of thyroid hormones, as is the case with Graves disease. Therefore, antithyroid medications are ineffective. The degree of hyperthyroidism in postpartum thyroiditis tends to be mild and transient. Symptoms can usually be effectively treated with a low-dose beta blocker with postpartum thyroiditis due to Hashimoto thyrotoxicosis. Patients with postpartum thyroiditis are also at risk for developing hypothyroidism at 4−8 months postpartum, which this patient previously described, from continued destruction of the thyroid. Although an I-123 uptake and scan can distinguish the difference between Graves (high uptake) and postpartum thyroiditis (normal or low uptake), this is usually not necessary and the patient would need to pump and discard her breastmilk for 48−72 hours. ^{131}I is contraindicated in pregnancy and breastfeeding given the half-life is ~8 days (up to 75 days to clear in circulation) and isotopes are concentrated in breastmilk. If the patient has TPO antibodies suggestive of Hashimoto, her hyperthyroid state is likely to resolve. Whether she develops the hypothyroid stage of postpartum thyroiditis at 4−8 months postpartum or whether her Graves relapses during the same time period is difficult to predict, and she should be referred to Endocrinology for close monitoring. If her TPO antibodies were negative and she appeared to have only a Graves relapse, a low dose of PTU or MMI should be used (either can be used in breastfeeding), but a dose of 150 mg twice daily is much higher than needed for her slight increase in free T4.

9. c. The first step in evaluating any thyroid nodule is to determine the thyroid status (i.e., hyperthyroid, euthyroid, or hypothyroid). If the TSH is suppressed at this gestation, it is possible she has a warm or hot nodule, which is rarely thyroid cancer and does not require any additional evaluation at this time. After delivery, an I-^{123} uptake and scan can be used to determine if the nodule itself actively takes up RAI and, if so, it is highly unlikely to be

malignant and can simply be monitored. However, if the TSH is normal or elevated, the nodule could be malignant. If the nodule meets radiologic criteria for recommended biopsy, most experts recommend a FNA at this gestational age (and LT4 treatment if the TSH is elevated) to make a cytologic diagnosis, even if the patient chooses to defer treatment until postpartum. The two major guidelines that stratify the risk of a nodule to be malignant and necessary for biopsy are from the American Thyroid Association and American College of Radiology, and there is no consensus over which appears to be more predictive. Molecular biomarkers have not been validated in pregnancy to improve the prediction of nondiagnostic follicular nodules. A calcitonin is rarely high and usually not helpful unless there is a clear family history of MEN2 or medullary thyroid cancer.

10. b. Patients with a history of RAI ablation, thyroidectomy for hyperthyroidism, remission of Graves, or TRAb positivity should have TRAb/TSI levels checked in early pregnancy. TRAb and TSI levels >3× the upper range of normal is associated with a higher risk for fetal or neonatal hyperthyroidism with rates of 20% with high levels. TRAb or TSI levels should be repeated in midtrimester (20−24 weeks) if early gestation antibody levels are elevated or the patient is taking ATDs because they may fall with the immunosuppression of pregnancy and pose much less of a risk. Patients with TRAb or TSI levels in this high-risk range at 20−24 weeks should be referred to a maternal-fetal medicine specialist with expertise in this area. Management includes serial ultrasound assessments of fetal growth and markers of fetal Graves disease and amniotic fluid volume, antenatal fetal surveillance, and repeat TRAb or TSI testing again at 30−34 weeks to evaluate the need for newborn monitoring. If the levels are low (<3× normal range) or undetectable in early pregnancy, repeat testing in midtrimester is of low utility. If it is difficult to ascertain the etiology of a fetal goiter (i.e., from fetal hyperthyroidism due to high levels of TRAB or TSI or fetal hypothyroidism from high doses of maternal MMI or PTU or if LT4 is required for mother but the fetus is showing

signs of fetal Graves), sometimes a percutaneous umbilical sampling (PUBS) from a highly experienced provider can be helpful to quantitate the degree of fetal hypothyroidism or hyperthyroidism and direct management, although this carries ~1% risk of major fetal complications. Patients with Graves and TRAb or TSI antibody positivity should notify the neonatologist at delivery and their pediatric provider to determine the appropriate postnatal assessments. Given that this patient is on a full replacement dose of LT4, the TSH should be checked every 4 weeks until 18 weeks because the fetus is dependent on maternal thyroid hormone until then, as well as due to increasing requirements of LT4, especially in the first 20 weeks of pregnancy. After 18 weeks the TSH should be checked every 4−8 weeks depending on its stability and whether dosing changes have been required.

11. c. Adequate iodine intake is often not sufficiently addressed. The maternal iodide pools are relatively lower in pregnancy due to increased maternal T4 synthesis by the thyroid gland, the placental transfer of iodine for fetal iodine requirements, and renal iodide clearance that nearly doubles. Consequently, an increased consumption of iodine (50-150 mcg/day for a total intake of 250 mcg/day) during pregnancy and lactation is required to maintain adequate T4 production. Reduced iodine intake leads to impaired fetal and maternal TH synthesis, affecting T4 more than T3 synthesis. Isolated hypothyroxinemia without an elevated TSH may be caused by iodine deficiency due to preferential synthesis of T3, which requires less iodine to form than T4 and which negatively feeds back on TSH. In this case, the T3 may be normal but the T4 slightly low. A slightly low FT4 in the setting of a normal TSH in the late second and third trimesters may occur in up to 60% of analog assays, which is much more likely to be due to assay limitations (laboratory error) and the lack of pregnancy-specific norms than due to hypothyroxinemia from iodine deficiency or central hypothyroidism. In the case of iodine deficiency, the patient should have an enlarged thyroid and a goiter can be extremely large with marked iodine deficiency. If the

hypothyroxinemia is due to mild iodine deficiency (more severe would cause both a decrease in T4 and T3 and an increase in TSH), the fetus is at risk for adverse perinatal outcomes and impaired offspring cognitive development. It is difficult to diagnose mild iodine deficiency by 24-hour urine iodine due to the changes in iodine consumption on a daily basis. Therefore, if iodine insufficiency is suspected, treatment with iodine and levothyroxine is recommended, recognizing that the fetus also requires iodine to synthesize thyroid hormone.

12. d. Patients on LT4 for previously diagnosed thyroid cancer will usually need close to a 30% dose increase in pregnancy with a goal to maintain the same preconception degree of TSH suppression during pregnancy (i.e., TSH <0.1 mIU/L with evidence of persistent structural disease or TSH = 0.1–0.5 mIU/L if recent treatment and no evidence of structural recurrence). The degree of TSH suppression depends on the risk of recurrence, but in all circumstances, the FT4 should not be allowed to rise above the normal range due to the possibility of excess LT4 exposure to the fetus, risk of suppression of fetal thyrotropes, and newborn congenital hypothyroidism. Patients with a history of successfully treated thyroid carcinoma, a negative prepregnancy ultrasound and undetectable TG levels do not have an increased risk for cancer recurrence with a subsequent pregnancy nor will pregnancy impact survival or overall thyroid cancer prognosis. The prepregnancy response to therapy is a strong predictor of progression in pregnancy, and those without structural disease are unlikely to progress, but those patients with persistent prepregnancy structural disease may experience progression or new cervical lymph nodal metastases. Ultrasound and TG monitoring should be performed in pregnancy among patients with an incomplete therapeutic response before pregnancy and recurrent or residual disease, but there is no reason to repeat ultrasounds every 12 weeks unless there is evidence of structural disease. This patient received her I-131 1 year ago, which has not been shown to have any long-term adverse effects in women desiring pregnancy. However, if it is given within 40 days

(7–8 weeks after LMP) of when the fetus begins to concentrate and synthesize TH at ~10–12 weeks' gestation, I-131 would be highly destructive to the fetal thyroid. Therefore, conception should be postponed after thyroid cancer is successfully treated and the stability of thyroid function has been achieved for at least 6 months after I-131 ablative treatment. Molecular markers are not helpful in this situation and have not been validated in pregnancy, and only medullary thyroid cancer is associated with an elevated calcitonin.

13. d. Illness can result in significant alterations in TH metabolism, resulting in nonthyroidal illness syndrome. In the acute phase of illness, serum T3 decreases secondary to decreased circulating binding proteins, decreased T4 to T3 conversion by deiodinases, and increased TH clearance. Severely ill patients can go on to further manifest lower serum FT4 with a low-normal TSH due to a loss of pulsatile TSH secretion and downregulation of the HPT-axis (i.e., decrease hypothalamic TRH expression), which is often further suppressed with the use of glucocorticoids and dopaminergic agents. In the recovery phase of nonthyroidal disease, the TSH rises (but rarely above 20 mIU/L) and FT4 normalizes. Diagnosing NTIS from true hypothyroid states can be difficult, especially in ICU patients. The presence of TPO antibodies or TSH >20 IU/L is more suggestive of true Hashimoto thyroiditis. Therefore, it is not recommended to routinely check thyroid function tests in critically ill patients unless there is a significant index of suspicion for true thyroidal disease.

14. b. TPO antibody positivity is a marker of decreased thyroid reserve due to Hashimoto thyroiditis. Among euthyroid persons with TPO antibody positivity, 20%–60% will ultimately develop mild elevations in TSH that require LT4 therapy over a number of years. The current evidence demonstrates an association of infertility with overt hypothyroidism and SCH, particularly in the setting of TPO antibody positivity. Treatment with LT4 is recommended for individuals desiring pregnancy with overt hypothyroidism or SCH. Treatment of mild SCH with LT4 generally show higher pregnancy and delivery rates

among those undergoing assisted reproductive technology. Individuals seeking pregnancy with assisted reproductive technology with overt or SCH should be treated with LT4 to achieve a TSH 0.5–2.5 mIU/L. However, euthyroid patients who are TPO antibody positive have not been shown through large randomized controlled studies to improve pregnancy outcomes with respect to live birth rates, miscarriage, preterm birth, or neonatal outcomes. Approximately 20% of women with TPO antibodies develop subclinical hypothyroidism (SCH; TSH ≥4 mIU/L) during gestation despite early normal TSH values. Therefore, euthyroid pregnant persons with TPO antibody positivity should be screened for developing abnormal TSH levels every 4–6 weeks through midgestation according to recent American Thyroid Association guidelines.

15. c. Patients with malabsorption, celiac disease, or taking medications that may interfere with absorption may require higher doses. Adequate absorption of most oral LT4 formulations requires dissolution under acidic gastric conditions. Hence, conditions such as atrophic gastritis can impair dissolution. Gastroparesis can also adversely affect LT4 absorption by delaying exposure of the drug to the intestinal mucosa and allowing an admixture of the LT4 preparation with gastric content. LT4 absorption tests are sometimes useful in determining whether there is a definite problem with absorption versus compliance. Tirosint is a gel-cap formulation of LT4 that is dissolved in glycerin, bypasses the need for gastric dissolution, and may result in better absorption among patients with malabsorption syndromes, a history of bariatric surgery, or gluten sensitivity or who are taking absorption-interfering medications. Medications and supplements such as ferrous sulfate, iron-containing prenatal vitamins, high-dose calcium, and soy products interfere with LT4 absorption and should be taken at least 4 hours apart from thyroxine therapy, which she has done. She has also appropriately increased her dose by ~25% due to the increased requirements in pregnancy. All of these issues could be operational in this patient's situation, but malabsorption from her bypass surgery is likely contributing the most and

should be considered before assuming the patient is noncompliant.

Chapter 62

1. c. During pregnancy, PTHrP levels rise as early as 3–13 weeks, accompanied by an increase in 1,25 dihydroxyvitamin D and a reduction in PTH. Because increases in 1,25 dihydroxyvitamin D enhance calcium and phosphorus absorption from the maternal gut, serum calcium and phosphorus levels remain within normal limits during pregnancy, despite high fetal demand and active placental calcium transfer.
2. a. This person has vitamin D insufficiency and evidence of anemia. It is important to exclude malabsorptive conditions like celiac disease and correct vitamin D insufficiency before conception. The Endocrine Society Clinical Practice Guidelines for the evaluation, treatment, and prevention of vitamin D deficiency recommend evaluating serum 25-$(OH)_2$-D_3 as the appropriate screening test for vitamin D adequacy, aiming to maintain 25-$(OH)_2$-D_3 levels between 50 and 125 nmol/L (20–50 ng/mL). Guidelines recommend that pregnant and lactating women take at least 600 IU of vitamin D daily and emphasize that for some women, intake of 1500 to 2000 IU per day may be required to maintain a serum level of greater than 75 nmol/L (30 ng/mL).
3. b. This woman has autoimmune polyglandular syndrome type 1. She presents with HypoPT and a clinical picture suggestive of adrenal insufficiency. She also has a background history of oral candidiasis. A careful evaluation of other autoimmune conditions is necessary. Diagnosis can be confirmed with DNA assessment of the *AIRE* gene.
4. b. This patient has modestly high serum phosphorus and a low normal serum calcium level, but no signs of hypocalcemia. Her calcium supplements should be taken with meals to act as phosphate binders and prevent hyperphosphatemia, which has been linked to extravascular calcifications as a long-term consequence in patients with HypoPT. It is vital to advise patients who take both L-thyroxine and calcium supplements not to take them at the same time, as calcium can interfere with L-thyroxine absorption, resulting in poor replacement.
5. b. This woman is likely suffering from pregnancy-related osteoporosis. However, before confirming the diagnosis, secondary causes for bone loss need to be excluded. Osteomalacia, PHPT, thyrotoxicosis, hypercortisolism, osteogenesis imperfecta, malabsorptive state (e.g., celiac disease), eating disorders, inflammatory arthritis, and inflammatory bowel disease are some examples. Chronic use of glucocorticoids, excessive thyroxine, anticonvulsants, GnRH analogs, selective serotonin reuptake inhibitor, and cytotoxic chemotherapeutic agents are also other contributing factors and need to be excluded.
6. c. This woman suffers from primary hyperparathyroidism. Although preeclampsia, pancreatitis, and fractures can all be caused by this condition during pregnancy, nephrolithiasis remains the most commonly reported maternal complication in the literature.
7. a. Pharmacologic intervention is severely limited during pregnancy because of the lack of long-term safety data with the available drug treatments. Calcitonin has, however, been used safely during pregnancy as it does not cross the placenta. Tachyphylaxis may develop with prolonged use of calcitonin. It is advised to ensure adequate hydration and consider parathyroidectomy in the second trimester. Bisphosphonates such as zoledronic acid cross the placenta and may be teratogenic. Cinacalcet has been used in several case reports, but it does cross the placenta. Animal studies have shown no adverse events in the offspring. Cinacalcet should be used with caution in pregnancy and only offered to symptomatic patients or those with corrected calcium levels above 2.85 mmol/L, in whom surgery cannot be performed. Denosumab has been reported to cause an osteoporotic-like syndrome in animal studies and should never be used in a pregnant patient.
8. b. Neck ultrasound remains the safest diagnostic tool during pregnancy and has a sensitivity of 69% and specificity of 94% at identifying parathyroid adenomas. Computed tomography and sestamibi scanning are both generally contraindicated during pregnancy and should be avoided when possible.
9. d. Evidence from case reports and case series suggest that even in women experiencing osteoporosis-related fragility fractures during pregnancy, there is spontaneous recovery of the associated bone loss in the following 6–12 months as assessed by BMD and qCT. Fractures occurring during pregnancy have a low risk of recurrence. Fractures do not appear to be associated with parity. The most frequent sites of associated fractures are the spine and hip.
10. b. There are limited data on effective treatment strategies in pregnancy-associated osteoporosis. Case repots describing the use of teriparatide and bisphosphonates have shown improvements in BMD.

Chapter 63

1. c. Vitamin B_6 is probably the best initial treatment for mild symptoms and has a low potential of side effects. Ondansetron has become the most frequently prescribed antiemetic in the United States, but there may be an ill-defined risk for fetal anomalies and it should not be considered a first-line agent. Metoclopramide should be reserved for moderate symptoms. Acupuncture has conflicting results regarding symptom improvement.
2. d. Thiamine deficiency should be screened and treated during the initial resuscitation, particularly before administering glucose solutions. A depressed thyroid-stimulating hormone is often seen but, usually, in the absence of a prior history of hyperthyroidism is not clinically significant. Intravenous fluid infusion and electrolyte replacement are important. Severe hyponatremia may be encountered, and sodium replacement should be judicious given the risk of central pontine myelinolysis.
3. e. An appendiceal diameter of >6 mm determined by either ultrasound, helical CT, or MRI is considered abnormal. Abdominal ultrasound is easily obtainable but is operator dependent, and often the appendix is not visualized. Helical CT, while not the preferred modality given the risk of radiation, is not contraindicated, particularly if MRI is not obtainable. Gadolinium should be avoided in pregnancy, unless the risks are outweighed by the benefits.
4. d. Intraabdominal pressure should be limited to 12 mm Hg to avoid

hypercapnia and subsequent fetal acidosis. Laparoscopy in experienced hands can be performed in all trimesters. Operative time for laparoscopy is often shorter than that for laparotomy. Initial port placement can be accomplished with either Hassan, Verres needle, or optical trocar, as long as the location is adjusted to the fundal height, previous incisions, and surgeon experience. Cervical manipulators are contraindicated during laparoscopy on viable pregnancies.

5. d. Both infliximab and sulfasalazine are considered to be appropriate therapies for inflammatory bowel disease in pregnancy. Sulfasalazine does not appear to be teratogenic. The 2016 Toronto Consensus Statement recommended that pregnant women on anti-TNF monotherapy for maintenance of remission should continue through the duration of pregnancy. Fluoroquinolone antibiotics should be avoided in pregnancy.

6. b. The most widely available screening test is the antiendomysial IgA test with a specificity of near 100%. The gold standard diagnostic test is small intestinal biopsy from the distal duodenum. Celiac disease is often underdiagnosed with a prevalence ranging from 1/80 to 1/300 individuals. Literature suggests that celiac disease, particularly poorly controlled, may be associated with prematurity, growth restriction, and miscarriage. However, whether celiac disease is causative or merely associated with adverse perinatal outcomes continues to be debated. Most patients with celiac disease are diagnosed before the age of 15.

7. b. Lifestyle and dietary changes should be initiated for mild symptoms. This would include screening for medication-use anticholinergics, calcium channel blockers, antidepressants, and antipsychotics, which may aggravate symptoms. EGD is rarely needed for diagnosis or management but should be considered for cases refractory to standard medical management. Antacids and histamine$_2$ receptor antagonists are usually the first-line medical therapies. Proton pump inhibitors such as omeprazole are used when there is poor response to H$_2$ blockers.

8. d. Fiber and bulk agents should be initially prescribed, followed by hyperosmolar laxatives. Stimulant medications may be considered for those who fail first-line therapies. However, prolonged use of hyperosmolar laxatives may lead to electrolyte abnormalities, and stimulant medications may result in tolerance. Therefore, prolonged use of both should be avoided. Lifestyle changes include education about increased fluid and fiber intake, exercise, and defecation in the morning or after meals when colonic activity is at its highest.

9. b. Rubber band ligation is effective for internal hemorrhoids that are reducibly prolapsed. Sclerotherapy can be considered, but 5% phenol is safe in pregnancy. Surgical hemorrhoidectomy is reserved for internal hemorrhoids that prolapse and incarcerate or have failed conservative therapy. However, surgery may be associated with postoperative bleeding and subsequent hypotension.

10. d. Results from small studies suggest that endoscopy and colonoscopy are safe in pregnancy. Risks relate to both the procedure itself (and may include perforation, bleeding and infection) and maternal sedation. The benefits of these procedures must be weighed against the risks of possible complications. Endoscopic ultrasound can be used in pregnancy to look for stones in the common bile duct because it is more sensitive than MRI. Small bowel wireless capsule endoscopy would not be a common procedure in pregnancy, as it is reserved for those with unexplained severed or recurrent gastrointestinal bleeding. Furthermore, pregnancy is considered to be a relative contraindication for capsule endoscopy. The American College of Obstetricians and Gynecologists and American Society for Gastrointestinal Endoscopy have published guidelines related to endoscopy in pregnant women.

Chapter 64

1. c
2. d
3. b
4. a
5. d
6. b
7. e
8. b
9. d
10. c
11. e
12. b

Chapter 65

1. d
2. c
3. a
4. c
5. c
6. a
7. c
8. b
9. c
10. e
11. d
12. c

Chapter 66

1. b. Carbamazepine is an enzyme-inducing anticonvulsant that interferes with the effectiveness of oral contraceptives. Several other anticonvulsants including clobazam, eslicarbazepine, felbamate, oxcarbazepine, perampanel, phenobarbital, phenytoin, primidone, topiramate, and rufinamide have a similar effect. Women with epilepsy prescribed these medications should be counseled about the reduced effectiveness of oral contraceptives, and an additional method of contraception should be discussed.

2. c. Valproic acid is the anticonvulsant associated with the highest risk of major congenital malformations and should be avoided in women of childbearing potential when possible. If feasible, monotherapy is preferred to polytherapy during conception and pregnancy because polytherapy confers an increased risk of congenital anomalies. Seizures pose a risk to the fetus, likely through transient hypoxemia, and patients with epilepsy who stop their anticonvulsants are at increased risk of developing status epilepticus. Folic acid may mitigate the risk of some congenital anomalies associated with anticonvulsants.

3. d. Noncontrast head CT is not indicated in patients with known epilepsy who have a breakthrough seizure where the semiology is consistent with previous seizures and when there has been no head trauma, there is no evidence of preeclampsia, and there are no risk factors for an intracranial process (e.g., history of brain tumor or lesion, coagulopathy, immunocompromise, focal neurologic findings). Anticonvulsant levels, especially that

of lamotrigine, can be lower during pregnancy and should be monitored before conception and throughout pregnancy, with dose adjustments to maintain adequate serum levels.

4. e. A new headache in a pregnant patient warrants head imaging and should raise the possibility of a cerebral dural venous sinus thrombosis. MRI is preferable to CT in pregnant patients to avoid any radiation exposure to the fetus. A magnetic resonance venogram can be obtained without contrast and is usually sufficient, when combined with a high-quality MRI, to rule out cerebral venous sinus thrombosis.

5. b. The patient is presenting 2 hours after last being seen normal. A noncontrast head CT must be obtained to rule out hemorrhage in order to determine eligibility for thrombolysis, and a CT angiogram must be obtained to determine eligibility for embolectomy. Both studies should be ordered simultaneously and obtained as quickly as possible in order to avoid any delay in treatment. MRI invariably takes longer than CT and is inappropriate in the evaluation of acute stroke unless an institution has a dedicated MRI scanner with a rapid imaging protocol for stroke patients.

6. c. Intravenous thrombolysis is approved in Europe for use up to 4.5 hours after stroke onset, which is defined as the time a patient was last seen at their neurologic baseline. In the United States, the Food and Drug Administration has approved tissue plasminogen activator for use up to 3 hours after stroke onset, although off-label use up to 4.5 hours is common.

7. b. When not related to streptococcal infection or other systemic illnesses or structural lesions, chorea gravidarum has a favorable prognosis and does not affect fetal outcomes.

8. b. Ankle dorsiflexion, eversion, and inversion are mediated by the L5 myotome, and the anterior, medial, and lateral leg below the knee comprises the L4 and L5 dermatomes. L5 nerve root compression due to a disk herniation is less likely to present after vaginal delivery than lumbosacral trunk compression. With sciatic and femoral neuropathy,

other muscle groups should be involved, and the common peroneal nerve does not supply the skin over the medial leg.

9. c. This patient has evidence of thiamine (vitamin B_1) deficiency due to hyperemesis gravidarum. Thiamine deficiency can cause peripheral neuropathy and Wernicke encephalopathy, both of which are apparent in this patient. If left untreated, and especially if glucose is administered before thiamine repletion, patients are at risk for developing Korsakoff dementia, a highly disabling—and preventable—state of permanent short-term memory loss.

10. d. Although 30% of patients with myasthenia may experience worsening of symptoms after delivery, an escalation in treatment is not indicated unless symptoms develop. Answers a, b, c, and e highlight important aspects of the peripartum management of patients with myasthenia.

Chapter 67

1. d
2. d
3. a
4. d
5. b
6. c
7. a
8. d
9. b
10. c
11. b
12. d

Chapter 68

1. e
2. d
3. a
4. e
5. b
6. c
7. d
8. d
9. b
10. a
11. e
12. a
13. b
14. b
15. a
16. b
17. e
18. d

Chapter 69

1. d
2. d
3. b
4. b
5. b
6. a
7. a
8. b
9. a
10. d
11. c

Chapter 70

1. d
2. b
3. a
4. d
5. e
6. b
7. a
8. d
9. d
10. a
11. b
12. a
13. d
14. b
15. b
16. b
17. b
18. b
19. a
20. e

Chapter 71

1. d. The PAC is an invasive intervention but is not contraindicated in pregnancy. The physiologic changes of pregnancy are similar to sepsis (increased cardiac output, reduced systemic vascular resistance), making assessment more difficult. Duration of insertion of the PAC is limited to a few days due to the risk of infection and mechanical trauma to cardiac valves and myocardium, and it is not suitable for long-term monitoring. Several studies have demonstrated an increased mortality in patients managed by PAC, making its use relatively uncommon. Cardiac output measurement via PAC usually requires an intermittent injection of cold saline for a thermodilution measurement.

2. b. Sepsis in pregnancy is more common in those at a low socioeconomic level. The diagnosis of sepsis is based on the

presence of life-threatening organ dysfunction with presumed infection, not requiring cultures. Cesarean delivery, particularly after the onset of labor, is a significant risk factor for sepsis. Initial treatment should be with broad-spectrum antibiotics, planning to deescalate to a narrower spectrum when cultures are available. In the presence of septic shock, inotrope therapy may be necessary to maintain blood pressure and organ perfusion (including the placenta).

3. a. Early antibiotics are essential, with an increase in mortality documented for every hour of delay. The usual criterion for crystalloid bolus is 30 mL/kg, but often less is given in pregnancy. There is no clear role for colloid administration in the management of sepsis. Initial antibiotics administered are broad spectrum, not based on cultures. PACs are now infrequently used in the management of sepsis.

4. c. ARDS is more common in pregnancy than the nonpregnant population. Pregnancy is not associated with an increase in respiratory rate, and $PaCO_2$ plays no role in ARDS diagnosis. Amniotic fluid embolism is a cause of ARDS, likely related to the acute inflammation state induced by amniotic fluid contents. There is no evidence that delivery improves the respiratory state in a pregnant patient with respiratory failure, and delivery should be based on usual obstetric indications. The calculation of tidal volume in the management of ARDS used "predicted body weight" based on height rather than actual body weight.

5. c. IVC diameter is obtained from point-of-care ultrasound measurements. CVP is measured with a central venous catheter or pulmonary artery catheter. SVR is calculated from parameters obtained from a PAC (cardiac output, right atrial pressure) and mean arterial pressure. Pulse contour analysis requires an arterial waveform (i.e., arterial cannulation).

6. a. After cardiac arrest, patients should be admitted to the ICU. The scenario in b is appropriate if sepsis may be

present or evolving, and higher-acuity monitoring is indicated rather than general ward care, but an intermediate-care or high-dependency unit is set up for higher levels of monitoring. Similarly, c and d are situations in which additional monitoring, drugs, or blood products are required but life-support interventions are not.

7. b. Imaging studies should be performed as would be indicated in any other case. Neuroimaging does not deliver high doses of radiation to the fetus even when ionizing radiation is used. Teratogenesis is a first-trimester problem, of no import at this gestational age: a is clearly incorrect. Data on the outcome of pregnancies after maternal ICU admission are limited, but less than half of women admitted to an ICU in several small case series have been reported to have a spontaneous abortion; c is, to the best of our knowledge, incorrect. Because the family may be at odds about whether the pregnancy should be continued or interrupted, and neurosurgical intervention such as aneurysm repair needs to happen quickly, d is incorrect.

8. c. The q SOFA score, which does not take pregnancy physiology into account, is based on assessment of:
   • Systolic blood pressure ≤100 mm Hg
   • Respiratory rate >22/min
   • Altered mental status
   This patient has two of these criteria, so organ dysfunction should be considered. Sepsis is a possibility.

9. d. Impending respiratory failure is not an indication for emergent delivery. Options a and b are noninvasive modes of additional respiratory support; high-flow oxygen via specialized nasal cannula, like CPAP or BiPAP, may provide enough support to stave off mechanical ventilation. Giving 100% O_2 via nonrebreather will probably fail in severe cases but may be tried, and if intubation is to be considered, it is helpful in preoxygenation. Option c is a standard approach to hypoxemic respiratory failure.

10. d. There is a paucity of knowledge about long-term outcomes after maternal ICU admission. We do not know whether these women are at higher or lower risk for the usual quality-of-life outcomes compared with other ICU survivors. Information obtained from qualitative analysis suggests that women struggled with separation from the newborn, with expectations of being able to cope, and with other issues peculiar to parenting after critical illness.

Chapter 72

1. f
2. a and c
3. c
4. c
5. b
6. c
7. b
8. a
9. a
10. a
11. c
12. a
13. a
14. d
15. a
16. c
17. a
18. a

Chapter 73

1. c
2. a
3. e
4. b
5. a
6. d
7. a
8. e
9. b
10. d
11. a
12. c
13. c
14. d
15. a
16. c
17. b

Page numbers followed by *f* or *t* indicate figures and tables, respectively.